Examination of the Newborn and Neonatal Health

Examination of the Newborn and Neonatal Health

A Multidimensional Approach

Second Edition

Edited by

Lorna Davies, RN, RM, BSc (Hons), PGCEA, MA PhD
Academic Manager
Nursing, Midwifery and Allied Health
Ara Institute of Canterbury, Christchurch
Canterbury
New Zealand

Sharon McDonald, RN, RM, BSc (Hons), PGCEA, MA, PGCE, PFHEA, DClinPrac
Public Health Midwife Smoking Cessation and Healthy Lifestyle Lead
Family and Women's Services
Princess Alexandra Hospital
Harlow, UK

Foreword by

Stephanie Michaelides
Programme Leader Graduate/Post Graduate Certificate in Neonatal Care
School of Health and Education
Middlesex University
Hendon, London, UK

ELSEVIER

Notices

Practitioners and researchers must always rely on their own experience and knowledge in evaluating and using any information, methods, compounds or experiments described herein. Because of rapid advances in the medical sciences, in particular, independent verification of diagnoses and drug dosages should be made. To the fullest extent of the law, no responsibility is assumed by Elsevier, authors, editors or contributors for any injury and/or damage to persons or property as a matter of products liability, negligence or otherwise, or from any use or operation of any methods, products, instructions, or ideas contained in the material herein.

Senior Content Strategist: Robert Edwards
Senior Content Development Specialist: Kirsty Guest
Content Coordinator: Heather Killian
Project Manager: Srividhya Vidhyashankar
Design: Patrick Ferguson
Illustration Manager: Narayanan Ramakrishnan

Printed in Poland

Last digit is the print number: 9 8 7 6 5 4 3 2 1

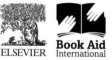

Working together to grow libraries in developing countries

www.elsevier.com • www.bookaid.org

CONTENTS

FOREWORD

I was delighted to be invited to write the foreword for this important book for midwives, student midwives and neonatal nurses, to equip them with the knowledge and skills for examining the newborn baby, supported by research and evidence.

The assessment of the newborn is now a central role of the midwife as well as the neonatal nurse practitioner. The inclusion of the full examination of the newborn within the midwife's practice enables holistic care to be given to the mother and the newborn, utilising a multi-disciplinary team approach in order to provide high-quality, seamless care to the newborn and their family.

It is important to note that the full examination of the newborn is a comparatively new addition to the role of the midwife. In the early 1990s, there was a combination of factors, including the reduction in junior doctors' hours, and also the recognition that expanding the midwife's skills to include this examination would be appropriate in line with caseload and group practice midwifery. I was able to design and develop the first examination of the newborn course in the UK, the Neurobehavioral Physical Assessment of the Newborn (NBPAN); and this has now increased throughout the country, and has informed postgraduate as well as undergraduate midwifery curricula. Following the development of the NBPAN in 1994, the Newborn and Infant Examination (NIPE) Screening Tool was developed and published in 2008, focussed on four areas of screening: the eyes, heart, hips and testes. I therefore have a huge interest in resources for practitioners which can support them in their role and provide direction for further information and research that they may need access to.

The new United Kingdom Nursing and Midwifery Council (NMC) education standards (NMC 2020) have recognised the importance of the holistic examination as a "top to toe" assessment – distinguished from the screening tool – Newborn and Infant Examination (NIPE), which focusses on the examination of the eyes, heart, hips and testes. The holistic examination enhances the information accessed by the midwife, and shared with the mother and family, in understanding better the physiology and the needs of the newborn baby.

This unique textbook provides a strong foundation to enable the practitioner to undertake the full examination of the newborn, with the understanding that in some areas the NIPE assessment is viewed as the priority area of assessment. The full holistic examination enables far more information to be gained and shared with the mother and family, and informs better care planning for the baby. The four areas of screening within NIPE are included within the top-to-toe assessment; however, where NIPE concentrates on the screening of the eyes in regard to cataracts the holistic assessment reviews the eyes to exclude infections, subconjunctival haemorrhages, jaundice, syndromes and other congenital abnormalities which include cataracts.

A better understanding of her baby can support maternal–infant interaction and enable the mother to form a partnership with the professional providing the care, and this is likely to ensure safe care to the baby and thus reduce morbidity and mortality.

Actions that the practitioner undertakes in the assessment can only be validated as normal if this is based upon a deeper underpinning knowledge of physiology, pathology, social, cultural, religious, psychological and educational needs. This knowledge enables the practitioner to give the appropriate support to women by using the correct terminology for her and her family to understand the information imparted to her. The information in regard to the baby's wellbeing should begin in the antenatal period to support decisions made in the postnatal period.

This book provides the guidelines and structure for the whole assessment, through 15 chapters written by experienced practitioners, recognising the importance of the top to toe assessment stated within the new NMC standards. Chapters including the NIPE screening of the four areas (eyes, heart, hips and testes) and also other elements of the full assessment including neonatal skin, neurological behaviours and growth, and the actual practical aspects of the whole assessment.

Throughout the book the baby and his/her parents are recognised as individuals. It recognises the importance of embryological development, transition to post-natal life and the subsequent changes and how deviations can be recognised and referred appropriately.

The structure of the book takes the reader logically through all aspects of the assessment. This includes a strong foundation of embryology and normal physiology to build knowledge and understanding of the development of the fetus, the transition to neonatal life, plus the wider aspects that need to be considered such as the impact of social and health inequalities. The importance of the initial interview with the woman as a starting point for data gathering in relation to the health and wellbeing of the neonate is highlighted. History may not in itself provide a diagnosis but is essential in any assessment of the newborn, and this chapter guides the practitioner to focus on specific areas of assessment, for example, a history of rubella, cardiac anomalies or eye conditions such as cataracts. It also suggests the specific tests that need to be undertaken to exclude the abnormalities.

The reader can also find information on antenatal and neonatal screening, new screening techniques and tests. It also addresses what tests are currently offered and takes into account both legal and ethical implications of practice in neonatal care. An important chapter is on assisting parents in making decisions using a scenario/case study approach, which enables the practitioner to have some experience of what the parents' perspective might be. It well illustrates how the practitioner can assist parents to make decisions and validate normality through the knowledge of normal physiology.

The thorough approach to this care is demonstrated by the inclusion of the importance of record-keeping to support both continuity of care and the development of individualised care in the future. The emphasis on the education of parents will enhance sound follow-up care when parents are left to manage their own baby.

The physical examination is critical in recognising the normal baby, using the knowledge of normal physiology to aid in the formation of a diagnosis. This is essential in recognising which baby should be referred for follow-up care.

This book will be such an important resource for students and for qualified practitioners; it will add to the repertoire of knowledge in the holistic assessment of the newborn, and motivate practitioners to continue to read and gain further new knowledge to enhance the care of the newborn and his/her family.

Stephanie Michaelides

PREFACE

The first edition of *Examination of the Newborn and Neonatal Health: A Multidimensional Approach* offered a departure from similar existing publications when it was published in 2008. This was accomplished by taking a more holistic approach, viewing the baby as a sentient being within a social context. In this new edition, we have continued to place the baby, its mother and its family within this social milieu even when there are factors that lead to complexity and challenge for the newborn/infant. The stories and photographs generously provided by parents of babies facing a range of challenges bear testimony to this intention, by introducing their babies and these challenges in a real-world family setting.

This latest edition has been updated to reflect changes and developments in both evidence, care and treatments available. Our knowledge around concepts such as epigenetics and the microbiome has increased exponentially in the last decade, and so these have been included. Likewise, our understanding of both maternal and infant mental health and neurohormonal contribution has attracted considerable attention in recent years, and therefore these areas are expanded within this edition. The book continues to introduce the normal anatomy and physiology that the practitioner would expect to find during the routine newborn assessment, as well as variations of normal and deviation from normal. Again, these 'classifications' are presented within a spectrum rather than delineated framework.

This edition is still aimed primarily at midwifery, nursing and medical students and qualified healthcare professionals, although allied health professionals such as complementary practitioners and childbirth educators may find aspects of the book useful for their practice. The revised and updated text is supported and illustrated with a rich array of newly drawn figures, photographs and micrographs.

We are always pleased to receive feedback from readers, which informs future editions, ensuring it continues to meet the learning needs of students in an evolving educational environment.

LIST OF CONTRIBUTORS

The editor(s) would like to acknowledge and offer grateful thanks for the input of all previous editions' contributors, without whom this new edition would not have been possible.

Jacqui Anderson, RGN, RM, MMid
Midwifery Advisor
National Office
New Zealand College of Midwives
Christchurch
New Zealand

Penny Champion, RGN, RM, ADM, MSc
Specialist Midwife Practice Development
Women's Health
Basildon and Thurrock University Hospital
Basildon, Essex
UK

Lorna Davies (editor), RN, RM, BSc (Hons), PGCEA, MA PhD
Academic Manager
Nursing, Midwifery and Allied Health
Ara Institute of Canterbury, Christchurch
Canterbury
New Zealand

Angela Deken, BN, BM, MM
Midwife
Women and Children's Health
Canterbury District Health Board
Christchurch
New Zealand

Martina Donaghy, BSc(Hons), MA, PGDip, DipHE, DipAS (Nursing)
Senior Lecturer in Midwifery
Faculty of Health, Education, Medicine and Social Care
Anglia Ruskin University
Chelmsford, Essex
UK

Sarah Fiadjoe, RGN, RGM
Antenatal and Newborn Screening Co-ordinator
Family and Women Services
Princess Alexandra Hospital NHS Trust
Harlow, Essex
UK

Elaine Jefford, PhD, MSc, PG Teaching and Learning, BSc(Hons), Midwifery, BSc(Hons) Nursing
Research Lead
Southern Cross University
Lismore
Australia

Sharon McDonald (editor), RN, RM, BSc (Hons), PGCEA, MA, PGCE, PFHEA, DClinPrac
Public Health Midwife, Smoking Cessation and Healthy Lifestyle Lead
Family and Women's Services
Princess Alexandra Hospital
Harlow, UK

Andy McVicar, BSc, PhD
Professor of Stress and Health Sciences
School of Nursing and Midwifery
Anglia Ruskin University
Chelmsford, Essex
UK

Maggie Meeks, MB, ChB, MHealSc (Hons), MD, DipED, FRCPCH, FAcadMEd, FRACP
Consultant Neonatal Paediatrician
Neonatal Intensive Care Unit
Canterbury District Health Board (CDHB)
Christchurch, Canterbury
New Zealand

Corinne Neville, RGN, DipHE (Midwifery)
Infant Feeding Lead Midwife
Princess Alexandra NHS Hospital Trust
Harlow, Essex
UK

Sanjay Raina, MBBS, MRCPCH, FRCPCH
Consultant Paediatrician
Paediatrics Department
Princess Alexandra NHS Hospital Trust
Harlow, Essex
UK

Julie Richards, RM, RCpN, MMid, DTLT
Nelson/Marlborough Midwifery Lecturer, Third Year
    Coordinator
Te Hoe Ora ki Manawa
Department of Health Practice
Christchurch
New Zealand

**Lindsey Ann Rose, BSc(Hons) Midwifery, MSc
    Medical and Healthcare Education**
Senior Midwifery Lecturer
School of Nursing and Midwifery, Cambridgeshire
Anglia Ruskin University
Cambridge
UK

John Siderov, PhD, MCOptom, FAAO
Professor of Optometry
University of Huddersfield
Huddersfield
UK

Sharon Trotter, BSc Advanced Studies in Midwifery
Founder and Director, TIPS Ltd,
Troon, UK

Eshita Upadhyay MBBS
Specialty Trainee Doctor Paediatrics
Luton and Dunstable University Hospital
Luton
UK

ACKNOWLEDGEMENTS

Editing a second edition of a textbook feels initially like less of a challenge than a first edition. However, as we learned, it brings its own trials and tribulations. For that reason we have a long list of people that we need to thank in this section. Once again we would like to acknowledge our appreciation of our families, friends and colleagues for their faith, encouragement and support during the development of this edition. We would like to offer thanks to our partners Tom and Chris for their patience and quiet encouragement; to all of those who dutifully read drafts and shared their expertise: you know who you are; to the chapter authors who have made the time to contribute and who have helped us to view the forum of neonatal health from many different perspectives. We would especially like to express our gratitude to the parents who generously offered to share the stories of the challenges that they and their children had faced. We are extremely grateful to the team at Elsevier for their support and expert advice during the 'gestation' of the book. Finally, to anyone else we may have forgotten to mention, we offer thanks for your invaluable help and support, without which this book would not have been written

Lorna Davies
Sharon McDonald

Introduction

Lorna Davies and Sharon McDonald

CHAPTER CONTENTS

It is over 10 years since we published the first edition of this book, and in that time things have changed considerably. Treatments have changed, screening methods have changed, resuscitation techniques have changed, and even some aspects of our understanding of physiology have changed. Knowledge and skills relating to the newborn assessment have also been refined, and attitudes to who carries out the assessment have mellowed. In many ways, the midwifery role in relation to the practice has come of age. The Newborn Infant Physical Examination (NIPE) programme has been running for more than 20 years in the UK. The course name and assessments may have changed, but the programme continues to be one of the most popular post-registration courses available. The performing of the NIPE by the midwife is now a far more accepted and routine part of postnatal care in the UK where Sharon resides, although it has not reached the same level of universality as in New Zealand, where Lorna is based.

In the UK the skills associated with the procedures involved are now viewed less as advanced skills performed within an extended scope of practice. Many universities in England and Wales have incorporated a module into their undergraduate midwifery programmes, although in Scotland, universities have not to date followed suit. In New Zealand, where Lorna is based, midwives are frequently self-employed, caseload-holding practitioners, and the examination is seen as an incorporate part of their remit. The student midwife receives preparation to meet the requirements for carrying out the full examination and to undertake the screening of the newborn as part of the pre-registration curriculum. This means that the new graduate midwife is able to carry out the assessments from the first day of registration.

CONTEXTUALIZING THE NEWBORN INFANT EXAMINATION

Traditionally, the midwife carries out the initial newborn check at birth, performing a top-to-toe assessment but without the four screening areas (eyes, heart, hips, testes) associated with NIPE. The newborn assessment would hopefully determine any obvious reasons for immediate referral to a paediatrician. The first NIPE programmes were known as the Neuro Behavioural and Physiological Assessment of the Newborn (NBPAN) and were introduced in the UK in the 1990s following the changing childbirth report and a reduction of junior doctors' hours in practice. Midwives extended their role to embrace some of the former duties of their medical colleagues, including the physical examination of the normal, healthy term baby within 72 hours of birth. The introduction of the programme and its completion by qualified midwives offered a new dimension to the examination. Midwives, who often had an established relationship with the mother and her family, were able to make a much more holistic assessment than the doctors, who are usually only presented with an opportunistic snapshot view of the baby and its parents.

In 2004, Townsend et al. estimated that only 2% of babies in England were examined by a midwife, even though 44% of midwifery units had midwives with the requisite skills and qualifications. In 2019 we do not have accurate data to confirm if the number of midwives undertaking the assessment in the UK has increased, or whether more midwifery units are offering this service. However, the perception is that there has been a substantial increase (Lomax, 2015) and a study undertaken by McDonald (2018) clearly identified that, at least in the south of England, the number of midwives with the required skills has increased and midwives continue to maintain their skills. However, there are still challenges, mainly related to allocation of midwives' time to undertake NIPE (McDonald, 2008; McDonald et al., 2012), and in those areas where there is a lack of mentorship and clinical support for students to undertake the assessments. Arguably, if NIPE were part of the normal scope of practice (as seen in New Zealand), it may not present such a problem. National population screening programmes in the UK are implemented in the NHS on the advice of the UK National Screening Committee (UK NSC) (Chapters 4 and 8), which first introduced the NHS Newborn and Infant Physical Screening Programme Standards and competencies in 2008; this was followed by a published review in 2016–17 and the standards were updated in 2019 (PHE, 2016).

There has been a perceptible shift towards an acceptance of the value of midwives undertaking NIPE. The EMREN trial (Wolke et al., 2002) found that 'from the mother's perspective, the quality of midwife examination is at least as satisfactory as that of junior paediatricians'. In 2019 the perception is that while mothers are still happy with the quality of the examination performed by either midwives or doctors, it would appear that they view midwives as more thorough when carrying out the newborn infant physical examination (McDonald et al., 2012; McDonald, 2016).

Another benefit of midwives undertaking NIPE is that it has been proven to generate substantial cost savings for the health service by reducing the length of stay for women and their babies. However, this has come at a cost because NIPE is frequently performed in midwife-led clinics and midwives are allocated to daily or weekend rotas to undertake the assessment. Sadly, this does not reflect the initial concept of the first programmes, where the emphasis was on a holistic service

with continuity of carer (McDonald, 2018). For parents, it may not be an ideal situation and may place unnecessary demands on their families at a time when they should be at home relaxing and getting to know their baby. Some women may be unable to return to clinic because of logistical problems such as childcare or transportation. We are however, beginning to see a change in the way care is delivered in the UK. The National Institute for Health and Care Excellence (NICE) guidelines on postnatal care (2006, updated in 2015) emphasize the importance of having a named health care professional to coordinate and implement individualized care to meet the needs of the mother–infant dyad. Since the publication of Implementing Better Births in 2017 (NHS England, 2017) the focus of UK maternity services is on the introduction of a continuity of care model, which it is anticipated will only serve to improve birth outcomes and the provision of holistic care for mothers and babies (RCM, 2017). In New Zealand, where a continuity of care model already exists, the same midwife generally carries out three assessments in the 6-week period following birth.

WHEN IS THE NIPE PERFORMED?

In the UK, the required standard of the Public Health England Screening Programme is that the NIPE must be completed within 72 hours of birth and a second assessment within 8 weeks of birth (PHE, 2016). It may be carried out by a midwife, paediatrician, health visitor or general practitioner. Conversely, in New Zealand, the partnership model which underpins delivery of care means that the Lead Maternity Carer (LMC)—who is usually a midwife, though occasionally a GP or obstetrician— will continue to provide care for both the woman and her baby until 4–6 weeks postpartum. The LMC therefore carries out the three required assessments, as determined by the Ministry of Health, thus ensuring continuity of care.

These differences in delivery of care have led us to consider the advantages and disadvantages of both systems. An involvement in helping to develop the educational standards for practice has also influenced the way in which we now view the newborn assessment. The provision of education relating to the newborn assessment in the rest of the world would appear, anecdotally at least, to be a more ad hoc affair, left to the discretion of the educational institution.

Although the newborn assessment forms the major focus, the book is far more than an account of how and why we carry out the examination. It is, in fact, an exploration of a continuum of health, from the antenatal period through to the neonatal phase and beyond—sometimes way beyond, into adulthood. The examination does, however, act as the pivot—that is, as the point where the subjects addressed within the book converge. As a point of clarification, the terms *newborn* and *neonate* will be used interchangeably within the book to refer to babies in the first month of life. From 1 month to 1 year, the term 'infant' will be used.

From the outset, we recognized that we did not necessarily want to restrict the contents of the book to the physical examination of the baby. We felt that we needed the health and well-being of the baby to be viewed from a holistic perspective. This means taking into consideration all of the cogent influences that can impact on the brand new world of the neonate, including those of an emotional, social, environmental, cultural and spiritual quality.

Many of the existing textbooks have a tendency to focus on pathology and abnormality. While we fully recognize the need for the midwife to detect any abnormalities and to refer appropriately, it is equally important that she/he approaches the newborn baby from a perspective of normality; this was a vital consideration for us.

The book is primarily aimed at UK undergraduate and postgraduate midwives who are undertaking the newborn infant physical examination programme, but we anticipate that it will equally be of use to student midwives, medical students, health visitors, neonatal nurses, parents and others involved in caring for the newborn baby. We also believe that it will be of use to practitioners in other countries.

Within the book, we have brought together many authors who are specialists in their own fields, to share their wealth of knowledge and expertise. The contributors come from a range of disciplines and include midwives, neonatologists, cardiologists, physiologists, optometrists and parents. This has resulted in a book with a broad range of styles which we feel enables us to offer a truly multidimensional approach to the subject. We feel that the book remains at the cutting edge, because it still approaches the examination of the newborn from a more inclusive and holistic standpoint than has been attempted elsewhere. Although it

acknowledges the micro-perspective and values the importance of the finer points in relation to, for example, anatomy and physiology, it equally offers the reader the challenge of the macro-perspective and seeing the bigger picture.

As we have previously stated, the practical examination of the newborn is the cornerstone of this book. In Chapter 2, Sharon presents a clear and comprehensive account of the newborn infant physical examination which lays the foundation for the remaining structure of the book. She explores the development of the examination and the evidence for broadening the scope of practice for the midwife and other practitioners to take on the responsibility for the assessment. She also explores in depth where, when and how the examination of the newborn should be carried out, and who is best placed to perform it. She considers what the practitioner needs to know before commencing the examination, what preparations they need to make and finally how to carry out a thorough and methodical physical examination. Emphasis is placed on the importance of gaining consent from the parents and ensuring effective communication and accurate documentation, with an understanding of the circumstances in which referral is necessary. She also considers the future development of the examination in the light of ever-evolving health care provision, from an educational as well as a practice-based perspective.

In the book, we have included what we believe is a comprehensive coverage of fetal and neonatal anatomy and physiology that will meet the needs of novices as well as experienced practitioners. Where possible, we have attempted to relate newborn anatomy and physiological functioning to the practical aspects of the examination.

In Chapter 3, Andrew McVicar outlines the important stages of embryological development and introduces the reader to genetic influences on the development of the embryo and fetus. This, in turn, informs many of the other chapters. In Chapter 6, Julie Richards and Lorna Davies introduce the structure of the fetal heart and outline the changes that follow birth. This is followed up in Chapter 9 by Eshita Upadhyay and Sanjay Raina, who explore structural anomalies of the heart in the newborn and discuss an extensive range of cardiac conditions and how they present in the newborn and infant. In Chapter 7, Penny Champion talks about the physiology of respiration and applies this to the resuscitation of the newborn. In Chapter 8, Sharon and Lindsey Rose explore the neurological system and explain the purpose of specific reflex testing during the assessment, as well as applying the principles to gestational dating of the newborn. John Siderov explores eye examination in the newborn in Chapter 10 and includes a discussion of visual function as well as screening for ocular disorders. Jacqui Anderson and Lorna Davies, in Chapter 11, use information on genetic inheritance to inform a discussion on congenital abnormality. We hope that these and other similar inclusions will help practitioners to gain a deeper understanding of the anatomy and physiological processes that relate to the examination of the newborn.

We have also included chapters that do not necessarily provide comprehensive lists of causes and effects in relation to areas such as fetal development or intrapartum influences, but take a much broader, more holistic and sometimes longer-term perspective. For example, Chapter 5, which explores prenatal effects on neonatal, child and adult health, challenges us to make a paradigm shift in our thinking by concentrating on a narrow range of influences to illustrate the broader issues at stake.

Jaundice is a regular occurrence in many newborn babies. In Chapter 12, Ange Deken and Maggie Meeks present the viewpoint that we are too ready to pathologize a condition that may offer significant long-term health benefits. Though acknowledging that pathological jaundice can, if left untreated, pose life-threatening conditions for babies, they offer a counterperspective which challenges existing knowledge and practice using the most up-to-date sources of evidence available. Sharon Trotter (Chapter 13) takes a brave stance and hypothesizes that commercial skin care products, freely distributed to parents during both pregnancy and the postnatal period, have the potential to cause a range of skin conditions. She provides an extensive range of literature and research to support her claims. This, too, may challenge some practitioners and parents.

Throughout the book, we have aimed to provide the reader with the most recent evidence available. In Chapter 6, Lorna Davies and Julie Richards introduce us to findings relating to the transition from intrauterine to extrauterine life, including the relatively new field of the microbiome. Chapter 4, written by Sharon and

Sarah Fiadjoe, updates issues relating to neonatal health in antenatal screening and aims to offer a comprehensive view of the tests currently offered in pregnancy. The chapter contains the most up-to-date recommendations from the UK NSC and identifies the timing and significance of these tests. The newborn screening and immunization chapter (Chapter 14) by Sharon and Lindsey Rose also uses material from the UK NSC and discusses current and potential future trends in newborn screening tests and methods.

One of the other significant features of the book is the inclusion of parents' stories. We are immensely grateful to those parents who have agreed to contribute in order to offer practitioners the opportunity to share their experiences. They serve to offer us insight into what it is like to be on the receiving end as a parent both during pregnancy and postnatally, when informed that there may be problems with the baby, or when asked to make important decisions regarding its care.

In the final chapter (Chapter 15), academics and midwives involved in public health initiatives come together to explore issues such as breastfeeding and co-sleeping (Martina Donaghy), tongue-tie (Corrine Neville), smoking and Vitamin K administration within a framework led by Elaine Jefford, an expert in the area of decision-making. The chapter considers how practitioners may help parents in their decision-making processes by deconstructing some of the attitudes and behaviours that may be observed in relation to the thornier issues around infant health.

The book is not an attempt to address every issue relating to neonatal health and the examination of the newborn; that would be an unrealistic quest. There are undoubtedly areas that receive less attention than you may think they deserve, and some that are not addressed at all. What we have attempted to do first is to offer an overview of the examination and ways in which it may be effectively performed using an evidence-informed approach. Second, we have offered the opportunity to gain a more in-depth understanding of some of the procedures within the examination, such as listening to the heart, examining the hips or carrying out a visual screening test. Finally, we have endeavoured to raise awareness of broader issues around the continuum of health within the life cycle by encouraging readers to look beyond the physical state of the baby. As Kharitidi (2001) states, 'the human being is a dual being and in the scientific paradigm of physics today, he is both particle and wave'. The whole is the sum of its parts; if we are unable to look beyond the biophysical profile of the newborn, then we are missing out on hugely significant factors that may promote (or, conversely, militate against) a positive state of health for the baby and possibly its future well-being.

We will leave you to explore the other chapters with a few words from a midwife who completed the newborn infant physical examination programme some years ago now. The sentiment expressed is partly what set us on the journey to create this book. We simply hope that our approach enables you, as reader, to view the area of newborn health with greater clarity.

Probably above all else, the Examination of the Newborn programme has left me with a rekindled respect for the newborn. I have always considered myself to be a 'woman-focused midwife'. A year or so ago, I was involved in a discussion about whether midwives perceived themselves to be 'woman focused' or 'baby focused', and I parked myself firmly with the 'woman focused' camp. I now realize that such a division is just that—divisive. The mother–baby dyad cannot be separated and I now consider myself a much more holistic practitioner as a result.

REFERENCES

Kharitidi, O., 2001. The Master of Lucid Dreams. Hampton Roads, Charlottesville, p. 225.

Lomax, A., 2015. Examination of the newborn: an evidence-based guide, 2nd edition. Wiley-Blackwell: West Sussex.

McDonald, S., 2008. Examining a newborn baby are midwives using their skills. British Journal of Midwifery 16(11): 722–724.

McDonald, S., 2018. Integration of the examination of the newborn into holistic midwifery practice: a grounded theory study. Evidence Based Midwifery 16(4)128–135.

McDonald, S., Allan, H., Brown, A., 2012. Perceptions of changing practice in the examination of the newborn, from holistic to opportunistic. British Journal of Midwifery 20(11):786–791.

NHS England, 2017. Implementing Better Births: Continuity of Carer. Available from: https://www.england.nhs.uk/publication/implementing-better-births-continuity-of-carer.

National Institute for Health and Clinical Excellence, 2015. CG 37 Postnatal Care: Routine Postnatal Care of Women and Their Babies. London, NICE. Available from: www.nice.org.uk. Accessed March 2019.

Public Health England, 2019. Antenatal and Newborn Screening Timeline-Optimum Times for Testing. Available from: https://assets.publishing.service.gov.uk/government/uploads/system/uploads/attachment_data/file/768805/ANNB_Timeline_v8.4.pdf 2018. Accessed January 2019.

Public Health England 2016 Newborn and Infant physical examination (NIPE) screening programme handbook (updated 2019) Available from: https://www.gov.uk/government/publications/newborn-and-infant-physical-examination-programme-handbook/newborn-and-infant-physical-examination-screening-programme-handbook. Accessed March 2020.

RCM, 2017. Continuity of Carer. Available from: https://www.rcm.org.uk/continuity-of-carer-0. Accessed March 2019

Townsend, J., Wolke, D., Hayes, J., 2004. Routine examination of the newborn: the EMREN study. Evaluation of an extension of the midwife role including a randomised controlled trial of appropriately trained midwives and paediatric senior house officers. Health Technology Assessment 8:14

Wolke, D., Dave, S., Hayes. J., et al., 2002. Routine neonatal examination: effectiveness of trainee paediatrician compared with advanced neonatal nurse. Archives of Disease in Childhood—Fetal Neonatal 85(2)100–104.

2

The Practical Examination of the Newborn

Sharon McDonald

This chapter aims to offer a comprehensive and holistic guide to the practicalities of the newborn infant physical examination (NIPE), from gathering maternal history to record-keeping and imparting information to parents. It serves as the foundation of the book, providing the background to all of the chapters that follow and which, in turn, link back to the examination and assessment of the newborn.

The purpose of the examination is to confirm normality, thereby reassuring parents and carers, and to identify and act upon any abnormalities (PHE, 2018a).

The four screening areas of NIPE are as follows:

- **Eyes:** about 2 or 3 in 10,000 babies have problems with their eyes that require treatment.
- **Heart:** around 1 in 200 babies may have a heart problem. Overall the incidence of congenital heart defects is 4 to 10 per 1000 live births, ranging from non-significant to major and critical lesions. Critical or major congenital cardiac malformations are found in approximately 2 to 3 per 1000 live births and are a leading cause of morbidity and mortality in the neonatal period and beyond.
- **Hips:** about 1 or 2 in 1000 babies have hip problems that require treatment. A proportion will have a positive screening test and will require specialist ultrasound screening within 2 weeks of birth. A further percentage will have a negative screening test but will have identified risk factors and will require specialist hip ultrasound before 6 weeks of age.
- **Testes:** about 1 in 100 baby boys have problems with their testes that require treatment.

WHEN SHOULD THE NEWBORN INFANT PHYSICAL EXAMINATION BE CARRIED OUT?

The UK National Screening Committee (UK NSC) policy for NIPE is that all eligible babies will be offered screening and a conclusive screening result will be achieved within 72 hours of birth. Screening may be delayed if a baby is unwell or too premature (PHE, 2018b) (Fig. 2.1).

A second examination is required at 6 to 8 weeks when the general practitioner or health visitor will continue the recommended screening.

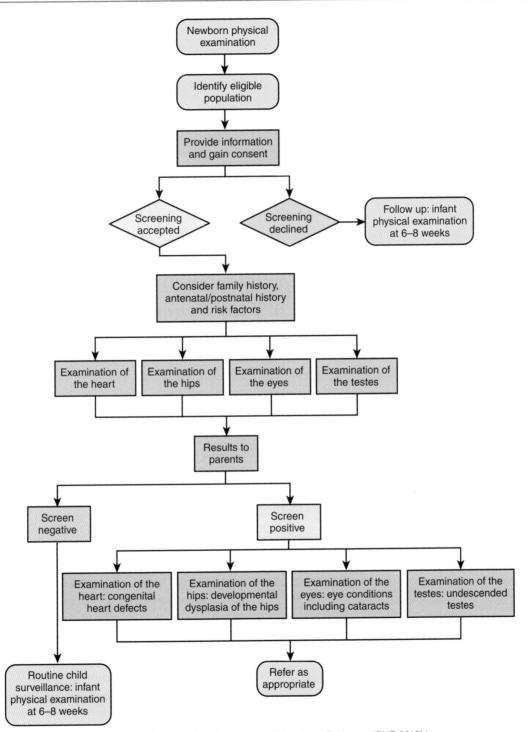

Fig. 2.1 NIPE Screening Programme: Newborn Pathway. (PHE 2018b)

PRACTICAL EXAMINATION OF THE NEWBORN

This section of the chapter aims to give a comprehensive guide to the practicalities of the NIPE. While it is beyond the scope of the chapter and book to provide a detailed discussion of all the variations and abnormalities listed, some insight is offered where possible. Practitioners are encouraged to undertake further reading as required, and where indicated in the text.

It is a legal and ethical requirement that valid consent should be gained from the parent(s) prior to examining the newborn/infant. It is recommended that practitioners should familiarize themselves with the Department of Health Reference guide to consent for examination or treatment (DoH, 2009). Good, effective communication is essential when discussing the issues of informed consent and the options for examination and treatment, as is an understanding and awareness of different cultural and traditional practices, values and beliefs (Reshma and Sujatha, 2014). It is essential that the practitioner gives information that is clear and comprehensible in a verbal and, if appropriate, written format (ensuring the mother can read and is able to understand English), and, if necessary, employing the services of a suitable translator.

The practitioner must fully acknowledge their responsibilities and limitations within the Nursing and Midwifery Council (NMC) Code (or appropriate regulatory bodies in other countries) and acknowledge their sphere of practice; they must initiate referrals for further investigations and/or treatments appropriately (NMC, 2018).

Record-Keeping: Reporting

Significant advances in the recording of NIPE have taken place in the UK, with the introduction of an IT management system for recording and reporting. In April 2019 the current system, NIPE Smart, was replaced with a new system, SMaRT4NIPE (S4N).

In addition, those undertaking NIPE should record the findings in the Personal Child Health Record books; the 'Red Book' has been used in the UK for many years and similar paper-based systems for sharing information between health professionals and parents are available across the world. Online versions are also being developed. Midwives are also advised to record in the mother's notes that the NIPE has been completed. An improved method for referral documentation is available via the SMaRT4NIPE (S4N) system. An aim of the new system is to instigate a reduction in the number of babies being diagnosed late with congenital medical conditions.

Environment

Ideally, the environment in which the examination is carried out should be warm, well lit (but not too bright) and peaceful. The parents should be present and be made comfortable, and reassurance should be given that their baby's welfare is of paramount importance. At the end of the examination, time should be taken to answer any questions and to provide advice. Chapter 15 highlights some of the key concerns parents may have in relation to decision-making.

Equipment

If the examination is being undertaken on a postnatal ward, the use of the Resuscitaire (overhead heater) ensures warmth and a firm base on which to examine the baby's hips. Alternatively, a cot can be used, though this is not ideal as it may not offer adequate stability or room for manoeuvres (Jones, 1998). In the home setting, a changing unit or another covered hard surface can be utilized. A last resort in either setting would be the use of a changing mat on a bed; the hygiene implications must be considered, as well as the practitioner's need to prevent back strain due to poor posture.

Other equipment should include:
1. Thermometer to assess neonatal temperature
2. Ophthalmoscope
3. Light source (pen torch) for visualizing the soft and hard palate
4. Neonatal stethoscope
5. Disposable tape measure for head circumference
6. Measuring mat for accurate length measurement

The Lasso-O measuring tape allows the head circumference to be measured to the nearest millimetre. A measuring mat is preferable to a tape measure for a more accurate supine length.

History Gathering

Prior to undertaking the NIPE, it is vital that a thorough and comprehensive history is obtained from both talking to the mother and briefing the maternal notes in a systematic appraisal of social history, family and maternal medical history, obstetric history, current pregnancy, investigations, labour and delivery, concluding with the newborn history. This will provide the practitioner with relevant information to inform the physical examination and to aid the practitioner in giving accurate information, support and advice (Tappero and Honeyfield, 2018; Gill and O'Brien, 2007). Even when the midwife knows the woman within a continuity of care model, this important information should be revisited. Anecdotal evidence suggests that, even though women are asked during the antenatal period about any family history of note, they need to be asked once again prior to the neonatal examination about family history, especially related to sight, heart, hearing and hip problems. Table 2.1 provides an indication of some areas to consider, but reference should also be made to other chapters as appropriate.

Physical Examination

Hand washing (following universal guidance) is an absolute prerequisite before commencing a physical examination (NICE, 2014).

The practitioner is likely to adopt their own way of examining a baby. However, a top-to-toe approach is recommended to ensure that a methodical and thorough approach is taken (see Box 2.1). To an extent the examination is opportunistic. Therefore if the baby is quiet, examination of the heart and lungs would be advised; alternatively, if the baby is crying and the practitioner can visualize the palate and elicit the suck, swallow and gag reflexes, they would be wise to do so, hopefully calming the baby to enable them to continue with the examination.

It is recommended that practitioners should always recheck the head circumference and temperature (axilla) prior to undertaking the assessment. The ideal axilla temperature for a term neonate is 36.5–37.3°C. If the temperature is within the normal range, the examination can be commenced. The practitioner should undress the baby to allow for adequate observation at all times and to facilitate the full range of movement required, for example during the hip examination.

TABLE 2.1 History Taking

Social History	Family Medical History	Maternal Medical History
Ethnic group	Diabetes	Hypertension
Single/partner/marital status	Tuberculosis (TB)	Diabetes
Family support	Congenital anomalies	Epilepsy
Type of occupation	Heart	TB
Smoking	Hearing (30% of hearing loss is related to family history)	Congenital anomalies
Safeguarding issues and referrals	Hip problems	Heart, hearing or hip anomalies
Social Service referrals	Other significant illnesses	Medication
Alcohol and recreational drug use	Health status of maternal, paternal and newborn's siblings	
		Other significant illnesses
Previous Obstetric History	**Current Pregnancy**	**Most Recent**
Parity	Gestation	Haemoglobin (Hb)
Antenatal history	Ultrasound scan reports: dating scan/anomaly scans	Mean cell volume (MCV)
Intrapartum history	Maternal blood group	Any other significant serology results, for example, sickle cell trait, thalassaemia, G6PD
Postnatal history	Rhesus factor	
Health status of newborn's siblings	Rubella status	
	Hepatitis status	
	HIV status	

Continued

TABLE 2.1 History Taking—cont'd		
Other Investigations	**Labour and Delivery History**	**Neonatal History**
Midstream specimen of urine (MSU)	Gestation	Weeks gestation:
	Onset	Age of exam (days/hours)
High/low vaginal swabs	Spontaneous/induction	Sex
Further considerations if required dependent on history:	Date and time of delivery	Immediate neonatal period:
Blood group	Amniotic fluid colour	Any resuscitation required
Full blood count	Membranes ruptured/hours prior to delivery	Any medication given
Rhesus factor for anti D immunity		Apgar: 1 minute
Direct Coombs	Length of 1st stage	Apgar: 5 minutes
Antibodies present	Length of second stage	Cord gases
Bacillus de Calmette-Guérin (BCG)	Complications of labour	Placenta or cord abnormalities
Microbiology	Complications of delivery	Well/not well
Swabs taken at birth	Type of delivery	Vital signs: temperature, Apex and respirations
	Management of third stage of labour	Elimination: passed meconium and/or urine
	Drugs administered during labour and time	Complete centile chart: weight, head circumference, length
	Anaesthesia administered: type and time	Breast feeding or artificial feeding
		Note the time of first feed, and length of feed

BOX 2.1

The examination of the neonate should always commence with observation, followed by a combination of palpation and auscultation of each system.
- **Observation**: Accurate observation incorporating the visual and auditory skills will alert the examiner to carry out a more thorough examination of a system.
- **Palpation**: Using touch to assess both superficial and deeper body characteristics.
- **Auscultation**: Listening to the sounds produced by the body, by either direct auscultation (practitioner's ear) or indirect auscultation (stethoscope).

Observation

It is important to observe the baby before commencing the physical examination. A great deal of information may be elicited from skilled observation of the newborn's general appearance in relation to colour (ethnicity), position, posture, tone, spontaneous activity, facial dysmorphia and body proportions. The examiner should be noting, for example: Is the baby alert, awake or asleep (see Chapter 8)? Are there any signs of nasal flaring and sternal recession? Does the baby have its fists clenched or are they relaxed?

Cry

Is the baby crying or not? Note the type of cry and ensure that normal symmetry of the facial features can be seen. In term neonates a loud lusty cry is described as normal.

ABNORMALITY

High-pitched cry is associated with, for example, intracranial pressure, infection (meningitis) and pain; if accompanied by a shrill and incessant screaming, cry (and irritability) is associated with drug withdrawal (Siney, 1999).

Weak and whimpering: unwell, ill and premature newborn

Cat-like cry: cri-du-chat syndrome

Tone

When the practitioner handles the baby, they should be able to determine normal limb movements and muscle tone. Term babies will generally lie with their limbs in a flexed position, described as an 'attitude of flexion'. The term 'floppy' is sometimes used to describe a neonate with reduced tone, which may be related to reduced gestational age or may suggest a hypotonic state where there is possibly some muscle weakness or neurological impairment.

Skin

Once the baby is undressed, the practitioner will be able to assess the overall health of the baby and the condition of the skin; they should note the colour, perfusion, texture, tone and turgor of the skin and the presence of birth marks. Neonatal skincare and implications for practice are explored further in Chapter 13, but some examples of common skin variations, abnormalities and birth marks follow.

COMMON VARIATIONS NOTED WITH SKIN OBSERVATION/EXAMINATION

Superficial peeling of the skin	Often seen in the newborn, particularly in babies born post-term; no treatment is necessary.
Acrocyanosis	Usually seen at birth, this benign condition is exacerbated by low temperatures and presents in the newborn as a bluish discoloration of the hands and feet. It should improve or disappear within the first 48 hours.
Circumoral cyanosis	This is seen as a bluish discoloration around the mouth. It should improve or disappear within the first 24 hours.
Erythema toxicum neonatorum	Small white or yellow papules or vesicles which have an erythematous base. This benign neonatal rash can be found anywhere on the neonate's body and is often exacerbated by handling, heat and irritation caused by clothing. If the spots do not disappear within 48 hours or have white heads, consider infection and swab accordingly (Fig. 2.2).
Epstein pearl's and milia	Epstein's pearls are seen in the mouth and milia (white pimples) are seen on the nose, brow and cheeks. These are epidermal cysts which are caused by blocked sebaceous gland secretions. They resolve spontaneously and are seen in a high proportion of newborns.
Lanugo	Presence of fine hair.
Vernix caseosa	Creamy white greasy material. It covers the fetus and reduces with gestational age. This should be noted if present but not rubbed off or removed; it will dissolve into the skin.
Dry patches	Commonly seen in post-term babies, particularly around the ankles and wrists.
Jaundice	A yellow discoloration of the skin, common between 3 and 5 days of life (neonatal jaundice, see Chapter 12).
Permanent pigmented skin lesions	These are due to abnormal development of the melanin cells which produce pigment; the melanocytes infiltrate the dermis, causing a discoloration of the skin (grey-blue, blue-black or deep brown).
Hyperpigmented macule	The most common birthmark, seen in an estimated 90% of Asian, Hispanic and African American infants and around 10% of Caucasian infants. Still described by some practitioners as a 'Mongolian blue spot' (named by 19th-century German anthropologist Erwin Bälz, who frequently found this birthmark on his 'Mongolian' patients), it is a benign congenital birthmark, flat with wavy borders and an irregular shape. It normally disappears 3 to 5 years after birth, and almost always by puberty (Figs 2.3 and 2.4).
Bruising	Usually due to birth trauma. However, if extensive or petechial skin haemorrhage is seen, investigate further.

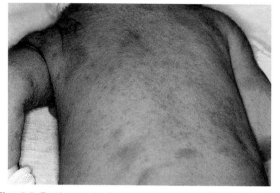

Fig. 2.2 Erythema toxicum neonatorum. (Reprinted from Thomas R & Harvey D, Paediatrics and Neonatology in Focus 2005, with permission from Elsevier Ltd.)

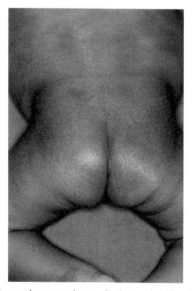

Fig. 2.3 Hyperpigmented macule: buttocks. (Reprinted from Thomas R & Harvey D, Paediatrics and Neonatology in Focus 2005, with permission from Elsevier Ltd.)

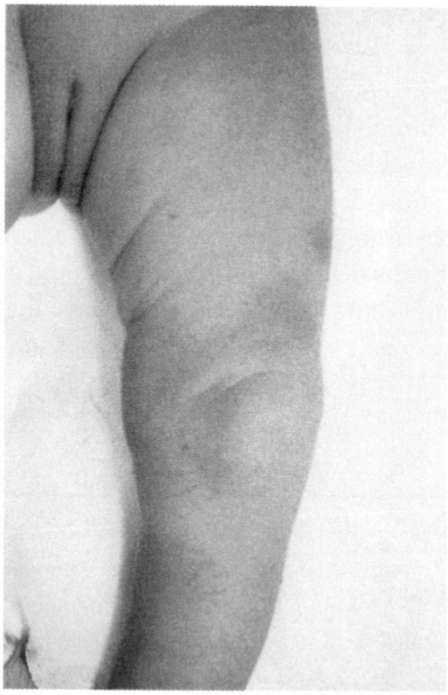

Fig. 2.4 Hyperpigmented macule: knees. (Reprinted from Thomas R & Harvey D, Paediatrics and Neonatology in Focus 2005, with permission from Elsevier Ltd.)

Plethora	Red coloration of a newborn infant's skin. Facial plethora can be caused by an unusually high proportion of erythrocytes per volume of blood, familial polycythaemia or drug reactions, and can occur following delayed cord clamping. Treatment of facial plethora follows diagnosis of the underlying condition; with treatment of the cause, facial plethora will fade automatically.

ABNORMALITY

Jaundice	If baby is less than 24 hours old, consider pathological jaundice (see Chapter 12).
Cyanosis	Due to hypoxia. If central cyanosis is observed, particularly in the mucous membranes, consider cardiac anomaly.
Pallor	May indicate a shocked baby, but also linked to anaemia (normal haemoglobin for the neonate is 16–18g/dl).

BIRTH MARKS These may be either vascular naevi (capillary) or haemangiomas (cavernous); they are caused by an abnormal development of tiny blood vessels which can be temporary or permanent.

Naevus simplex	Common superficial capillary naevi, known as 'stork bites', they are often seen on the eyelids, forehead and nape of the neck (naevus flammeus).

Superficial cavernous haemangioma	A haemangioma is usually bright red, slightly raised and sharply defined. It is commonly called a strawberry birth mark. This is not usually seen at birth but appears within the first week, gradually increasing in size (variation) until about 6 months when it starts to regress; it disappears by the time the child is 5–7 years old.
Capillary haemangioma	This is larger and darker than the naevus flammeus and can appear anywhere on the body, though frequently seen on the face (port wine stain).
Café au lait spots/ patches	Often seen in the axilla and viscera. If larger than approximately 3 cm or greater than six in number, consider cutaneous neurofibromatosis (von Recklinghausen disease, in which tumours form on the peripheral nerves).
Birth trauma	The skin should also be observed for lesions due to trauma caused by fetal scalp electrodes, forceps, ventouse extraction and other less common conditions.
Sucking blisters	Often seen on lips and fingers.
Cutis aplasia	A congenital abnormality in which layers of the skin are absent. This is not a common condition; it can occur anywhere on the body though is more often seen on the scalp.

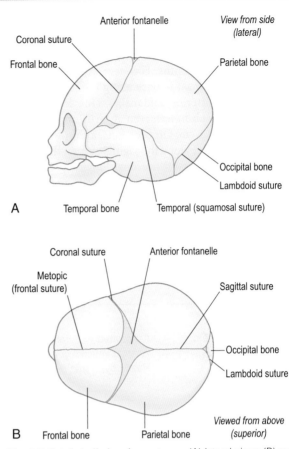

Fig. 2.5 **Fetal skull showing sutures.** (A) lateral view; (B) superior view.

cephalohaematoma or forceps disortion, as it is likely to be less than accurate (see Box 2.2).

Palpation

Feel the suture lines from the frontal (metopic) suture upwards to the anterior fontanelle. The size of the

Head (Fig. 2.5)

Head circumference
Vault of head for shape and symmetry: skull depressions or irregularities
Anterior fontanelle
Posterior fontanelle
Palpate sutures
Hair presence and texture

Observation

Assess shape and symmetry. The head measurement taken on the first day should not be used as a point of reference unless there is no moulding, caput,

---

BOX 2.2

To measure the head circumference (occipital-frontal circumference), place the tape measure around the head from the occipital prominence, to the level of the helix of the ear, to the middle of the forehead. It is advised to check and recheck the position of the tape up to three times to ensure accuracy of the reading, which should be to the nearest 0.5 cm. The head measurement will be dependent on mode of delivery, gestation and size. The average is considered to be 35 cm at term although measurements range between 33 and 37 cm (10th and 90th percentiles).

anterior fontanelle varies between 1.5 and 5 cm in diameter; it is diamond shaped and should not be depressed or bulging. Closure of this fontanelle occurs around 12 to 18 months. Feel across the coronal sutures, then from front to back along the sagittal suture towards the posterior fontanelle. This fontanelle is sometimes difficult to feel, even at birth, and measures approximately 0.5 cm. On occasions, a third fontanelle may be felt midway along the sagittal suture; this can be an indicator of Down syndrome. Finally, palpate the lambdoidal suture. Note the absence or presence of hair and feel the texture of the hair, which should be soft with a normal hairline observed at the front and back. Note the presence of and number of hair whorls (Fig. 2.6).

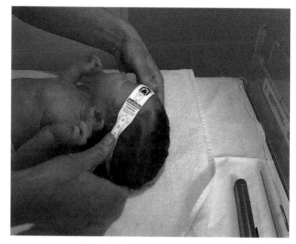

Fig. 2.6 Head measurement.

VARIATIONS

Bruises/lacerations to face	Associated with forceps delivery/caesarean delivery, face presentation/compound presentation/nuchal cord/shoulder dystocia.
Moulding	Head shape that results from pressure on the head during birth.
Caput succedaneum	Caused by pressure on the head in prolonged labour which results in accumulation of serum above the periosteum. Crosses the suture lines and often accompanied by bruising and petechiae. The oedema usually disappears within 48 hours of birth.
Hair whorls	Up to two is normal. More than two, with an abnormal hairline, brittle texture and an increased quantity of hair, are associated with abnormal brain growth and/or congenital abnormalities (Tappero and Honeyfield, 2018).
Asymmetry (other than postural asymmetry)	Caused in utero, should resolve.
Cephalohaematoma	Can occur spontaneously following normal birth, although there is an association with assisted delivery. Friction during birth causes blood vessels between the periosteum and the skull to rupture and blood accumulates below the periosteum. Swelling is contained within the suture lines but may be unilateral or bilateral. Develops during the first 24 hours of life. May lead to pronounced jaundice (Chapter 12). If no coagulation disorder is present, most are benign and treatment is rare. Prognosis is excellent; usually resolves spontaneously by 3 months of age.
Birth injury	Scalp lesions from amniotic hook, fetal scalp electrode, fetal blood sampling, forceps or ventouse cap. Suturing is sometimes required for lacerations. Observe for infection.
Tense and bulging fontanelle	Due to intracranial pressure.
Sutures	Open, wide, fused or overriding.
Hydrocephaly	Enlarged head caused by excess of cerebrospinal fluid within the ventricles of the brain.
Macrocephaly	Excessively large head—may be familial or due to hydrocephaly. Also associated with achondroplasia.
Microcephaly	Small head—may be a normal variation, familial or due to perinatal hypoxia, chromosomal disorders or a severe metabolic disorder.
Craniotabes	Soft skull bones; common along the margins of the sutures. However, it can be a sign of rare disorders, for example osteogenesis imperfecta, if not confined to the suture margins.

Craniosynostosis	Premature fusion of the sutures; incidence estimated at 1 in 10,000 births. May require surgery due to risk of raised intracranial pressure (Fish and Lima, 2003) Associated with hyperthyroidism (metabolic disorder) and genetic syndromes: Apert (estimated incidence 1 in 65,000–85,000 newborns) and Crouzon (1.6 per 100,000).
Brachycephaly	Flattening to the back of the cranium; the head appears distorted, wide and short.
Plagiocephaly	Distortion of the cranium due to restricted intrauterine posture, premature birth and congenital torticollis.
	Can be exacerbated postnatally by a prolonged static position in the cot, therefore the importance of noninvasive repositioning techniques to reduce the risk of positional plagiocephaly should be discussed with parents. The current recommendation from the Lullaby Trust (2019) includes advice to parents to give babies supervised 'tummy time' to reposition the head, and to reduce the amount of time a baby spends in a car seat. Car seats should only be for transporting; the recommendation is that, if well, baby should only be in a car seat for a maximum 2 hours in a 24-hour period, and observed during this time (see Table 2.3). Cranial remoulding orthoses to remould and control skull growth may be required in moderate to severe cases of positional plagiocephaly diagnosed after 3 months of age.
Skull fractures	Associated with forceps-assisted delivery. May be linear or depressed. Associated with both extracranial and intracranial haemorrhages. The baby may demonstrate abnormal neurological signs, such as poor tone, decreased activity, or poor feeding. If treated early, both types have excellent prognoses as long as there is no indication of underlying brain injury (Figs 2.7 and 2.8).

Face and Forehead

The forehead makes up one-third of the face; observe for symmetry (shape) and determine that there are no dysmorphic features. Observe for trauma from delivery. For example, forceps can cause facial palsy, bruising and abrasions; face or brow presentation can lead to bruising and petechiae; fetal scalp electrodes can cause abrasions. Babies delivered by non-elective and elective lower segment caesarean section should be examined for scalpel marks.

> **VARIATION** Malformations of the newborn and/or dysmorphic features—can be an isolated finding in an otherwise normal individual.

> **ABNORMALITY** Dysmorphic features or syndromes associated with congenital disorder, genetic syndrome, or birth defect.

Eyes (Fig. 2.9)
Presence of eyelashes and eyebrows
Epicanthal folds
Two eyes
Pupils
Bilateral red reflex
Lacrimal process
Sclerae

Observation

The normal features of the eye that are visible on external inspection are the eyelids and eyelashes, the cornea, the sclera and conjunctiva (a thin, semi-transparent membranous coat), the iris, the anterior chamber, and the pupil. Elicitation of the red reflex (Box 2.3) should always be attempted. There should be two eyes, centrally placed and equally spaced; they should be symmetrical from the bridge of the nose with eyebrows which do not meet in the middle. Track from the inner canthus of the eye to the outer canthus, drawing an imaginary line to the posterior fontanelle. Note the presence of eyelashes which curl out and up at the top and outwards at the bottom. The sclera should be white and clear, and the iris should form a complete circle around a black pupil.

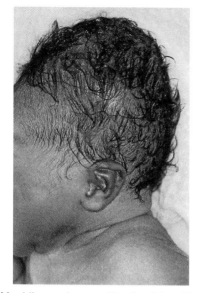

Fig. 2.7 Moulding and caput. (Reprinted from Thomas R & Harvey D, Paediatrics and Neonatology in Focus 2005, with permission from Elsevier Ltd.)

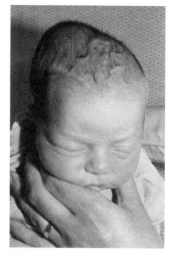

Fig. 2.8 Parietal cephalhaematoma. (Reprinted from Thomas R & Harvey D, Paediatrics and Neonatology in Focus 2005, with permission from Elsevier Ltd.)

BOX 2.3

Practitioners must elicit the red reflex to exclude congenital cataracts. To perform the test, an ophthalmoscope must be used. Sometimes it can be difficult to perform this test. If possible, dim the lights; alternatively, elevate the baby's head or ask the mother to hold the baby over her shoulder as this position sometimes aids examination. The pupils should react to the light and there should be no clouding of the cornea. This examination is discussed in detail in Chapter 10.

Conjunctival and subconjunctival haemorrhages	Rupture of small capillaries within the conjunctiva due to elevated venous pressure in the head and neck. Often observed after normal birth but frequently when tight nuchal cord present. No treatment is required.
Strabismus	See Chapter 10.
Epicanthal fold	A vertical fold of skin which can be seen from the corner of the eye up towards the eyebrows. Characteristically seen in Asian individuals but also 20% of non-Asians and in babies with Down syndrome.
Brushfield spots	Whitish spots seen on the edge of the iris; these are a normal variation in some ethnicities but are also seen in babies with Down syndrome.

VARIATION

Blocked nasolacrimal duct	The nasolacrimal duct may not be fully patent up to 7 months of age; consequently, fluid will often not drain sufficiently. Advice should be given to parents on how to keep eyes clean, including gentle cleansing from the inner eye outwards with water and cotton wool (preferably pads so that there are no loose fibres), one eye at a time; alternatively gentle lacrimal massage can be effective. Prompt referral made if signs of infection or pus (exudate) are observed.

ABNORMALITY

Retinoblastoma or retinopathy of prematurity—if the red reflex is absent a white pupillary reflex will be seen. Absence of red reflex (leukocoria) may indicate a severe ocular problem.

Absence of eye(s), asymmetry of the eyes, bushy eyebrows, very long or absent eyelashes.

Setting sun sign, where the sclera is visible above the iris, can be observed with intracranial pressure and hydrocephalus.

Squint or nystagmus—eye muscle imbalance.

Jaundice.

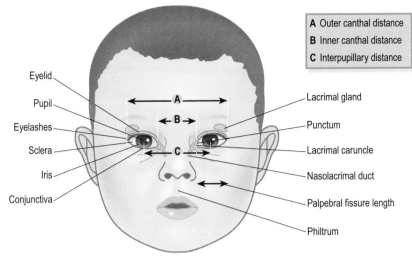

Fig. 2.9 Newborn eyes.

Ears (Pinna) (Fig. 2.10)

Two ears
Symmetrical/alignment
Shape
Patent meatus

Observation

Two ears—we use the term 'complicated ears', which refers to the folds of the ears. The size and shape of all newborns' ears will vary.

Examination

To look at the position of the ears, we draw an imaginary line from the inner canthus of the eye to the outer canthus, along an imaginary line to the posterior fontanelle. The helix of the ears should be on this imaginary line and no more than a third above or a third below it. Ensure that there is natural recoil of the helix as this is a sign of normal gestational age. It is vital to look behind the ears to check for skin tags and preauricular nodes or sinus. Visualize just inside the ear canal with a light source to check for a patent meatus. Hearing screening is most often undertaken prior to discharge from the hospital, but practitioners should check for any hearing anomalies as part of the initial history gathering and advise parents that they will be offered hearing screening (PHE, 2016) (Fig. 2.11). Universal hearing screening is discussed further in Chapter 14.

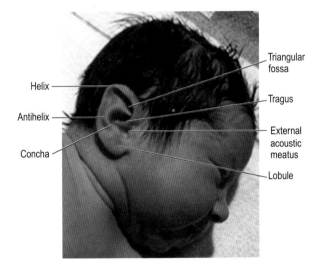

Fig. 2.10 Newborn ears.

VARIATION

Preauricular sinus is a common birth defect which generally appears as a tiny skin-lined hole or pit. It can be found unilaterally or bilaterally, usually on the upper part of the ear where the cartilage meets the face. It does not cause problems unless it becomes infected (requires antibiotics or surgery to remove the sinus).

Overly prominent ears.

Absent or poorly formed helix.

Darwinian tubercle—small nodule on upper helix.

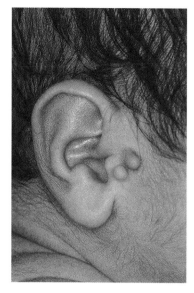

Fig. 2.11 Accessory auricles. (Reprinted from Thomas R & Harvey D, Paediatrics and Neonatology in Focus 2005, with permission from Elsevier Ltd.)

> **ABNORMALITY**
> All or part of the ear is absent.
> The ear is large and flabby.
> Abnormal placement/attachment—seen in some chromosome disorders, e.g., trisomies 13 and 18.

Nose

Size
Placement—vertically in the midline
Symmetry
Patency of two nares

Observation

Observation of the nose takes into consideration the above features. In addition, check that the two nares are centrally placed and confirm nasal patency by observing the newborn breathing. Practitioners are reminded that babies are obligate nose breathers and normal sneezing is common; excessive sneezing is not.

> **ABNORMALITIES**
> Nasal flaring.
> Nasal grunting.
> Inspiratory wheezing.

Respiratory distress (see Chapter 7).
Choanal atresia.
Injury to nasal structure—associated with forceps delivery. Damage can range from slight abnormality to complete dislocation of the septum. Severe cases can significantly compromise breathing for infants, who are obligate nose breathers.

Philtrum

The philtrum is the indented area between the nose and mouth.

> **VARIATION**
> A flat philtrum and thin lips may alert the practitioner to fetal alcohol syndrome (see Chapter 5).

Mouth

Symmetrical grimace
Lips/gums
Tongue
Arched palate
Uvula
Pink mucous membranes
Suck, swallow and gag reflexes

Observation

Lips should be pink and bow-shaped.

Examination

Examination of the mouth to exclude a cleft palate: the RCPCH guidance (Hunter and Habel, 2014) states that examination of the baby's hard and soft palate should be carried out by visual inspection only digital inspection is no longer advocated unless the palate cannot be visualized. A torch and method of depressing the tongue should be used to visualize the whole palate and to observe the colour of mucous membranes (pink). Parents should be informed if the whole palate (including the full length of the soft palate) has not been visualized during the first attempt, then a further attempt at visual examination should be made within 24 hours. While this is the guidance from RCPCH and should be undertaken in clinical practice, it is acknowledged by many clinicians that, due to clinicians' time constraints and parents' wishes for early discharge, the reality is that if you are unable to visualize the hard and soft palate with a light source during the initial NIPE, a digital examination will be undertaken to ensure the palate is examined; any referrals will be undertaken in a timely manner.

If you have been unable to visualize and observe fully, then with the mother's permission and gloved hands, do the following: feel along the alveolar ridges (gums) to exclude early dentition; elicit the sucking, swallow and gag reflexes (as the gag reflex is activated, the uvula may be seen); note the shape, size and colour of the tongue; exclude ankyloglossia (tongue-tie) by noting the position of the frenulum (the band of tissue running from the floor of the mouth to the base of the tongue) and movement of the tongue.

VARIATION

Epstein's pearls—white cysts seen on the palate.
Sucking tubercle—blistered area on the lips.
Premature dentition (1 in 2000 births).
Ranuli—benign bluish mucous cysts found under the tongue (Fig. 2.12).
Bifid uvula—associated with a submucous cleft palate; the cleft, covered only by a thin membrane of tissue, may involve just the soft palate or extend to the hard palate.
Tongue-tie—the lingual frenulum is abnormally tight and anchors the tongue tip to the floor of the mouth, restricting the newborn's ability to protrude the tongue (NICE, 2005; Johnson, 2006; Chapter 15).

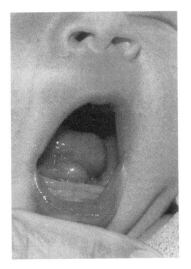

Fig. 2.12 Ranula. (Reprinted from Thomas R & Harvey D, Paediatrics and Neonatology in Focus 2005, with permission from Elsevier Ltd.)

ABNORMALITY

Asymmetry—may indicate facial palsy.
Cleft palate (see Chapter 11).
High-arched palate.
Thrush.
Macroglossia—large protruding tongue.
Profuse saliva—exclude tracheoesophageal fistula.

Chin
Observation

Note the presence of the chin and its size and shape. It should not be abnormally large (macrognathia) or abnormally small (micrognathia, often seen in Pierre Robin sequence).

Neck

Shape
Masses
Movement
Tonic neck reflex

Observation

It is important to lift the head to visualize the neck, to palpate both the back of the neck and underneath the chin to check for webbing, and to exclude torticollis.

Palpation

Feel for any unusual lymph glands or nodes around and in the skin folds. Feel for the carotid pulses; make sure there are no thrills felt.

ABNORMALITY

Webbing—associated with Turner syndrome.
Torticollis—shortening of neck muscle; results in an involuntary spasm of the musculature of the spine in the neck. Treatment involves stretching the shortened neck muscle. Prognosis is good.
Cystic hygroma—a soft fluid-filled sac resulting from a blockage in the lymphatic system. The most common neck mass (1 in 800 pregnancies, 1 in 8000 live births). Most often benign but can be linked to chromosomal abnormalities (e.g., Turner syndrome, Edwards syndrome, Down syndrome) and Noonan syndrome. Many disappear before birth or regress spontaneously; others require surgical resection. They can cause problems with breathing and eating depending on size and placement.

Sternomastoid tumours—can be found in the middle third of the sternomastoid muscle. They are caused by a difficult birth but often do not present until days or even weeks later.

Dermoid and thyroglossal cysts—uncommon occurrences.

Lymph node enlargement—not a common occurrence; generally indicates infection.

Skeletal System

Careful examination of the musculoskeletal system involves inspection and palpation (Fig. 2.13).

While it is beyond the scope of this chapter to explore all of the variations and anomalies associated with the musculoskeletal system, a comprehensive assessment of the prenatal history (particularly review of ultrasonography assessments) will alert the practitioner to any potential effects on the development and maturation of the musculoskeletal system (and subsequently the fetus). The assessment should include any changes to the uterine environment, and the perinatal history including duration of labour and type of delivery which may have resulted in birth trauma or neurological insult (Table 2.1).

The skeletal system is the internal framework that provides the body with support and the ability to move. It consists of bones, joints, supportive and connective tissues. The human skeleton consists of the axial skeleton—the vertebral column, rib cage, skull and other associated bones—and the appendicular skeleton, which is attached to the axial skeleton and made up of the shoulder and pelvic girdle in addition to the bones of the upper and lower limbs. At birth, we have

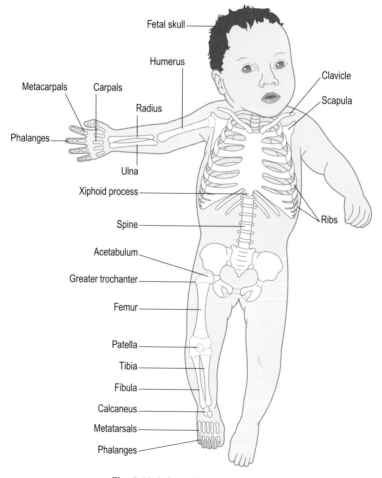

Fig. 2.13 Infant skeletal system.

approximately 270 bones; this total will decrease to around 206 by the time we reach adulthood following the fusion of some bones. Bone mass reaches maximum density around the age of 21. The skeletal system protects the brain and spinal cord, produces red and white blood cells and stores minerals, especially phosphorus which works with calcium to help build bones. The bones of the newborn are soft and flexible, the joints are elastic and the muscles should be firm. Their shape is smooth; no swelling or muscle wasting should be seen or felt. The process of ossification occurs rapidly during the first year of life.

Upper Extremities

Clavicles
Shoulders
Arms: length and movement
Hands and fingers/thumbs: length and movement
Nails
Grasp reflex
Axillae

Observation

Two arms which are of equal length and symmetrical movement.

Palpation and Examination

Feel along the clavicles to exclude fractures, along the upper extremities to the shoulder joint, along the humerus and the elbow joint, then the radius and ulna. Move the pivot joint in the wrists gently backwards and forwards; greater wrist flexion is seen in term infants. Check there are only four fingers and a thumb on each hand, with intact nails, no skin tags or webbing, and two palmar creases. Note any acrocyanosis. Fingers are usually flexed into a fist with the thumb positioned under the fingers. Obtain the grasp reflex by placing your finger in the palm of the neonate's hand and gently lifting upwards; the baby should grasp the finger (Fig. 2.14). Observe and palpate under the arms (axillae) for enlarged glands or masses.

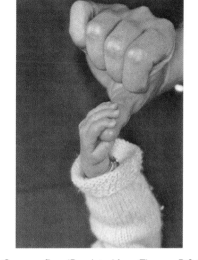

Fig. 2.14 Grasp reflex. (Reprinted from Thomas R & Harvey D, Paediatrics and Neonatology in Focus 2005, with permission from Elsevier Ltd.)

ABNORMALITY

Fractured clavicles—consider the possibility of fractured clavicles if the baby is unsettled or cries when you palpate the clavicles or shoulders. Consider the maternal history and mode of delivery, particularly shoulder dystocia or other difficult birth. Note if there is any crepitus, swelling or tenderness and whether the baby has restricted, abnormal or absent movement of one or both arms, or absent or poor grasp reflex in either hand. The majority of fractures require no treatment.

Fractured humerus—during a difficult or breech birth, forced traction on the limbs may fracture or dislocate the humerus or femur. Treatment includes immobilization by either traction or casting. These injuries generally heal without complications.

Abnormally shaped digits and nails and abnormally positioned digits.

Absence of nails—seen in some congenital syndromes, for example Turner syndrome and trisomies 13 and 18 (see Chapter 11).

Fisted hands where the newborn's fists appear clenched—associated with cerebral palsy.

The following apply to hands and feet:

Webbing of digits.

Paronychia—infection of nail beds. Usually caused by *Staphylococcus aureus*.

Polydactyly—extra digits.

Syndactyly—fused digits. Also seen in Apert syndrome.

Clinodactyly—incurved digits.

VARIATIONS

Simian creases—there are usually two palmar creases on each hand. A single crease can be present and most are of no consequence. However, one palmar crease is also a 'soft sign' present in babies with Down syndrome.

Chest

Shape
Breasts
Examination of the chest involves observation, palpation and auscultation of the heart, lungs and bowels.

A good neonatal stethoscope will allow for more accurate monitoring of the heart and lungs. The diaphragm will pick up high-frequency sounds, while the bell is used for low-frequency sounds. The choice of which part of the stethoscope is used will vary, although the heart can be heard with both parts of the stethoscope, while the breath sounds are more clearly heard with the diaphragm.

Observation and Palpation

The chest should rise and fall with inspiration and expiration of breath. There should be no signs of sternal or rib recession. There should be two nipples, equally spaced, with breast tissue (approximately 1–2 cm of palpable breast tissue is normal); note any engorgement (result of maternal oestrogen) or discharge (witch's milk) or swelling (mastitis with discharge—this is rare) of the breasts.

VARIATION

Shape of the chest and muscle development—variations may be scaphoid (sunken) or protruding. An indented sternum (pectus excavatum) is seen in 1–8 per 1000 newborns and is most often of no significance. However, some cases can restrict breathing and cause pain. Concave, barrel-shaped, pectus carinatum (pigeon chest), where the sternum protrudes outwards, is seen more often in males; it can be described as a funnel-shaped chest and is seen in Noonan and Marfan syndromes. The lower part of the sternum is depressed but the degree and severity vary.

Placement of nipples—they can occur anywhere along the mammary ridge, which is in line with the armpits, down to the groin.

Supernumerary nipples with or without breast tissue.

Breast engorgement—this can be normal and resolves within a few days.

ABNORMALITY

Poland syndrome—absence of the pectoralis major muscle, plus rib defects and upper limb hypoplasia.

Signs of sternal and rib recession—an indication of respiratory distress.

Cardiac Examination

The embryological development of the heart is outlined in Chapter 3 and the transitional adaptation of the newborn and adjustment to extrauterine life are explored in Chapter 6. A comprehensive explanation of the pressures within the heart and their significance, particularly in relation to some of the more common cardiovascular conditions and their presentation in the neonate and infant, are described in Chapter 9.

Assessment of the cardiovascular system continues to cause a degree of anxiety among practitioners who are new to the examination; a systematic description of the practical physical examination has therefore been included to lead the learner through the process step by step. There are, additionally, a vast number of websites which practitioners can access to hear how the normal and abnormal heart sounds. One of these is Stanford Medicine: https://med.stanford.edu/newborns/professional-education/photo-gallery/heart.html.

The cardiac examination is best performed early in the assessment in order to take advantage of the quiet state of the newborn.

Cardiovascular assessment of the newborn requires the skills of observation, palpation and auscultation. It is important to auscultate the precordium in a systematic way, covering all four valve areas (Fig. 2.15). Anatomically, the precordium is the portion of the anterior chest wall over the heart and lower chest. It is therefore usually on the left side, except in dextrocardia, where the individual's heart is on the right side.

It is important to recognize how the normal heart sounds. The two obvious but discrete heart sounds which should be heard are the first and second sounds, heard as a 'lub dub'. The sounds represent the closure of the heart valves and demarcate systole from diastole. The pressure during systole is much greater in the left ventricle than the right, which means that the mitral valve closes before the tricuspid in the S1 sound. Similarly, the aortic valve closes before the pulmonic valve in S2, because pressure at the start of diastole is much higher in the aorta than in the pulmonary artery. When a valve is damaged or stenotic (narrowed), the resultant abnormal blood flow produces a murmur (see Box 2.4).

Heart

Colour of infant
Point of maximum impulse
Rate

Observation of the Newborn's General Activity	Palpation	Auscultation (Heart Sounds)
Activity of the precordium—the precordium in the term newborn is quiet; however, in the first few hours of life a visible impulse may be seen along the lower left sternal border. If seen after the first few hours of life, this is not normal in a term newborn and may indicate heart disease. Breathing. Cry. Colour: pink or cyanosis.	Peripheral perfusion (capillary refill): press down centrally with one finger on the upper chest, and release; colour should return to normal 'pink' within 3 seconds. Feel across the chest for the point of maximal impulse (PMI, also described as the apex beat), normally located at the fifth intercostal space. Heaves and thrills. Femoral pulses. Palpate the brachial pulse at the same time as listening at the PMI, feeling for equal rate, rhythm and volume.	When performing the cardiovascular assessment, it is recommended that practitioners should listen for a full minute at the PMI and for approximately 30 seconds at each valve. The two heart sounds should be heard in all areas and there should be no extra sounds heard.

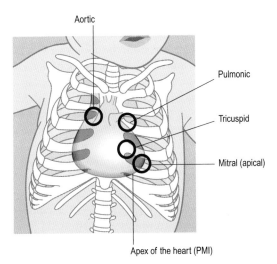

Fig. 2.15 Position of the heart within the chest cavity, showing four auscultatory areas.

Rhythm
Central perfusion
Peripheral perfusion
Capillary filling time
Presence, quality, symmetry of brachial and femoral pulses

Observation and Palpation

- Observe baby's colour, which should be appropriate for its ethnicity.
- Observe the chest for symmetrical movement; there should be no sternal recession and the chest wall should appear equal on both sides.
- Check for capillary refill by placing one finger in the middle of the chest, pressing down and releasing; the skin colour should return to normal within 2 or 3 seconds.
- Place one hand across the chest at a right angle to feel for the point of maximal impulse (PMI). This is also described as an apical impulse or apex beat, but may not always be in the same place. Feel for any heaves and thrills with the palm of your hand; a heave is a distinct lifting movement of the chest and is associated with volume overload. A thrill is a continuous palpable sensation and feels like a cat purring; thrills are indicative of a palpable murmur. For any vibratory sensations, place the side of your hand along the sternal wall and across the PMI; the PMI (apex beat) should be felt just below the left nipple, between the fourth and fifth intercostal spaces (between the mitral and tricuspid valves).

- Listen to the two heart sounds by placing the stethoscope (diaphragm) at the appropriate intercostal spaces:
  - *Mitral* valve: fifth intercostal space just to the left of the mid-clavicular line, below the left nipple.
  - *Tricuspid* valve: fourth intercostal space, lower left sternal angle.
  - *Aortic* valve: second intercostal space, right sternal angle.
  - *Pulmonic* valve: second intercostal space, left sternal angle.
- While listening to the heart, simultaneously feel the right brachial pulse for equal rate, rhythm and volume.
- Note the heart rate, which is usually around 110–160 beats per minute (bpm). A heart rate of 80–90 bpm can be heard in babies who are asleep or very relaxed; a heart rate above 160 bpm may be heard in babies who are distressed.
- The femoral pulses should be palpated bilaterally, assessing for equal rate and rhythm, followed simultaneously by one femoral (left) and the right brachial pulse (the right subclavian artery is preductal). If the pulses are absent or weak, this is abnormal and may indicate decreased aortic blood flow as seen in coarctation of the aorta or aortic stenosis. Bounding pulses are found in patent ductus arteriosus (PDA). Referral for four-limb blood pressures and further assessment is indicated.
- Some practitioners will feel for femoral pulses at this time or may wait until they are examining the genitalia. as discussed below.

Lungs

Respirations—rate, rhythm, depth, type of breathing: recessions, periodic, shallow
Shape and symmetry of the chest
Symmetrical expansion

ABNORMALITY

Colour change—particularly central cyanosis.
Clubbing of fingers—indicative of cyanotic heart disease.
Visible pulsations over precordium—these are not uncommon in the newborn.
Bradycardia—defined as a heart rate less than 90 bpm.
Tachycardia—defined as a heart rate over 160 bpm.
Presence of extra heart sounds—if a murmur is present, you may hear an abnormal heart beat or unusual

---

noises; for example, ejection clicks and a whooshing sound caused by turbulent blood flow.
Systolic murmur—if present, more often heard along the left sternal border (Gill and O'Brien, 2007: 58).
Hepatomegaly—enlarged liver, seen in cardiac failure.
Abnormal location of PMI—may be due to pneumothorax or diaphragmatic hernia.

Observe the chest for symmetric, diaphragmatic respirations, and examine mouth and nose for oral and nasal secretions (fetal fluid cleared by the lungs). Normal oral secretions can be clear, white, frothy mucus; if yellow or green, consider meconium; if blood-tinged, may indicate maternal blood was swallowed.

Auscultation of the lungs should be carried out in a systematic and symmetrical way, listening to six areas at the front of the chest and the same on the baby's back. Working from right to left, start from the mid-axilla line. Listen at the second, the fourth and finally the sixth intercostal space. (If you place the stethoscope slightly further outwards from the midline at the sixth intercostal space, it is often possible to hear the respirations in the lower lobes.)

By placing the stethoscope (bell) over the aortic valve (second intercostal space, to the right of the mid-clavicular line), and counting the respirations for one full minute in this area, practitioners should be able to hear the respiratory rate quite clearly as a soft muffled sound (Fig. 2.16). A respiratory rate of 30–60 is considered 'normal' in the newborn who is not distressed (20–30 in the infant). In all areas of the chest the sounds heard should convey that the baby has clear airways and good inhalation and expiration breaths. The assessor should compare one side with the other and there should be no extra noises, crackles or wheezing.

ABNORMALITY

Asymmetric chest movement—exclude diaphragmatic hernia, cardiac anomalies, pneumothorax, phrenic nerve damage.
Dyspnoea—laboured or difficult respiration.
Tachypnoea—respiratory rate greater than 60.
Depending on the maternal history, you may hear the following adventitious sounds:
Nasal flaring—could mean that the newborn is attempting to clear fetal lung fluid or airway obstruction.
Inspiratory and expiratory grunting—this noise is made by expiration against a partially closed glottis as the

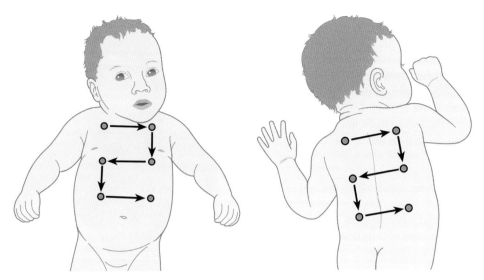

Fig. 2.16 Sequential placement of stethoscope to listen to breathing.

newborn attempts to increase laryngeal airway resistance and functional residual capacity in the lungs, and stabilize the alveoli.

Rhonchi—associated with secretions; more commonly heard after a Caesarean section birth. Bubbling, gurgling sound heard on expiration.

Rales—commonly known as crackles. A popping, discontinuous, wet sound, more often heard on inspiration. Depending on location and sound, can be associated with infection and significant amounts of secretions, or be an early sign of heart failure.

Wheezes—due to air moving through a narrowed airway. Associated with obstruction, this sound is high pitched, squeaking and continuous. It is mainly heard on expiration but seldom heard in the newborn.

Retractions—airway obstruction.

Inaudible breath sounds.

Stridor—indicates partial obstruction of the airway and presents as a high-pitched, hoarse sound, produced at the larynx or upper airways and heard during inspiration and expiration.

Abdomen

Colour/shape/size

Bowel sounds

Umbilical cord central insertion: contains two arteries and one vein and covered in Wharton's jelly to protect the vessels

Liver

Spleen

Kidneys

Bladder

Examination

Auscultate for bowel sounds in each of the four quadrants of the abdomen.

Gather information from the mother related to the baby's elimination history, noting the passage of urine within the previous 24 hours and the passage of stool within 48 hours (MacGregor, 2008). Table 2.2 gives an indication of what is considered to be a normal pattern for newborns, irrespective of their feeding method.

TABLE 2.2	**Elimination in the Newborn**		
Day	Urine Passed	Bowels Open	Colour
1–2	2 plus	1 plus	Meconium stools are sticky in consistency. Green/brown/black.
3–4	3 plus	2 plus	Changing stools. Green/brown.
5–6	5 plus	2 plus	Softer consistency. Pale brown/yellow.
7 plus	6 plus	2 plus	Soft consistency. Yellow.

In the first 48 hours, urates may be present in the nappies of males. These are salts in the urine and they look like a brick red paste deposit. In females, a very light bleed (pseudomenstruation) can occur as a result of circulating maternal hormones. Both are harmless, but parents should be informed that they may occur as otherwise this can cause anxiety. There is an increased risk of Hirschsprung disease in babies who fail to pass meconium within the first 48 hours.

Observation

Observe the abdomen for peristaltic action and note the abdominal shape and colour; this is normally flat and smooth although mild distension is common. There should be no obvious signs of infection around the umbilicus, or any presence of hernias.

Palpation

Palpate around the cord to exclude hernias.

Palpate the four quadrants of the abdomen to exclude masses; this is made easier as the baby breathes in.

To carry out a deeper palpation of the internal organs, bend the left leg to relax the abdominal muscles and palpate deep into the groin while using the right hand in a down-and-upwards motion as the baby breathes in and out. Fingers should maintain contact with skin at all times. Practitioners should not be able to feel right to the ribs.

The fingers should stay in contact as palpation is carried out on the left side to feel for the spleen. This may require a slightly deeper palpation than on the right (practitioners generally are not able to palpate the spleen, although its tip can sometimes be felt).

Carry out the same action on the right side; bend the right leg with your left hand to relax the abdominal muscles and palpate deep into the groin using the right hand as before. Palpate from the groin upwards to feel for the liver, the edge of which may be felt 1–2 cm below the fifth costal margin (Figs 2.17, 2.18 and 2.19).

When the baby is relaxed:
- Palpate the right kidney by placing the right hand under the baby's back. Feel towards the spine for the lumbar notch. Once the notch is located, apply gentle pressure upwards with your fingers only. Keeping the back of your hand on the flat surface, with two fingers of the left hand from above, ballotte the kidney by rolling gently downwards and backwards.
- Palpate the left kidney by placing the right hand again in the lumbar notch and with the left hand

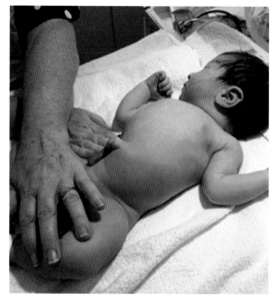

Fig. 2.17 Abdominal palpation: liver.

directly above, gently attempt to ballotte the kidney. Generally, practitioners seem to find it easier to palpate the right kidney than the left.

If possible, visualize and gently palpate for the bladder 1–4 cm above the symphysis pubis. Feel along the inguinal canal for hernias. Feel along the groin for the femoral pulses which should be equal in volume, rate and rhythm. Simultaneous palpation of the femoral pulse on the left and the right brachial pulse should reveal equal rate, rhythm and strength. If the pulses are unequal or bounding, consider coarctation of the aorta (see Chapter 9). Palpating the femoral pulses can be difficult but must always be done and is a key element of the NIPE (Fig. 2.20).

Advise parents to keep the cord clean and dry; there is no need to apply any lotions or cream to aid separation as this will occur spontaneously—usually within the first week, though some cords will remain attached for up to a month (see Chapter 13). With boys, advise parents to angle the penis downwards when putting on a nappy.

> **VARIATION**
> Diastasis recti—abdominal muscle is parted; resolves spontaneously.

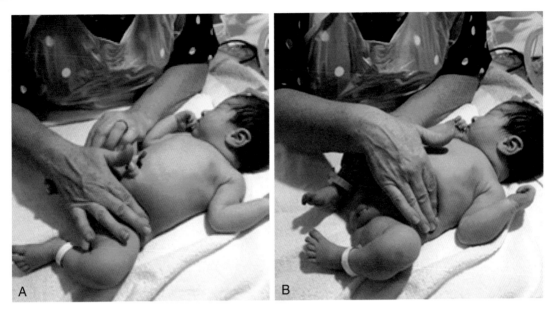

Fig. 2.18 Abdominal palpation: spleen.

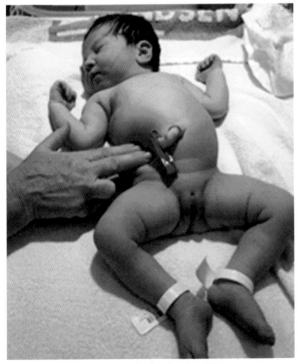

Fig. 2.19 Abdominal palpation: kidneys.

ABNORMALITY

Distended—may be due to bowels not having been open, but need to recognize risk of underlying pathology.

Gross distension—if at birth, linked to tumours.

Organomegaly—enlarged spleen (splenomegaly) may indicate infection. Enlarged liver (hepatomegaly) associated with infection, haemolytic disease or congenital heart disease.

Scaphoid (sunken)—seen with diaphragmatic hernia.

Tenderness.

Umbilical discharge—indicates infection

Umbilical hernia—common in infancy, particularly in the preterm infant (Fig. 2.21). Usually resolves without surgery.

Abdominal wall defects—omphalocele, gastroschisis, exstrophy of the bladder.

Inguinal hernia—more common in males and the preterm infant (Fig. 2.22)

Compression of the abdominal cavity, particularly during breech manoeuvres, may involve the spleen, the adrenal glands, or the liver. A haematoma develops on the affected organ, carrying the risk of rupture and major haemorrhage into the peritoneal cavity. Baby may present with pallor, abdominal distension, or unexplained anaemia. Treatment of abdominal organ haemorrhage is based on severity. Mild haemorrhages require only observation and/or transfusion; more severe haemorrhages may require surgery to achieve haemostasis.

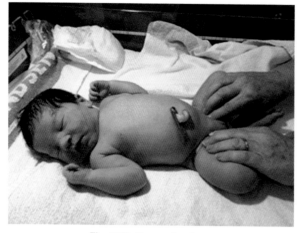

Fig. 2.20 Femoral pulses.

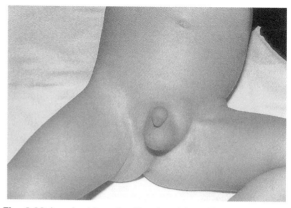

Fig. 2.22 Inguinal hernia. (Reprinted from Thomas R & Harvey D, Paediatrics and Neonatology in Focus 2005, with permission from Elsevier Ltd.)

or nonpalpable in the scrotal sac at the 6- to 8-week check. Surgery for undescended testes is recommended before the infant is 2 years old (see Chapter 11).

Male

Male genitalia
Size/shape
Penis
Foreskin (prepuce)
Urethral opening
Scrotal sac
Testes ×2

Observation

Appropriate genitalia, shape and size of the penis. The penis should be in the midline.

Examination

Bring the prepuce (foreskin) forward to check for a central meatus. Do not retract the foreskin, as it is adherent to the glans and should cover it completely. Check that the baby has passed urine and the type of flow seen. Urine should not spray and the foreskin should not fill with urine when the baby is voiding. By feeling along the inguinal canal, practitioners can feel down for a testis. To confirm that the testes are in the scrotal sac, palpate from the top on both sides of the scrotum downwards with the thumb and index finger. It is important to detect and record undescended testes.

The scrotum will vary in size; often it will appear swollen at birth and bruising can occur with breech

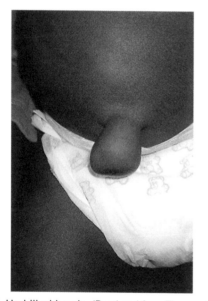

Fig. 2.21 Umbilical hernia. (Reprinted from Thomas R & Harvey D, Paediatrics and Neonatology in Focus 2005, with permission from Elsevier Ltd.)

Genitalia

These should be appropriate for gender. It is important to scrutinize the genitalia to confirm gender; ambiguous genitalia should always be referred for further investigation. As part of the newborn examination, practitioners will examine the male genitalia and palpate for descended testes. The UK NSC emphasizes the importance of detecting the presence of testes in the newborn period and the need for prompt referral if testes remain undescended delivery. The scrotum is covered by rugae (folds and wrinkles) at term.

Female

Labia majora
Labia minora
Clitoris
Hymen
Vagina

Examination

It is important to part the labia majora as they cover the labia minora in the term infant and anatomical accuracy must be confirmed. The clitoris is located at the junction of the labia minora, above the urethral meatus and the vagina. The perineum is the area between the vagina and the anus. By parting the labia, it should be possible to visualize a mucoid hymen covering the vaginal opening and to detect any masses, swelling or abnormal discharge.

Anus

The anus should appear in the midline. Confirm the passage of meconium to exclude anorectal anomalies. A digital examination should not be undertaken for routine examination of the newborn.

Lower Extremities

Legs
Feet
Toes
Movement
Hip movement

Observation and Examination

Ensure that there are two legs that move freely. Feel along each leg for the femur and to the knees for the hinge joint, then along the tibia and fibula down to the ankle joint and feet. Check for five toes with intact nail beds. Encourage the ankle joint and foot to relax, then perform the closed window manoeuvre which involves bending the toes and foot back (without force) onto the front of the ankle. There should be plantar creases on each foot. At this time, we recommend practitioners test the plantar reflex by placing the index finger at the base of the toes; toes should curl inwards (Fig. 2.23). The Babinski reflex can be determined by running a finger

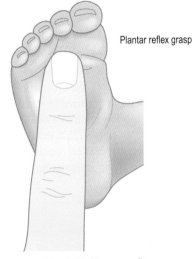

Plantar reflex grasp

Fig. 2.23 Plantar reflex.

VARIATION AND ABNORMALITIES

Male	Female
Priapism—adherent foreskin.	Mucoid (white) vaginal discharge, small bleed secondary to maternal hormone withdrawal.
Epispadias—the urethral meatus is on the dorsal surface (top side) of the penis; rare.	
Hypospadias—the urethral meatus is on the ventral aspect (underside) of the penis (Lissauer and Clayden, 2017).	Vaginal and hymenal skin tags. Enlarged clitoris—may be indicative of congenital adrenal hyperplasia.
Chordee—ventral curvature of the penis.	Pseudohermaphroditism—genitals at birth appear masculine.
Hydrocele—larger than average testes.	
Undescended testes—occurs in approximately 10% of infants; usually resolves within 2–4 weeks of birth in term babies.	
Torsion of testis—presents with hardness, pain and discoloration of testes. Not common.	

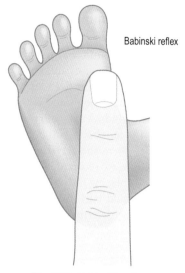

Babinski reflex

Fig. 2.24 Babinski reflex.

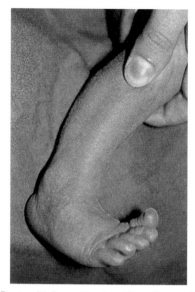

Fig. 2.25 Postural talipes. (Reprinted from Thomas R & Harvey D, Paediatrics and Neonatology in Focus 2005, with permission from Elsevier Ltd.)

along the outer edge of the foot, making the toes splay outwards (Fig. 2.24). There should be no extra digits, overriding toes or webbing of the toes; to exclude these, a thorough examination is required by parting all of the toes. The condition is often familial. Postural talipes can be a normal variation (Fig. 2.25); gentle massage or referral to physiotherapist may be required.

Observe and feel for skin integrity and dryness.

ABNORMALITY

Talipes equinovarus—talipes refers to the ankle; *equini* is turned down and *varus* means inwards. Otherwise known as club foot (Fig. 2.26).

Metatarsus adductus—more common than club foot; the metatarsal bones in the foot adduct (point inward).

Syndactyly—abnormal fusion of digits (Fig. 2.27).

Rocker-bottom feet.

Disproportionately short limbs—seen in achondroplasia

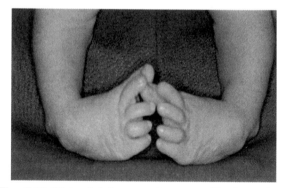

Fig. 2.26 Bilateral talipes equinovarus. (Reprinted from Thomas R & Harvey D, Paediatrics and Neonatology in Focus 2005, with permission from Elsevier Ltd.)

Back

Spinal curve (trunk incurvation/gallant reflex)
Spine integrity
Anal patency
Gluteal folds

Turn the baby over to observe and feel tone. Look at head movement and ensure that the hairline is appropriate. There should be two shoulders which are symmetrical with a straight spine and no apparent curvatures, and no clefts or tufts of hair. Gently work down the length of the spine, feeling the vertebrae to ensure there are no abnormal curvatures, no open clefts, dimples or sinuses.

Listen to the respiratory system while the baby is on its front.

Check for symmetry of the gluteal folds, although asymmetry is not considered to be a definitive marker for developmental dysplasia of the hip (DDH) in newborns (Jones, 1998). With the baby still on its front, observe for the crawl reflex and attempt to elicit a step reflex (Fig. 2.28).

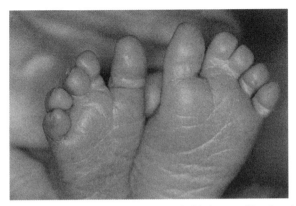

Fig. 2.27 Syndactyly of second and third toes. (Reprinted from Thomas R & Harvey D, Paediatrics and Neonatology in Focus 2005, with permission from Elsevier Ltd.)

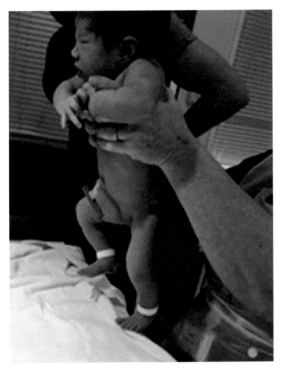

Fig. 2.28 Step reflex.

VARIATION

Sacral dimples—a fairly common occurrence, usually benign with no associated neurological deficit. The dimples are blind-ending pits; the practitioner must be sure that they can see the base of the dimple.

ABNORMALITY

Cysts, dimples, hair tufts—may indicate a spina bifida occulta.

Pilonidal sinus—a 'hole' with no visible end at the base of a sacral pit. If moisture is present, consider the possibility of a meningocele.

Scoliosis—curvature of the spine. Usually consists of two curves, the original abnormal curve and a compensatory curve in the opposite direction; there are three variations:

Idiopathic scoliosis—this is the most common. May be transmitted as an autosomal dominant or multifactorial trait.

Functional or postural scoliosis—this usually occurs as a result of a discrepancy in leg length and corrects when the patient bends towards the convex side.

Structural scoliosis – associated with vertebral bone deformities; does not correct with posture changes.

BOX 2.5

Risk factors for developmental dysplasia of the hips (DDH) are considered to be:

- Family history
- Female sex
- First born
- Breech presentation
- Oligohydramnios
- Large for gestational age (LGA)

Hip Examination

This part of the assessment is generally the last procedure performed as part of the NIPE (Box 2.5). The role of the hip screening examination is primarily to identify hips that are truly dislocated by undertaking the Barlow and Ortolani manoeuvres, and to refer appropriately based on finding (as discussed later and in Chapter 14). The two manoeuvres are most often undertaken as a combined test. During the review of this chapter, it became apparent that while many of us in the United Kingdom have been undertaking the Ortolani manoeuvres before the Barlow manoeuvres, in New Zealand the practice has always been to perform Barlow first. Cognisant of this information, expert opinion was sought from the UK NSC. Via personal correspondence in June 2019, the expert panel of consultant paediatricians and orthopaedic surgeons confirmed that they would *'advise everyone always did Barlow (dislocate) and then*

Ortolani (to relocate)'; they concur that *'no harm will be caused irrespective of the order of manoeuvre and that they do not hurt, nor do they damage the hip. In general Barlow is a provocation test, therefore once the adduction and posterior force is stopped, the hip will reduce; in a true Barlow the hip will not remain dislocated once the hip is placed in a more natural position. Therefore in this order practitioners do not have to worry about how best to relocate the hip'.* On detection of a dislocated hip (Barlow), some practitioners currently will perform an Ortolani manoeuvre to put the hip back in place; others will simply lift the leg up in a sort of reverse Barlow. The UK NSC panel advised that *'a dislocatable hip will normally go back on its own, and a dislocated hip will either stay dislocated (which it will probably return to after Ortolani abduction is released) or it may spontaneously relocate itself'.* They stated that *'the Ortolani manoeuvre (reduction of a dislocated hip) is the more important of the two tests. The majority of Barlow positive will stabilize spontaneously (a reduced hip which is dislocated posteriorly through axial/adduction force)'.* It could be argued that if the Ortolani is the key manoeuvre and is positive, there is no need to undertake a formal Barlow test; it follows that this should not be our first manoeuvre as is current practice for many clinicians. The literature is sparse with reference to the procedures and often the Ortolani manoeuvre is the first one to be explained. Another perspective given by not only the UK NSC experts but other clinicians is that 'it's the way they were taught' but we must ensure the underpinning evidence is in place before we commit our practice. It is apparent that the debate will continue.

Undertaking the Examination

Prior to commencing the hip examination (for both the newborn and the 6- to 8-week check), ensure the infant is relaxed and in the supine position. If the infant is distressed, they will generally tense their muscles, specifically around the hip joint. This can make diagnosis of an unstable hip joint very difficult and attempting the procedure will only cause more distress to the infant and parents. As previously stated, the hip examination should always be carried out on a firm surface with the baby completely undressed to facilitate the required manoeuvres.

The diagnosis of DDH is made by performing two manoeuvres: the Ortolani manoeuvre to see if the hip is

dislocated and, if so, whether it can be reduced; and the Barlow manoeuvre to determine if the hip is dislocatable. If a low-pitched clunk sound is heard during either of these manoeuvres, it is described as a positive Barlow and/or positive Ortolani manoeuvre. During the Ortolani manoeuvre, the 'clunk' sound heard is caused by the dislocated femoral head moving outside of the acetabulum. This same sound during the Barlow manoeuvre is caused by the femoral head sliding over the posterior rim of the acetabulum. The 'clunk' sound is distinct from the higher-pitched clicks which can be elicited with flexion and extension of the hip and represent normal movement of the ligamentum teres in the acetabulum in newborns. The practitioner must also distinguish between these and a subluxable hip, in which the hip is not in alignment and the joint more mobile; the femoral head manoeuvres may cause further distress and may move within the acetabulum without actual damage by dislocating the hip.

Hips

Leg length
Allis (Galeazzi) sign
Barlow manoeuvre
Ortolani manoeuvre

Observation

Observe the limbs for movement, normal abduction to 75 degrees and adduction to 30 degrees; observe for discrepancies in leg length and asymmetrical skin folds in the thighs and buttocks.

Examination

- Check the hips are symmetrical and that the legs are of equal length by straightening the legs out.
- Perform the Allis sign, whereby the soles of the infant's feet are placed together on a flat and firm surface and the knees gently flexed. The heels should be brought towards the buttocks and the knees observed (Fig. 2.29). They should be at the same height; if they are not, it may signify unequal leg length. However, this sign is not considered to be as effective from 2 months of age.

Ortolani manoeuvre (Fig. 2.30)
- With both the baby's knees flexed to the right angle and its heels against the buttocks, position your thumbs on the inner aspect of the thighs and your fingers along the outer aspect of the thigh. Slightly

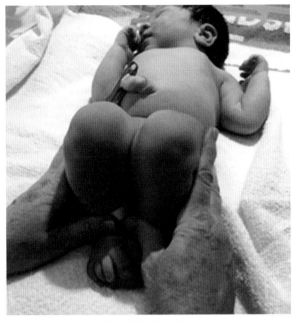

Fig. 2.29 Allis sign.

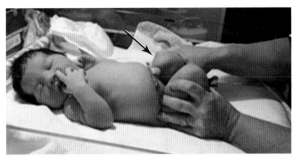

Fig. 2.31 Barlow manoeuvre: abduct leg towards the middle and telescope downwards.

while the flexed leg is held in place by the palm of the hand. One hip at a time from an initial 90-degree flexion, gently apply pressure with your thumb slightly backwards. Simultaneously provide slight adduction towards the midline and telescope downwards (preferably twice only). If the femoral head can be felt being displaced backwards and upwards, then instability is evident. Reduce the hip with the Ortolani manoeuvre or by releasing pressure on the thumb.

If you suspect or detect a dislocated or dislocatable hip, the baby should be referred to a paediatrician. Do not repeat the manoeuvres due to the risk of avascular necrosis to the femoral head.

It is not advisable to carry out the Ortolani screening test at the 6- to 8-week check because of increased muscle tone.

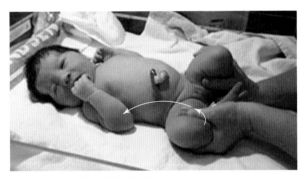

Fig. 2.30 Ortolani manoeuvre.

adduct (move inwards from the midline) the leg using the thumb, then apply pressure to the greater trochanter with the third and fourth finger. Without using excessive force, bring the flexed leg up to the midline and gently abduct (move away from the midline) the hip while lifting the leg anteriorly. With this manoeuvre, a 'clunk' is felt as the dislocated femoral head reduces into the acetabulum. This is a positive Ortolani sign.

Barlow manoeuvre (Fig. 2.31)
- Hips and knees should be flexed to the right angle. Position your thumb on the inner aspect of the thigh and your middle finger over the greater trochanter

---

VARIATION
Hips which have appeared stable at birth may well become dislocated; screening, both physical and observational, is therefore advised until the child is walking.
Subluxable hip.

ABNORMALITY
Developmental dysplasia of the hip.
Congenital dislocated hip.
Isolated dysplasia—due to abnormal development of acetabulum and/or the proximal femur. This condition is often associated with other abnormalities. Diagnosis is made by ultrasound.

Reflexes

The reflexes are tested in order to confirm normal neuro-logical development or to identify any problems. Some of the routine reflexes have been described briefly and will be addressed in more detail in Chapter 8; the red eye reflexes are outlined in Chapter 10. If a baby's gestational age is questioned or the baby is known to be preterm, then these can be performed and are discussed in Chapter 8.

Testing of the Moro reflex usually forms the very last part of the examination. This reflex is tested by bringing the baby forward until the chin rests on the chest. With one hand supporting the head, allow the baby to drop backwards into your other hand. As the baby falls back-wards, the normal reaction will be for them to flay their arms outwards and then bring them forwards towards the midline; this is the Moro reflex (Fig. 2.32). It is also possible to elicit the grasp reflex from this action, in ad-dition to assessing the baby's tone and ability to support its head. The startle reflex is very similar to the Moro, although the baby will not necessarily bring its arms forwards. However, this may be enough to satisfy the practitioner that the Moro reflex is not required.

> **VARIATION**
> Jittery.

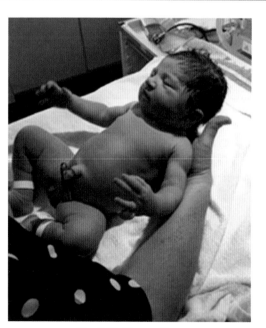

Fig. 2.32 Moro reflex.

> **ABNORMALITY**
> Absence of reflex or asymmetrical response.
> Floppy tone—drowsy or passive response, abnormal rhythmic sustained movements of extremities, e.g., seizures.
> For further neurological abnormalities, see Chapter 8.

Feeding

Pattern
Amount
Timing
Vomiting
Observation of a feed will confirm the suck and swallow reflexes. It is important to determine if the baby has fed and how often.

> **VARIATION**
> A reluctance to feed—may be due to maternal medica-tions, oral thrush, jaundice.

> **ABNORMALITY**
> Vomiting.

Growth

In April 2006 the World Health Organization (WHO) Child Growth Standards were introduced for children between 0 and 59 months of age. They represented nor-mal growth under optimal environmental conditions; introduced globally, they were adopted in most if not all countries. The charts and gestational age assessment are discussed further in Chapter 8.

'Correct measurement, plotting, and interpretation are essential for identifying growth problems' (WHO, 2008).

The average weight, length and head circumference of the healthy, term newborn are reported to be: weight from 2.6 to 3.8kg (5lb 11oz–8lb 6oz); average length from 45 to 55 centimetres (14–20 in); and head circum-ference between 32 and 35 centimetres (12.5–13.5 in). It is the responsibility of the practitioner to plot all mea-surements on the centile chart. This chart illustrates growth and development from birth and, although only approximate, provides a baseline for monitoring the infant. Importantly all findings should also be recorded in the Personal Child Health Record (known as the 'Red Book' in the UK, see Chapter 8).

Weight

All newborn babies are weighed at birth; however, there is no consensus on how frequently babies should be weighed, and little discussion of the anxiety caused to parents by weighing too frequently, especially for breast-fed babies. The National Institute for Clinical Excellence (NICE) postnatal guidelines (published in 2006 and updated in 2015) state that 'Healthy babies normally lose weight in the first week of life. This weight loss is usually transient and of no significance, but may be exaggerated if there is difficulty establishing feeding or if the baby is ill'. Anecdotal evidence from practitioners suggests that babies are routinely weighed by the midwife at birth, and then on day five (normally at the same time as undertaking the newborn blood spot screening; see Chapter 14), then by the health visitor between days 12 and 14, and again at the 6- to 8-week check. Due to health care provision changes in the UK and privatization of health visiting, many new mums now attend weigh-in clinics at their local children's centre; depending on local provision (which can vary considerably), these facilities are available until the child is up to 8 years old. Midwives will re-weigh any babies who have lost over 10% of their birth weight and will consider referral to a paediatrician if they have any concerns regarding the baby's well-being.

An awareness of the presentation of weight loss and dehydration is an important part of the newborn assessment. Signs and symptoms include lethargy, poor feeding, sunken fontanelles, poor tone, loose skin and dry cracked skin.

A suggestion that has been made is that midwives should weigh the baby at birth and repeat only if the baby is unwell or appears dehydrated, then health visitors should weigh the baby at the first visit (approximately 11 days) and subsequently at the 6- to 8-week visit unless otherwise indicated.

Length

The Child Growth Foundation (2004) recommends that all babies should have their length recorded at birth, using an appropriate measuring mat. The length should be measured from the head (crown) to the heel with the newborn on a flat surface in a supine position. The baby's head will need to be held straight and their legs extended for an accurate reading. This is the practice in many areas, although in others the practice has ceased or practitioners are still using tape measures. The length of the baby gives a baseline measurement for the child's future growth and development. However, it can be argued that the newborn measurement is not wholly accurate, because the baby may not stay still, and that the measurement would be more usefully taken at the 6- to 8-week check.

Discussion with Parents and Information Sharing

The holistic perspective of the NIPE includes listening to parents' concerns and the sharing of information. Any discussion should obviously be linked to references which will support further exploration of the subject in question if necessary. It is impossible to expand on all of these here; however, Tables 2.3 and 2.4 refer the reader to chapters within this book and other sources covering some of the topics which often come up during the examination.

It is anticipated that the general practitioner or health visitor will carry out a thorough examination of the newborn at the 6- to 8-week check, possibly with the exception of the hip examination and some of the reflexes. In addition, they will explore many of the communication topics seen in Tables 2.3 and 2.4.

Information offered to parents should be tailored to meet their individual and specified needs. However, there are subjects—such as minimizing the risk of sudden infant death syndrome (SIDS) and car seat safety—where verbal discussion should take place with each parent. The handing over of information in leaflet form is not a satisfactory alternative. Good verbal discussion, utilizing appropriate language in conjunction with written material, is the most appropriate way of ensuring that information is received and absorbed by women and their partners.

Referrals

Some anomalies will be detected antenatally and others will be detected at birth; however, it is sometimes the case that the baby is a few hours or even days old before the anomaly is detected—often by the mother. In all these situations, effective communication is vital and interprofessional working at this sensitive time essential. Never underestimate the anxiety that can be caused by a pause or puzzled look on the practitioner's face. It is always hard to communicate unanticipated news; remember that many professionals find this extremely difficult. This issue is explored further in Chapter 6. It is important to inform parents that the initial examination represents only part of the screening process and further screening will be offered, i.e., the blood spot screening and 6- to 8-week check.

TABLE 2.3 Communication Topics: Newborn Examination

Topic	Chapter	Links
Breastfeeding	Chapter 15	www.babyfriendly.org.uk
Skin & cord care	Chapter 13	
Co-sleeping	Chapter 15	http://www.cosleeping.org/ http://www.lullabytrust.co.uk
Sudden infant death syndrome (SIDS) statistics		https://www.lullabytrust.org.uk/?s=statistics
Hearing testing	Chapter 4	http://hearing.screening.nhs.uk/cms.php?folder=63
Jaundice	Chapter 12	
Newborn screening	Chapter 14	http://www.ich.ucl.ac.uk/newborn/resources/delivery. htm#parents
Vitamin K	Chapter 15	http://www.aims.org.uk/
Postnatal depression	Chapter 5	https://www.mind.org.uk/ https://www.nice.org.uk/guidance/CG192 Antenatal and postnatal mental health: clinical management and service guidance. Accessed 2018
Smoking cessation	Chapter 15	https://www.nice.org.uk/Guidance/pH26 Smoking: stopping in pregnancy and after childbirth June 2010 Accessed March 2019.
Safety issues i.e., car seats, smoke alarms		Lullaby Trust www.lullabytrust.org.uk https://www.nhs.uk/ conditions/pregnancy-and-baby/child-car-seats-and-child-car-safety/car seats The Royal Society for the Prevention of Accidents (ROSPA) https:// www.childcarseats.org.uk/

TABLE 2.4 Communication Topics: Antenatal and 6- to 8-Week Examination

Topic	Resource
Baby massage	http://www.iaim.org.uk/
Domestic abuse	https://www.gov.uk/government/publications/domestic-abuse-a-resource-for-health-professionals https://www.gov.uk/search?q=DOMESTIC+ABUSE
Growth and development monitoring	http://www.childgrowthfoundation.org/
Immunization programme	https://www.nhs.uk/conditions/vaccinations/childhood-vaccines-timeline/ https://www.nct.org.uk/baby-toddler/postnatal-checks-and-immunisations/baby-immunisations-and-vaccinations
Maternal and infant bonding	https://www.familylives.org.uk/
Nutrition: mother and baby	https://www.nct.org.uk/ https://www.laleche.org.uk/ Human Growth Foundation (2019) http://hgfound.org/
Smoking cessation	https://www.nhs.uk/smokefree https://www.nice.org.uk/guidance/PH26 https://www.nhs.uk/conditions/pregnancy-and-baby/smoking-pregnant/

In conclusion, practitioners are encouraged to remember that you are accountable for your own practice, but all need to work together as a multidisciplinary team. This allows all practitioners to learn from each other and to develop guidelines and policies which meet the needs of mothers and babies from a perspective of normality (McDonald, 2018; NMC, 2018; McDonald et al., 2012).

KEY POINTS

- The midwife's role as examiner is well established and the service that they offer is valued by clients and other health professionals.
- The optimal time to carry out the NIPE is within the first 24–72 hours after birth.
- It is a legal and ethical requirement that valid consent should be gained from the parent(s) prior to examining the newborn/infant.
- It is vital that a thorough and comprehensive history is obtained both from talking to the mother and by briefing the maternal notes.
- An accurate record of the examination findings is crucial. In addition, any referrals should be noted in the maternal notes.
- Information offered to parents should be tailored to meet their individual and specified needs.
- Practitioners need to work together to develop guidelines and policies which meet the needs of mothers and babies from a perspective of normality.

REFERENCES

Child Growth Foundation 2004 Growth and Growth Disorders series 1. Available from: https://childgrowthfoundation.org/wp-content/uploads/2018/07/01_Growth_and_Disorders-1.pdf. Accessed March 2020.

Department of Health, 2009. Reference Guide to Consent for Examination or Treatment, second ed. Available from: https://assets.publishing.service.gov.uk/government/uploads/system/uploads/attachment_data/file/138296/dh_103653__1_pdf. Accessed March 2019.

Fish, D., Lima, D., 2003. An overview of positional plagiocephaly and cranial remolding orthoses. J. Prosthet. Orthot. 15 (2), 37–45 Available online https://journals.lww.com/jpojournal/pages/articleviewer.aspx?year=2003&issue=04000&article=00002&type=Fulltext. Accessed March 2019.

Gill, D., O'Brien, N., 2007. Paediatric Clinical Examination Made Easy, fifth ed. Churchill Livingstone, Edinburgh.

Hunter, L., Habel, A., 2014. RCPCH Palate Examination: Identification of Cleft Palate in the Newborn, a Guide for Parents and Carers. October 2014 Great Ormond Street Hospital, London. Available from: https://www.rcpch.ac.uk/sites/default/files/2018-04/2015_palate_examination_-_best_practice_guide.pdf. 2014. Accessed May 2019.

Johnson, P.R.V., 2006. Tongue-tie—exploding the myths. Infant 2 (3), 96–99.

Jones, D.A., 1998. Hip Screening in the Newborn. A Practical Guide. Butterworth Heinemann, Oxford.

Lissauer, T., Clayden, G., 2017. Illustrated Textbook of Paediatrics, fifth ed. Elsevier, Edinburgh.

Lullaby Trust, Safer sleep for babies, Support for families 2019. Available from: https://www.lullabytrust.org.uk. Accessed May 2019.

MacGregor, J., 2008. Introduction to the Anatomy and Physiology of Children, second ed. Routledge, London.

McDonald, S., 2018, Integration of the examination of the newborn into holistic midwifery practice: a grounded theory study. Evid. Based Midwifery 16 (4), 128–135.

McDonald, S., Allan, H., Brown, A., 2012. Perceptions of changing practice in the examination of the newborn, from holistic to opportunistic. Br. J. Midwifery 20 (11), 786–791.

National Institute for Clinical Excellence, December 2005. Division of Ankyloglossia (tongue-tie) for Breastfeeding. Available from: https://www.nice.org.uk/Guidance/IPG149. Accessed March 2019.

National Institute for Health and Clinical Excellence, 2014. Infection Prevention and Control. Available from: https://www.nice.org.uk/guidance/qs61/chapter/quality-statement-3-hand-decontamination. Accessed March 2019.

National Institute for Health and Clinical Excellence, 2006. CG 37 Postnatal Care: Routine Postnatal Care of Women and Their Babies. London, NICE. Available from: www.nice.org.uk. Accessed March 2019.

Nursing and Midwifery Council, 2018. The Code. London, NMC. Available from: https://www.nmc.org.uk/globalassets/sitedocuments/nmc-publications/nmc-code.pdf. Accessed March 2020.

Public Health England, 2016. Newborn Hearing Screening Programme Overview. Available from: https://www.gov.uk/guidance/newborn-hearing-screening-programme-overview. Accessed March 2019.

Public Health England, 2018a. Our Approach to Newborn and Infant Physical Examination Screening Standards. Available from: https://www.gov.uk/government/publications/newborn-and-infant-physical-examination-screening-standards/our-approach-to-newborn-and-infant-physical-examination-screening-standards. PHE Gateway number 2017867. 2018a. Accessed March 2019.

Public Health England, 2018b. NHS Newborn and Infant Physical Examination Screening Programme Handbook. Available from: https://www.gov.uk/government/publications/newborn-and-infant-physical-examination-programme-handbook. Accessed March 2019.

Reshma, R., Sujatha, R., 2014. Cultural practices and beliefs on newborn care among mothers in a selected hospital of Mangalore Tauluknitte. U. J. Health. Sci. 4 (2), 21–26. Available from: http://nitte.edu.in/journal/June2014/21-26.pdf. Accessed May 2019.

Siney, C., 1999. Pregnancy and Drug Misuse, Elsevier, England.

Tappero, E.P., Honeyfield, M.E., 2018. Physical Assessment of the Newborn: A Comprehensive Approach to the Art of Physical Examination, sixth ed. Springer Publishing, New York.

World Health Organisation, 2008. Training Course on Child Growth Assessment. WHO, Geneva. Available from: https://www.who.int/childgrowth/training/module_a_introduction.pdf?ua=1. Accessed March 2019.

Websites

https://www.clapa.com/. Accessed May 2019

https://www.gov.uk/government/publications/guidance-for-health-professionals-on-domestic-violence. Accessed March 2019

https://www.lullabytrust.org.uk/. Accessed March 2019

https://www.steps-charity.org.uk/. Accessed May 2019

https://www.unicef.org.uk/babyfriendly/. Accessed March 2019

Women's environmental network- Green Baby https://www.wen.org.uk/. Accessed March 2019

3

From Gametes to Fetus: A Chronology of Embryo Development

Andrew McVicar

CHAPTER CONTENTS

INTRODUCTION

The chapter provides an overview of the nature of genes and the principles of inheritance; insights into the process of fertilization of the ovum; description and explanation of the critical stages of embryo development before and after implantation in the endometrium; the significance of the development of embryonic membranes and placentation; and insights into how congenital errors of development may arise. The development of the embryo after conception—a period characterized by initial determination of the basic body plan and the subsequent differentiation of tissues and organs, directed by selective genetic activities—is explored chronologically including selected examples which provide an overview of processes of organ differentiation and functional maturation; a more detailed account is not within the scope of the chapter. However, if you gain a sense of wonder at what takes place and a desire to know more, then its aim has been achieved!

OVERVIEW OF GENES, CHROMOSOMES AND INHERITANCE

To illustrate the role of genetics in embryo development, it is necessary to set the scene with an overview of genes and their inheritance. Technological advances since the 1980s have enabled science to study the genes that are critical to human embryos; this is opening up new directions for research but also raises some challenging ethical, moral and legal issues that have a significant potential impact on society. However, these are not explored here.

What Are Genes and Chromosomes?

Gaining an understanding of the roles of genes and chromosomes in embryological development is central to the learning arising from this chapter. Genes are identified in all forms of life and determine the appearance and physical functioning of every organism. Some genes linked to development have been conserved throughout evolution and have roles even in humans that are recognisable today. For example, a tiny nematode worm found in soil, *Caenorhabditis elegans*, represents evolutionary advance towards a 'complex' organism. It is comprised of only around 1000 cells, yet it has provided insights into the genetic control of some of the fundamental mechanisms of tissue differentiation. Research into the genetic control of development in more complex animals led to the recognition that many genes of relevance to human development are also present in very similar forms in other organisms.

Genes and the Genetic Code

In 1866 Gregor Mendel (1822–1884), a scientist and monk, published his observations on the hybridization of peas he grew in the abbey gardens. He recognized that although the inherited characteristics of the plants (e.g., plant and seed forms, flower colours) appeared random, there were patterns. He deduced that these patterns arose because 'units of inheritance' were being passed between generations. This groundbreaking work on the basic principles of inheritance was not acknowledged scientifically until some 30 or so years later, but the observations remain significant today. We now refer to those units of inheritance as 'genes'.

Genes are sections of a molecule of deoxyribonucleic acid (DNA), found mostly within the cell nucleus, that contain the information for cells to produce proteins needed for cell structure, critical cell functions, or for secretion into the extracellular fluid. Thus the *genetic code* encapsulated within the chemical composition of DNA provides a 'blueprint' for an individual's biological construct. Precisely how that plan operates is touched upon later, but at this point it is of note that despite most of our own trillions of cells having the same genetic code, there is a breadth of form and function. This means that the genetic code must be translated differentially in different cells.

The Genetic Code: From Gene to Protein

The genetic code is comprised of just four 'letters': A, T, G and C. Each represents a chemical called a base (**A**denosine, **T**hymine, **G**uanine, **C**ytosine); bases are also referred to as 'nucleotides' because they predominantly occur as constituents of nuclear DNA. There are over 3,000,000,000 nucleotides in our DNA, and nucleotide sequences of many thousands in length comprise our genes. The sequence of bases is 'translated' by organelles called *ribosomes* in the cell's cytoplasm (i.e., outside the nucleus) into a sequence of amino acids which is specific to that code. That sequence of amino acids in turn determines the final three-dimensional shape of the protein molecule, which is crucial to its function. The range of possible combinations of just four different nucleotides within such lengths of DNA is huge and the potential range of distinct proteins reflects this; our cells collectively have the potential to produce over 100,000 different proteins. Some of these will be found in most or all cells but others exist only in specific cell types. For example, a particular cell type may produce the hormone calcitonin when triggered to do so, but those cells are only located within the thyroid gland. Other cells do not ordinarily secrete the hormone, but their DNA retains the capacity to do so, because the DNA content of all cells is the same; breast cancer cells, for example, are known to activate the genes for calcitonin production and secretion. Because this is not a normal role of breast cells, they are unlikely to be subject to the usual regulatory mechanisms that operate in the thyroid gland; this can lead to calcitonin excess and potential complications of calcium imbalance.

Gene Mutation

A genetic *mutation* occurs when the nucleotide sequence within a gene is altered; this may or may not change the size and/or shape of the resultant protein, but potentially a different protein can be generated by changing just one nucleotide, and hence one amino acid within that protein. Geneticists refer to such changes as point mutations; the most frequent type is called a single nucleotide polymorphism (SNP) and is the commonest form of gene variation (and of alterations in non-gene sequences). Caution needs to be exercised here as the term 'mutation' is usually viewed entirely negatively—yet an altered gene may do no more than alter our capacity to roll our tongue, or perhaps change the shape of an earlobe, or contribute to hair colour. Most SNPs have no effect at all. In other words, the genetic change may have no major consequence for well-being, and may not be of consequence at all unless it confers a functional advantage. For example, it is now clear that small numbers of individuals are resistant to HIV infection; this would never have been recognized if the virus had not appeared as it did. Sometimes, however, the effects of a new protein—or perhaps loss of the 'usual' one—arising from a gene mutation can be profound; see Box 3.1.

Chromosomes

Most of our DNA, and hence our genes, lies within the cell nucleus, with only a few genes being found elsewhere in the cell (in the mitochondria, where they are primarily engaged in energy metabolism). A nucleus viewed through a microscope appears granular but otherwise almost featureless, with no indication that there is over a metre of DNA within it (a typical cell nucleus is of the order of just 10 micrometres, or 1/100 mm, in diameter). There are actually several separate DNA molecules within the nucleus, as becomes evident when the cell prepares to divide, either to support tissue growth or replacement or to generate sex cells. Then the DNA molecules fold and coil to produce 46 discrete packages of DNA that can be visualized microscopically; these are the *chromosomes* (from the Greek for 'coloured bodies'). Look closely at Fig. 3.1 and you can see that each chromosome appears to have an 'X' shape. In fact, what has happened is that each DNA molecule has duplicated itself but the duplicates (referred to as *chromatids*) remain

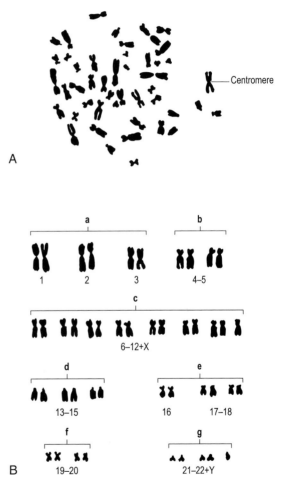

Fig. 3.1 Human karyotype. (A) Chromosomes stained for visualization under a microscope. (B) Male karyotype (note the presence of X and Y sex chromosomes) organized to show chromosome pairs. Further information on the genes found on each chromosome pair can be found on the web pages of the Human Genome Organisation (www.hugo-international.org last accessed 15.5.07; redrawn from Clancy J., McVicar A. *Physiology and Anatomy: A homeostatic approach*, 2nd ed, 2002, with permission from Hodder Education).

BOX 3.1 Examples of Disorders Linked to Single Gene Mutations

- In cystic fibrosis, an altered gene changes a transporting protein in the membrane of mucus-secreting cells, preventing the adequate transport of chloride ions into the cell. Consequently, cells secrete the thickened mucus that is symptomatic of the disorder.
- In phenylketonuria (PKU), an altered gene means that liver cells cannot produce the enzyme (protein) that converts the amino acid phenylalanine to tyrosine. Consequently, there is excessive phenylalanine in the blood; this interferes with uptake of the full spectrum of amino acids into brain cells. There is also a deficiency of tyrosine; this manifests as albinism, because tyrosine is necessary for melanin synthesis.
- In sickle cell anaemia, an altered gene changes the structure of the blood pigment haemoglobin. In normal adult haemoglobin, the sixth amino acid in the protein molecule is glutamic acid; in sickle cell anaemia, a slight genetic change leads to its substitution with another amnio acid, valine. This is enough to change the haemoglobin to make the red cells sticky and fragile, producing the vaso-occlusive and anaemic symptoms of the disorder.
- In achondroplasia, an altered gene causes an abnormality of cartilage (chondroitin) formation that results in shortened bones. Consequently, the person's stature is small and there is altered skeletal development. A detailed list of genes involved in ill health can be found on the Online Mendelian Inheritance in Man website, OMIM.org, accessed March 2020.

attached to each other close to the central region of the chromosome, called the *centromere*. The number and form of the chromosomes is referred to as an individual's *karyotype* (see Boxes 3.2 and 3.3).

Karyotype and Genotype

Karyotype refers to the size, shape and number of the chromosomes in a cell. A key point to note is that the 46 chromosomes in humans comprise 23 pairs (Fig. 3.1). These originate at conception when we inherit one complete set from each parent; our cells therefore actually

contain two genetic 'blueprints' and are referred to as *diploid* (*di* = two). All but one of the pairs are referred to as *autosomes*, numbered 1–22 according to size, and the remaining pair the *sex chromosomes*, also referred to as X and Y chromosomes. The X and Y chromosomes are visibly distinguishable from each other. In females the sex chromosome pair consists of two X chromosomes, which, like the autosome pairs, look identical at the microscopic level. In males the two chromosomes are visibly dissimilar; one is an X as in the female but the other, the Y chromosome, is much smaller. In addition to sex

---

BOX 3.2   Visualizing Individual Chromosomes, and How Many There Are in a Cell

Imagine a ball of wool that contains red, blue and white strands tangled together. You need to do something with the red strand, but untangling it is clearly going to take a long time, especially if there are multiple strands to disentangle. There are 46 strands (molecules) of DNA in a cell nucleus, but fortunately DNA molecules are not passive strands of wool; when they are about to divide, they are biochemically induced to fold and coil independently. In this condensed form, it is relatively easy for the cell machinery to shuffle and redistribute them during cell division as required.

Karyotype

We shouldn't read too much into the fact that human cells have 46 chromosomes. Chimpanzees have 48, as do hedgehogs and even potatoes! That is not to say that a humble vegetable has more genes than us, because much of the DNA does not translate as genes. Note, however, that this does not mean it is non-functional (see 'Epigenetics' later).

BOX 3.3   Chromosomal (Karyotype) Errors

Karyotype errors occur when a sex cell has excess DNA either because (a) the recombination of the chromosomes early in meiosis I resulted in a piece of chromosome breaking off and swapping places with a section of another chromosome (geneticists call this a *translocation*), adding genes to that chromosome's DNA and removing some of its original gene content; or (b) the whole chromosomes have not separated properly at the end of meiosis I. A common feature of both is the loss or gain of several genes.

An error in recombination may mean that too many or too few genes are inherited. Gene excess (through *duplication* gain of a chromosome, for example *trisomy*, or of part of a chromosome) is often too much to permit the survival of an embryo, but this is not always the case if the duplicated region is small. For example, in some cases of *Down syndrome*, which is usually the result of having three separate whole copies of chromosome 21, the baby inherits the usual two copies but also an additional segment of chromosome 21 that has attached to another chromosome. The loss of a segment of chromosomal material (*deletion* of a whole chromosome, hence *monosomy*) during recombination could mean a detrimental deficiency of genes; again,

these losses are often incompatible with survival, but small deletions are survivable and give rise to recognizable syndromes. For example, *cri-du-chat syndrome* arises because of the loss of part of chromosome 5.

When *nondisjunction* occurs for an entire chromosome pair, both copies pass into the same sex cell; this would also mean the formation of a sex cell deficient in a whole chromosome. This usually compromises survival at an early stage of intrauterine development, but there are instances when losses or gains of smaller chromosomes or sex chromosomes are viable. For example, in the usual form of *Down syndrome* there are three copies of chromosome 21 because two copies have been inherited in one parent's sex cell (usually the ovum) and one, as normal, from the other. Similarly, in *Klinefelter syndrome*, two X chromosomes and one Y chromosome are present, usually because two copies of the X chromosome are inherited from the mother plus one Y from the father. *Turner syndrome*, in which the karyotype has 45 chromosomes with a single X, arises from nondisjunction which results in the lack of a whole chromosome in one of the parental sex cells (inheritance of just a Y chromosome is not viable).

determination, the difference in gene content between the X and Y chromosomes also has consequences for the inheritance of characteristics, as described below.

Most genes in a cell are found on the autosomes, which are generally involved in functional activities other than sex determination. The autosomes are also termed *homologous pairs* (*homo* = the same; *logos* = reasoning or plan). This means that, if there is a gene at a specific location on, say, one member of chromosome pair number 1 then a copy of it will normally be found at exactly the same location on the other member of the pair. This consistency of location helps to ensure that all necessary genes are passed into new generations of cells but has also proved an essential aid for gene mapping because it allows scientists to pinpoint a particular gene on a specific chromosome. Scientists describe gene locations according to the chromosome number and the gene's position on the arm of the chromosome. Note that although chromosomes may be referred to as being shaped like an 'X', the centromere is usually not exactly at the midpoint of a chromosome and so the arms are of unequal lengths. The short arm of a chromosome is called the p-arm (from 'petite') and the long arm is the q-arm. For example, the gene responsible for cystic fibrosis is located at 7q31.2, that is, at a site designated 31.2 on the long arm (q) of chromosome 7.

The term *genotype* is used to refer to the complement of genes on the homologous chromosome pairs. Although the location of a gene is identical on each member of any given chromosome pair, the sequence of nucleotides that makes up the two copies may not be absolutely identical. In recognition that the two copies of a gene may not be the same, science uses the term *allele* to differentiate each 'version'; it is common practice to refer to a single genotype according to its two alleles. If the genetic code of the two alleles is identical then the genotype is said to be *homozygous* (*homo* = same) but if the two are different then it is *heterozygous (hetero* = different, variable).

In the heterozygous condition one allele, usually the 'normal' copy, assumes *dominance* over the other copy (which is then said to be *recessive*); the dominant allele will be the copy that determines the protein to be synthesized by the cell when the gene is active. The recessive copy will effectively be silent and is usually only expressed in any quantity if the genotype is homozygous (i.e., *both* alleles of the gene are of the recessive form); in this case the loss of the 'usual' protein, or the production of a different protein as a result of the altered genetic sequence, may change how the cell develops or functions. As noted

earlier, this is not necessarily detrimental, because it contributes to human variation—but occasionally the change in protein function may not be compatible with health or even survival. Examples of recessive alleles that produce health deficits commonly found in the UK are those for cystic fibrosis (located on chromosome 7), phenylketonuria (on chromosome 12) and sickle cell anaemia (on chromosome 11); these were described earlier in Box 3.1. Although someone with the heterozygous genotype will not be affected to a great extent by having a copy of the recessive (mutant) allele, reproduction with another individual might result in the child inheriting one recessive allele from each parent if both parents are heterozygous for the mutation; in this case, the child will have no 'normal' allele and will be affected by the related genetic condition. An individual with the heterozygous genotype is therefore referred to as a *carrier* of that recessive allele. We all carry recessive alleles of genes, including many that are potentially harmful. Being recessive, any effects of these will only become obvious when both forms of the allele are present, one inherited from each parent.

Rarely, the altered allele may actually be dominant to the normal one, and will be expressed even though it is only present in one copy. Again, this might not necessarily be detrimental, depending upon its impact on protein production, but might be highly influential; for example, achondroplasia, a form of dwarfism, results from the inheritance of just one copy of the mutant allele, which is sufficient for its expression.

The Chromosomes During Cell Division: Mitosis and Meiosis

In order for organisms to grow and reproduce, to make and repair organs and tissues, their cells need to replicate themselves. There are two methods of cell replication, both of which entail duplication of the cell's DNA content and its subsequent division into two new cells. These processes are mitosis and meiosis.

Mitosis

Growth and tissue replacement require the multiplication of cells. This occurs through a process of cell division called *mitosis*, in which two new 'daughter' cells are generated from the germinative (or 'parent') cell. One or both of these cells will assume the functions of that particular cell type. The number of chromosomes is preserved during the process and so the new cells continue to be *diploid*. Recall at this point that a chromosome typically has an 'X' shape because its DNA became duplicated into two chromatids during its preparation for cell division. During mitotic division, the two chromatids of each chromosome separate by breaking the proteins that have been binding the chromosome together at the centromere. One set of duplicates then becomes consolidated within one new nucleus, the other in another (Fig. 3.2) and a cell membrane forms between them, completing the production of two cells from the original one. By replicating (i.e., conserving) the genetic code of the duplicates in the first instance, the new cells are still capable of adopting all the functions of the original cell.

Meiosis

A different form of cell division occurs exclusively for the formation of sex cells—that is, spermatozoa in males and ova in females. Conservation of the normal diploid DNA complement in these cells would be disastrous since their fusion at fertilization would cause a doubling of the DNA in each successive generation. In contrast to cell division for growth or replacement, the production of sex cells requires germinative cells to reduce their nuclear DNA by half so that the full complement is restored at fertilization. This form of reduction cell division is called *meiosis* and has two stages, designated meiosis I and meiosis II.

In meiosis I, DNA duplicates are formed and the chromosomes appear, as in the first part of mitosis, but the two members of each homologous pair become 'tied' together by protein for a short while. The chromosome pair then swap a number of alleles in a process called *recombination* to produce a new and unique mix of alleles in the individual chromosomes. In this way we cannot inherit a set of chromosomes that are absolutely identical to those of our parents. We will still have genes for whatever character they produce but recombination means that the homologous chromatids may not now be identical; if a recessive allele has been swapped for a dominant one, the genotype will not now be the same on each half of that chromosome. This contributes to gene mixing between generations. Following recombination, the pairs separate and one of each pair will be consolidated into a 'daughter' nucleus (Fig. 3.2). The process of separating the pairs of chromosomes is referred to as *disjunction* (see also Box 3.4). Note here the distinction from mitosis, in which the chromatids separated and one copy went into each of the 'daughter'

cells, retaining the diploid DNA complement; at the end of meiosis I a whole chromosome (with both of its chromatids still intact) has passed into each new nucleus. Thus two new nuclei have formed but the number of chromosomes in each has been halved. At this stage, each chromosome is still comprised of two duplicates of its DNA, joined together at the centromere.

In meiosis II—a process analogous to mitosis—the centromeres break, and each DNA duplicate (chromatid) passes into a new nucleus, thus producing two new cells from each of the two nuclei formed in meiosis I.

Meiosis therefore produces four new cells from one original cell, but instead of 46 chromosomes (23 pairs), each nucleus now has just 23 single copies, half the usual complement, and is referred to as *haploid* in this respect.

Principles of Gene Inheritance

The division of the genetic material into new combinations during meiosis means that offspring inherit individual alleles more or less at random from their parents. There are two main categories of genetic inheritance: autosomal and sex-linked.

Autosomal Inheritance

For illustrative purposes, consider a hypothetical gene, which we will call gene B. Depending upon its DNA makeup, it could exist as the dominant allele, **A**, or as a recessive allele, **a**. Since each member of the homologous chromosome pair on which the gene is located has an allele, the genotype could be homozygous **AA** (each chromosome has allele A), heterozygous **Aa** (one chromosome has allele A, one a), or homozygous **aa** (each chromosome has allele a). If both parental genotypes are AA then the parents' sex cells will each have the A allele and so the baby will inherit the genotype AA (Fig. 3.3). Likewise, if both parents are of the aa genotype, then an aa genotype of the baby is inevitable.

However, in the heterozygous genotype, Aa, the individual is a *carrier* of the recessive allele; it is present but masked by the dominant allele A and so is not expressed (and the parent therefore may be unaware that they carry it). The outcome for the baby then becomes less predictable. Fig. 3.3 illustrates the various permutations. If both parents are heterozygous for this genotype, there are three possible outcomes. Firstly, the baby may be heterozygous **Aa**, inheriting allele A from one parent and allele a

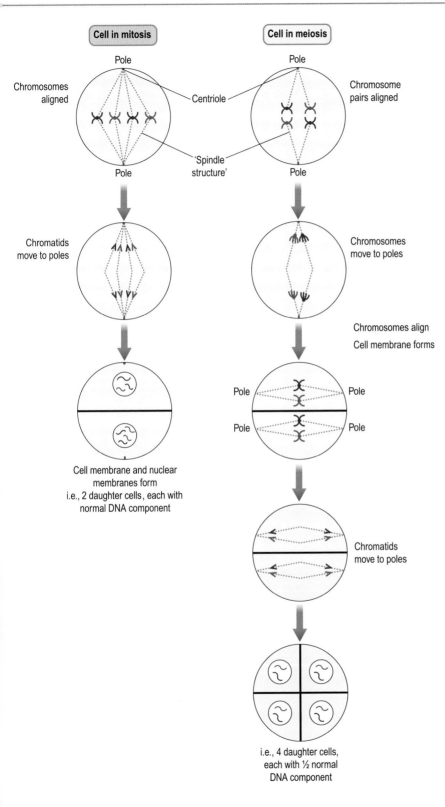

Fig. 3.2 Comparison of chromosome behaviour during cell division by mitosis and meiosis. Both processes are shown at metaphase (metaphase I in meiosis), the stage when the chromosomes first align themselves across the middle of the cell. In mitosis that alignment is haphazard; in meiosis the chromosomes are aligned in their pairs. (Redrawn from Clancy J, McVicar A *Physiology and Anatomy: A homeostatic approach*, 3rd ed, 2009, with permission from Hodder Education.)

from the other, in which case the baby will carry the recessive allele into the next generation as the parents had done. Alternatively, the baby may have inherited two dominant alleles (a **AA** genotype), eradicating the recessive allele altogether, or two recessive alleles (a bb genotype). In the latter instance the lack of a dominant allele means that the recessive form is likely to be expressed and so a characteristic, or *phenotype*, associated with that genotype will now be present. As noted, some—though by no means all—recessive alleles are detrimental to development or to later health. Statistically, if both parents are carriers of the recessive allele, there is a 1 in 4 probability that their baby will inherit two recessive alleles (aa), and a 3 in 4 probability that the baby will be either homozygous for the dominant A allele (AA) or heterozygous (Aa) (Fig. 3.3). It is important to note that the randomness of this process makes it impossible to predict which genotype will occur. Having one baby who is homozygous for the recessive allele, and perhaps has a disorder as a consequence, does not affect the statistical chance of a second baby also having that genotype, which remains 1 in 4. Please note that in rare instances the genetic code can arise spontaneously either in the parental gametes or early embryo through the actions of external factors, for example cosmic radiation or toxins, and so a baby may have an unexpected genotype with a new mutation.

Sex-linked Inheritance

Remember that in females the sex chromosome complement is XX, so in a female's cells each gene located on the X chromosomes will be present as a pair of alleles. This means that their mode of inheritance is generally very similar to that described above for autosomes, although it is actually a little more complicated because some portions of one X chromosome—areas that are specifically involved in sex determination—are inactivated by a 'masking' process referred to as *X-inactivation*. Sex differentiation is discussed later in the chapter.

There are some characteristics, for example colour vision deficiency (colour blindness), that appear predominantly in males. In males there is no concept of a homologous pair of sex chromosomes since the karyotype is XY, and the Y-chromosome, being much smaller than the X, has far fewer genes. This means that for a number of genes, only one allele is present, located on the X chromosome (Fig. 3.4). Without the possibility of an allele being masked by its partner, as observed in the autosomes, any allele might be expected to be expressed, irrespective of whether it is 'dominant' or 'recessive' (Fig. 3.4). This is why sex-linked recessive disorders—such as Duchenne muscular dystrophy, in which a membrane protein in muscle cells is altered, or haemophilia A, in which a clotting protein is deficient—predominantly affect boys but are associated with genes on the X chromosome.

Though unusual, it is possible for females to express an X-linked recessive condition by being homozygous for an inherited recessive gene on the X chromosome. Logically, this means she would have inherited one copy of the recessive allele on her maternal X chromosome—her mother being either heterozygous (i.e., a carrier) or homozygous (i.e., expressing the characteristic phenotype associated with the allele)—and one copy on the X chromosome from her father, who would also express that condition. A recessive allele with an innocuous consequence, say, colour vision deficiency (mostly identified in boys), does not confer reproductive constraints and so it is not unusual to find these traits expressed in females, albeit rarely when compared with their incidence in males. For inheritance of some recessive sex-linked conditions that are a threat to well-being, advances in clinical management have significantly improved the survival of affected males to beyond puberty and so in principle these individuals are capable of reproducing; if a resultant female child inherits a copy from both parents then she will have the associated disorder. It seems an unlikely scenario but there are a small

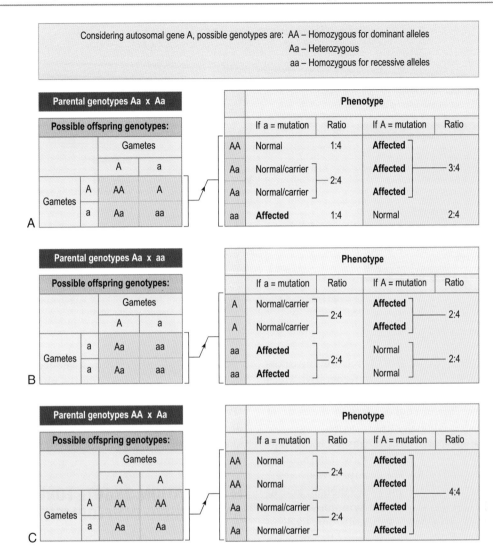

Fig. 3.3 Autosomal inheritance based on possible genotypes for gene A/a. In each case the phenotype (i.e., the characteristic associated with the gene) is shown if the recessive allele, a, or dominant allele, A, is responsible. Note how the statistical incidence of the inherited phenotype is influenced by the occurrence of recessive homozygosity, as is the likelihood of carriage of the allele in the recessive/dominant heterozygous state. Also note how asymptomatic carriage of a disease-causing allele would not be possible if that allele is dominant. (Redrawn from Clancy J, McVicar A *Physiology and Anatomy: A homeostatic approach*, 3rd ed, 2009, with permission from Hodder Education.)

number of instances worldwide where a girl has inherited, for example, haemophilia A.

Population Factors

Figs 3.3 and 3.4 clearly illustrate that the likelihood of a baby being born with a particular anatomical or functional characteristic depends upon the genotype of its parents and, in particular, their recessive alleles (dominant mutations of alleles are much rarer). It is usually the case that individuals are unaware they carry a recessive allele, but the likelihood that both parents carry the same recessive allele is increased if the parents are from the same locality or population.

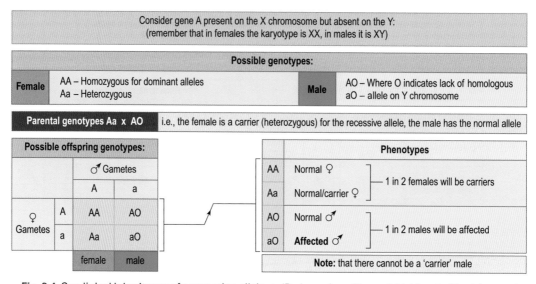

Fig. 3.4 Sex-linked inheritance of a recessive allele, a. (Redrawn from Clancy J, McVicar A. *Physiology and Anatomy: A homeostatic approach*, 3rd ed, 2009, with permission from Hodder Education.)

The local factor relates to familial relationships, possibly so long past that they are now unrecognized, which ensures a relatively high presence of the allele within the community. This of course refers to the issue of inbreeding which is taboo in most societies.

The population factor has contributed historically to the spread of alleles around the world. International travel is one reason for this. For example, *Huntington's chorea* is caused by a dominant allele (though, unusually, its expression is delayed and symptoms do not appear until well into adulthood) and seems likely to have been introduced into the Americas by European settlers. Other reasons for the geographical prevalence of recessive alleles are more speculative. For example, the sickle cell anaemia allele has a high incidence in people of African Caribbean, Asian and eastern Mediterranean descent (e.g., around 1 in 10 African Americans are carriers). This considerably raises the chances of a couple meeting and a subsequent baby inheriting two copies of the allele, one from each parent, and so the condition is particularly prevalent in those populations. However, carrying just one copy of the allele (i.e., a heterozygous genotype) appears to confer protection against malaria, common in Africa, Asia and parts of eastern Europe. Likewise, the autosomal recessive allele for cystic fibrosis has a high incidence in people of white European descent (around 1 in 25 are carriers), but it has been suggested that carrying just one copy of the cystic fibrosis mutation may confer resistance to tuberculosis and other conditions (Poolman & Galvani, 2006). A high carrier frequency of recessive alleles such as these does mean that the likelihood of the alleles being inherited will be higher in some communities.

FERTILIZATION, ZYGOTE FORMATION AND EMBRYO DEVELOPMENT

The *zygote* (= 'yoked together') is the product of *fertilization*, when the nucleus of a single male sex cell (*gamete*) fuses with the nucleus of the female gamete. Critical stages in forming the zygote can be categorized as:

1. Differentiation of the gametes in the parents, a process referred to as *gametogenesis*.
2. Ejaculation of the male gametes (spermatozoa) in semen in the cervix during sexual intercourse, and the survival and transit of the spermatozoa through the uterus.
3. Penetration of the female gamete (secondary oocyte) by a single spermatozoon.
4. Final differentiation of the secondary oocyte into an ovum and the fusion of its nucleus with that of the spermatozoon. This stage, fertilization, is usually viewed as the point of biological conception but

definitions of 'conception' can be confusing. Thus it is 'the point at which a woman becomes pregnant and the development of a baby starts' (Collins,) but, whereas embryo development commences very soon after fertilization of the ovum, pregnancy itself requires implantation of the embryo into the endometrium, an event that actually takes place several days after fertilization.

Each of these stages is described below. Readers interested in following them up in more detail, and how they might relate to infertility, will find a wide range of literature (e.g., Tosti and Menzo, 2016). However, the material can make for heavy reading and the more technically detailed general midwifery textbooks that also provide good insights, for example Blackburn (2018), may be preferable.

Gametogenesis

In both males and females, gamete formation commences with the generation of intermediate, or primary, sex cells from germinative cells within the gonadal tissues (i.e., the testis or ovary). Further meiotic cell division of the primary sex cells generates secondary sex cells that will form the actual gametes. Gender-specific terms for the process relate to the gametes produced. In males, the specific term is *spermatogenesis*, while in females it is *oogenesis*.

Spermatogenesis

Spermatozoa (*zoon* = life) are the specialized cells ejaculated in semen which characteristically can swim. They are produced in vast numbers, which means that germinative cells within the testes, called *spermatogonia*, must initially undergo rapid proliferation by mitosis. Some of the resultant *primary spermatocytes* (*cyte* = cell) then undergo cell division by meiosis to form haploid *secondary spermatocytes* (Fig. 3.5) and cannot divide again. At this stage they appear rounded and must undergo further gene-activated changes to complete their differentiation into spermatozoa:

- The nucleus of the spermatocyte becomes compacted and elongated.
- The cytoplasm is considerably reduced and the cell develops a 'tail' that will provide propulsion, and so enable the spermatozoon to swim.
- The mitochondria migrate to what becomes the midpiece connecting the 'head' of the spermatozoon with its 'tail'; they will help to produce the energy required for movement of the tail.

- The head section containing the cell nucleus develops a cap called the *acrosome* that contains digestive enzymes essential for the fertilization process.
- Other organelles in the spermatocyte lose their structure and form and degenerate, leaving the cell with a characteristic tadpole-like shape.
- The cells are now referred to as *spermatids*. In this state, they are not capable of fertilizing an ovum and so must remain located in the testis where they mature further in the *epididymis*, the tubular structure on the surface of the testis which eventually leads into the *vas deferens*, the duct that conveys semen to the penis during ejaculation.

Oogenesis

Oogenesis commences with the *oogonium*, a germinative cell located within what may become an ovarian follicle. As in the male, these cells increase in number via mitosis but, unlike in males (where spermatozoa are continuously generated throughout the individual's reproductive life), the population of oogonia within a woman's ovary is actually established before her own birth; there is no comparable continuous proliferation of germinative cells. Around the time of the woman's birth, the oogonia enter into a meiotic division (Fig. 3.5), but this process is suspended at the end of the meiosis I stage, with the pairs of chromosomes remaining attached to each other. The cell is referred to as a *primary oocyte* and it will remain in this state until puberty and beyond.

After puberty, some primary oocytes become 'reanimated' during each menstrual cycle and complete the first phase of the meiotic division. The chromosome pairs now separate, generating two haploid daughter cells with half the usual chromosomal complement; these new cells are referred to as the *secondary oocyte* and the *first polar body*. The second stage of meiosis I is suspended at this point; the polar body is discarded and subsequently degenerates. Ordinarily, a number of secondary oocytes will be produced within an ovarian follicle during a single menstrual cycle but just one will advance enough to be released at ovulation; the rest degenerate and are absorbed. At ovulation, this remaining secondary oocyte has grown to a diameter of about 0.1 mm, just about visible to the naked eye, and is released. Generation of the ovum itself, in the second phase of cell division (meiosis II), will not occur until *after* the oocyte has been penetrated by a spermatozoon. However, it has become a common

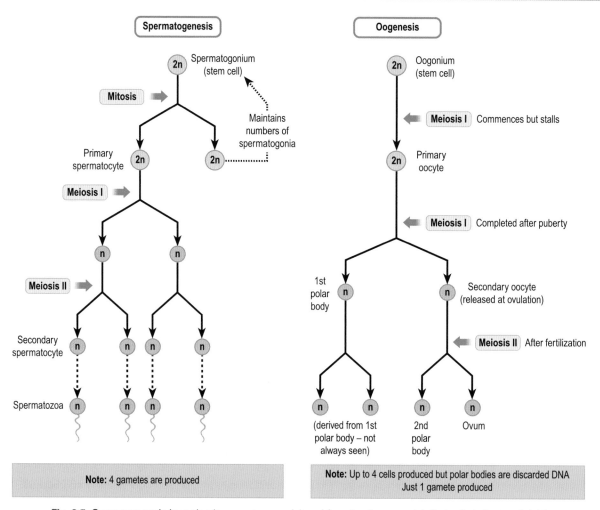

Fig. 3.5 Gametogenesis in males (spermatogenesis) and females (oogenesis). Note: *2n* indicates diploid cells; *n* indicates haploid cells.

(if somewhat inaccurate) practice to refer to the secondary oocyte itself as the ovum (or egg cell).

At ovulation, the secondary oocyte is surrounded by two protective layers: a thick protein coat, the *zona pellucida* (pellucid = transparent), and a mass of small undeveloped cells from the follicle arranged in layers that radiate outwards, called the *corona radiata* (corona = crown). The zona pellucida and corona radiata provide essential protection for the vulnerable oocyte as it drifts free in the fluid-filled fallopian tube towards the uterus. To access the oocyte during fertilization, the spermatozoa must find the means of penetrating these

protective layers. How they do this is explained later, but first we must consider how the spermatozoa traverse the uterus to arrive at the oocyte in the first place.

Transit of Spermatozoa Through the Uterus

In a male with normal fertility, there are at least 40 million spermatozoa per millilitre of semen; with an average ejaculate volume of 3 to 4 ml of semen, this means around 120 million spermatozoa are ejaculated. Only one of these may eventually penetrate the oocyte for fertilization to occur, but interaction with several hundred others in its vicinity is required if this is to happen.

Even so, that number of cells means that the rate of attrition has been exceedingly high:

- Many spermatozoa will not enter the cervix.
- Those that do will initially be adversely affected by the acidic cervical environment.
- Many will be destroyed by immune cells in the uterus that usually protect it against infection.
- Many will have undergone incomplete development and so are unable to swim adequately.

Mitigating against this, the survival and transport of spermatozoa to the oocyte is facilitated by the properties of semen:

- Not all of the semen remains in the vagina and so many spermatozoa fail to enter the cervix. However, semen coagulates at ejaculation and so a proportion of spermatozoa do remain close to the neck of the cervix. That semen then quickly liquefies, helping the spermatozoa to enter the cervix.
- Semen is alkaline and acts to neutralize the acidic mucus within the neck of the cervix, thus aiding survival of the spermatozoa.
- Semen is rich in fructose, a sugar that provides a source of energy for the swimming spermatozoa.
- Prostaglandins present in semen stimulate peristaltic muscle contraction of the cervix and uterine wall. These contractions are retrograde, that is they move away from the cervix, and so propel the spermatozoa towards and into the fallopian tubes, to the vicinity of the secondary oocyte released from the ovarian follicle.

Spermatozoa that do survive the journey remain functionally intact for 48 to 72 hours. But if we consider the uterus as being around 8 cm long (Egbase et al., 2000) and the velocity of swimming spermatozoa as 35 micrometres per second (2 mm or so per minute; Van den Bergh et al., 1998), then they should be capable of covering the distance to the ampulla in just 40 minutes. In reality, some spermatozoa may arrive at the oocyte in less than 20 minutes because the uterine muscle contractions have effectively increased their speed. Others may arrive after a couple of days as they 'escape' from the *cervical crypts*, having initially become caught up in these mucus-secreting glands. These two phases—rapid and slow—in the delivery of spermatozoa to the fallopian tube help to maintain a supply over a considerable period of time and so increase the likelihood of fertilization taking place.

Fertilization of the Ovum

On arriving at the fallopian tube, spermatozoa are directed towards chemical attractants secreted by the oocyte. As they approach it, the local chemical environment stimulates them to undergo *capacitation*, a process that modifies chemicals on their surface so that they can bind to complementary sites on the protective zona pellucida and later to the oocyte itself. Capacitation also enables the *acrosome reaction*, the release of digestive enzymes from the acrosome cap of the spermatozoa to facilitate penetration through the protective corona radiata and zona pellucida, a process which takes a few hours. A single spermatozoon cannot produce an acrosome reaction of sufficient magnitude to ensure penetration right through these layers to the oocyte, and thus the collective response of several hundred spermatozoa in the vicinity is required (see Box 3.5).

The first spermatozoon to reach the membrane of the oocyte binds to it. The respective cell membranes then fuse and the spermatozoon rapidly enters. Penetration

---

BOX 3.5 How Many Spermatozoa Are Required?

There is a vast attrition of spermatozoa ejaculated in semen:

- Those that are lost to the cervix, destroyed by acidity or ejected
- Those that, upon entering the vagina, are incapable of swimming normally due to not having developed properly
- Those that fall foul of maternal immune cells in the uterus
- Those trapped in uterine pits
- Those that enter the 'wrong' fallopian tube

Several hundred spermatozoa must reach the vicinity of the secondary oocyte in the fallopian tube. Such numbers are necessary to make the oocyte membrane below the zona pellucida coat accessible, even though only one spermatozoon will ultimately penetrate the oocyte membrane. Fortunately for the human race, a fertile male produces over 100 million spermatozoa in a single ejaculate! The requirement for such large numbers is illustrated by the threshold for diagnosing infertility: around 20 million spermatozoa per millilitre of semen. More information on male infertility can be found in Aitken (2006).

by further spermatozoa is prevented because that initial contact immediately triggers the *cortical reaction* in the oocyte; this is a release of granular contents which modify the oocyte membrane and act to make the zona pellucida more resistant to further acrosome reaction. Upon its penetration of the oocyte, the tail and midpiece of the spermatozoon degenerate, leaving the remaining nucleus to swell and form the *male pronucleus* (see also Box 3.6). In this state, it is now capable of fusing with the ovum, the final development of which is triggered when the spermatozoon penetrates the oocyte.

Although the spermatozoon has penetrated it, fertilization cannot be completed until the oocyte undergoes the second phase of division (meiosis II) to produce the ovum, because at fertilization the oocyte's chromosomes still have their duplicate chromatids. The nuclei of the spermatozoon and oocyte must therefore remain separate for a short while; the oocyte is around 50 times the diameter of the pronucleus of the spermatozoon, which is readily accommodated during this time.

In the secondary oocyte, the full meiotic division that commenced many years earlier is now completed, with the meiosis II stage generating the final two daughter cells – the *ovum* and the *second polar body*. As with the first polar body, the second polar body degenerates;

the nucleus of the ovum swells to form the *female pronucleus*.

Once both male and female pronuclei have formed, they fuse—i.e., fertilization occurs. As a result of this fusion, the new nucleus contains a full complement of 46 chromosomes, 23 from each pronucleus—it is now diploid. However, with half of its DNA coming from each parent, its genetic complement is very different from the germinative cells of either parent. The product is now referred to as the *zygote*.

Twinning

Should twinning take place, it usually occurs at or soon after fertilization of the ovum. As the second polar body does not have the capacity to be fertilized, twinning indicates either that two ova have been fertilized so forming two zygotes, or that one was released and fertilized as usual but the resultant zygote split into two early in development.

- If two ova (i.e., from two secondary oocytes released at ovulation) are independently fertilized then *fraternal* or *dizygotic* twins may result. Each ovum and fertilizing spermatozoon is genetically unique, so each embryo will be genetically distinct and will develop independently.
- *Monozygotic* twins develop when a single zygote divides into two and each new part develops into a separate embryo. Monozygotic twins are therefore genetically identical. Each embryo develops independently but if twinning occurs after the embryo has begun to differentiate, the pair may separate only partially, producing *conjoined* twins. The timing of twinning also has implications for development of the embryonic membranes, as discussed later in the chapter.

FROM FERTILIZATION TO IMPLANTATION (1–6 DAYS POST-FERTILIZATION)

The protective zona pellucida around the secondary oocyte remains intact during fertilization, despite its penetration by a spermatozoon; however, its presence around the ovum and early embryo would interfere with eventual implantation of the embryo into the endometrium and so it will eventually be shed. But because implantation will not occur for several days—during which the zygote/early embryo floats free within the fallopian tube—the continued presence of the zona pellucida helps to protect it during this vulnerable time.

BOX 3.6   Mitochondrial DNA

The organelles that generate metabolic energy for cells—the mitochondria—contain small amounts of DNA. Because the mitochondria are outside the cell nucleus, this DNA does not take part in the nuclear division process in either mitosis or meiosis. However, when the new daughter cells are formed, they do incorporate cytoplasm and hence mitochondria from the parent cell. By contrast, the process of fertilization requires the spermatozoon to shed all its cellular contents other than the nucleus. Consequently, the mitochondria in the zygote (and hence the embryo) are derived exclusively from the ovum; the small quantity of extranuclear DNA that we all carry within our mitochondria is derived entirely from our mother, and her mother, and so on. Such conservation of DNA from the maternal line has provided science with the opportunity to study lineages, including population and ethnic groups that may have dispersed thousands of years ago. The popular science book by Rutherford (2017) provides an accessible and fascinating read on this subject.

The Morula (0–4 Days Post-Fertilization)

Cell division (*cleavage*) of the zygote produces the first two new embryonic cells, referred to as *blastomeres* (= simple, undifferentiated cells) after about 30 hours. The blastomeres then continue to divide every 12 to 24 hours, remaining encapsulated within the zona pellucida which means that as they multiply, each daughter cell becomes progressively smaller than its predecessors. The zygote eventually becomes transformed into a ball of about 64 small, compacted cells; it is now referred to as a *morula* (named for its likeness to a mulberry). The morula arrives in the uterus about 3 to 4 days after fertilization (see also Box 3.7).

The Blastocyst (5–6 Days Post-Fertilization)

When the morula eventually arrives in the uterus, it begins to take in uterine fluid to form a fluid-filled cavity called a *blastocoele* (coele = cavity) at its centre. The formation of the cavity pushes the blastomeres outwards.

- At this point, the morula is still coated with the protective zona pellucida. Some of the cells are therefore flattened against the zona, forming a layer one cell thick which is now referred to as the *trophectoderm* (troph = nutrition; ecto = outer; derm = layer); the individual cells of this layer are referred to as *trophoblasts* and initially they will have a nutritive role when the embryo implants into the endometrium.

BOX 3.7   Karyotyping/Genotyping of Embryos

In *vitro* (literally 'in glass') fertilization of harvested secondary oocytes/ova will, if all is well, generate a small number of intact early embryos at the morula stage of development. Since blastomeres within the morula have not yet differentiated significantly towards the next step of development, it is possible to carefully extract one from an early morula without consequences for the later development of the embryo or baby. Such procedures may be applied to screen for chromosomal/genetic abnormalities before transference of the selected morula to the uterus. In the context of embryo development, the fact that the procedure can be performed also identifies that the genes responsible for specific tissue development have not yet been activated in cells of the morula stage.

Cells derived from this layer will eventually form the chorionic membrane.

- A small number of cells (12–15) form a crescent-shaped cluster towards one end of the blastocoele. These are referred to as *embryoblasts* and are destined to become the embryo proper. This tiny collection of cells is more simply referred to as the *inner cell mass*.
- The entire structure of trophectoderm, inner cell mass and blastocoele cavity is now referred to as a *blastocyst* (Fig. 3.6).

The blastocyst remains floating within the uterine fluid for about 2 days, and the trophoblast cells are activated to secrete digestive enzymes. Their actions enable the blastocyst to 'hatch' from its zona pellucida coat, giving it better access to nutrients in the surrounding fluid. Consequently, its size rapidly increases and it becomes positioned adjacent to the uterine endometrium in preparation for implantation.

Implantation (6–14 Days Post-Fertilization)

Chemical interactions between the blastocyst and endometrium promote complex processes which lead to the attachment of the blastocyst to the endometrial layer, followed by its implantation. The blastocyst is completely embedded in the endometrium by about the 12th day after fertilization (see Figure 3.6). The process also triggers another critical event, the early development of the chorionic villi, that occurs over the following 2 days and so is included in the timescale here. A more detailed exploration of molecular interactions that take place to ensure implantation occurs is provided by Aplin and Ruane (2017), but the critical stages are:

- Attachment and adhesion. The blastocyst secretes chemicals that remove barrier proteins from the surface of endometrial cells, which themselves are stimulated to secrete other proteins that promote adhesion of the blastocyst to them.
- Transmigration of trophoblasts. Upon adhesion, the layer of cells at the surface of the blastocyst (trophectoderm) differentiates into two distinct layers:
  - The outer layer, in contact with the endometrium, begins to fuse into a 'syncytium'—that is, a mass without the distinguishable membranes that had separated the cells; the cells of this layer are now referred to as *syncytiotrophoblasts*. This layer secretes enzymes that digest the nearby endometrial cells, so releasing nutrients stored within them,

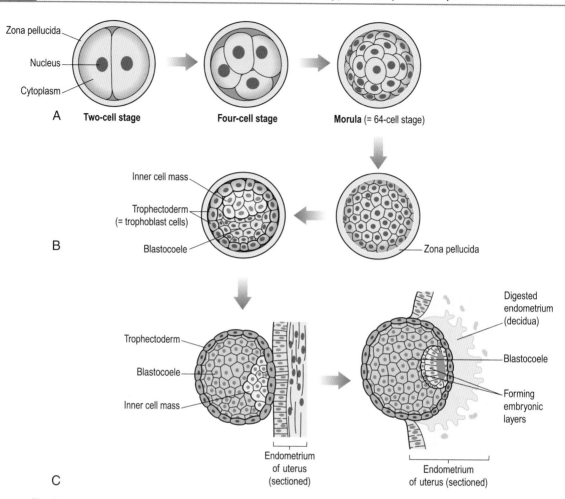

Fig. 3.6 Preimplantation development. (A) Development of the morula from the zygote. (B) The blastocyst, in section. (C) Implantation. (Redrawn from Clancy J, McVicar A. *Physiology and Anatomy: A homeostatic approach*, 3rd ed, 2009, with permission from Hodder Education.)

and also enabling the blastocyst to 'burrow in' and begin implantation.

- The other, lower layer of trophoblasts retain their individual cell structure; these cells are now referred to as *cytotrophoblasts* and function to maintain the syncytium above.
- The two layers grow and invade the underlying connective tissue layer of the endometrium, referred to as the *stroma*, and hence secure the implantation of the blastocyst. In doing so, they trigger the *decidual reaction*. This is the process by which stromal cells in the area become swollen with high-energy stores of glycogen and lipids to form a distinct nutritive region, the *decidua*, around the developing embryo. Continued invasion by the blastocyst releases nutrients from these decidual cells and so fuels the further growth of the blastocyst.

- The lacunar stage. Invasion of the decidua by the blastocyst causes fluid-filled spaces, or *lacunae*, to appear within it. These will have an important role in placentation, but at this early stage the trophoblast cells of the blastocyst block the spaces and prevent maternal blood from filling them. In this way, the embryo is not exposed to immune cells in maternal blood before placentation has taken place.

- The site where the blastocyst entered the endometrium is plugged, initially by a blood clot and then by the epithelium which quickly regenerates over the area. The early embryo is now fully implanted and physically isolated from the environment of the uterine fluid.

THE EMBRYO DURING AND AFTER IMPLANTATION (14–21 DAYS POST-FERTILIZATION)

Cell division in the embryo is now happening quickly and several developments occur over a short space of time. Embryo development from fertilization takes place over about 8 weeks in which time all tissues and organs are in place and most are functioning, albeit some only rudimentally. That distinction provides the transition point from embryo to fetus. Many of these developments occur simultaneously, but for convenience it is simpler to consider each development separately. The processes are extremely complex and are covered only in outline here; readers are referred to some of the more detailed textbooks (e.g., Rankin, 2017) for additional information.

The Embryonic Disc and 'Germ' Layers

Around the time that the blastocyst begins to implant, the collection of embryoblasts (or inner cell mass) within it flattens into a disc. By the end of 2 weeks after fertilization this disc will have become two-layered (*bilaminar*); one layer is called the *epiblast* (epi = upper), the other the *hypoblast* (hypo = lower). If we could look down directly on the flattened surface of the epiblast, we would see a thickened line of cells running along the middle of it. This line, called the *primitive streak*, is an indication of a very important change occurring. Underneath it, cells are forming and moving outwards to create a third layer of cells between the epiblast and hypoblast layers, and making the embryonic disc *trilaminar* (Fig. 3.7). This has significant implications for the next stage of development; but for the moment, note that the primitive streak has determined the head–tail alignment of the embryo, and also which parts of the disc will eventually form the left and right sides of the body. Disc formation and the primitive streak represent the first stage of differentiation (specialisation) of the embryo proper.

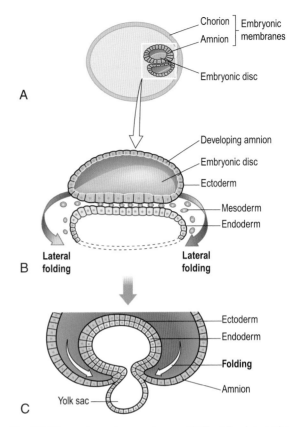

Fig. 3.7 The embryonic germ layers. (A) The trilaminar embryonic disc. (B) The growth of the amnion from the ectoderm layer. (C) Folding to internalize the endoderm. (Redrawn from Clancy J, McVicar A. *Physiology and Anatomy: A homeostatic approach*, 3rd ed, 2009, with permission from Hodder Education.)

The generation of the three layers is referred to as *gastrulation*. It is now usual to refer to the layers according to the specific terms used to identify the embryonic origins of cells and tissues within the baby; thus the epiblast becomes the *embryonic ectoderm* (ecto = outer; derm = layer), the hypoblast becomes the *embryonic endoderm* (endo = inner) and the layer that formed between them becomes the *embryonic mesoderm* (meso = middle). These terms will be more meaningful when the next event occurs.

At this point, the trilaminar disc is still two-dimensional with the cells arranged in those three layers, rather like a sandwich with a mesoderm 'filling'. However, early in the third week after fertilization, the edges of the disc begin to fold downwards and inwards along the axis formed by the primitive streak. Each layer fuses with its counterpart on the opposite side, transforming the two-dimensional 'sandwich' into a three-dimensional 'tube' with walls comprised of three concentric layers (Fig. 3.7). The ectoderm forms the outer layer of this tube, the endoderm the inner tube, and the mesoderm a layer between the other two. Some longitudinal folding also takes place, giving the embryo a 'bean' shape.

The embryo is tiny, still only about 0.2 mm long, but the significance of the trilaminar disc and subsequent gastrulation phase should not be underestimated; in forming the three-dimensional tube, the embryo has laid down the foundations for the basic layout of the body:

- The ectoderm will form the epidermis of the skin, but will also be associated with a variety of tissues including those of the nervous system.
- The endoderm, running centrally inside the structure, will give rise to the tissues and organs of the gastrointestinal tract and associated organs such as the liver and pancreas.
- The mesoderm will give rise to various tissues lying between the epidermis and gastrointestinal tract including the dermal layer of the skin, muscles of the body wall, lining tissues of the body cavities and blood vessels.
- The apertures formed at each end, where the inner tube of endoderm exits through the ectoderm, will form the mouth and anus, in accordance with the genetic 'decisions' taken earlier to locate the brain at one end (referred to as *cephalization*) and hence to establish the basic regionalization of the body.

Extraembryonic Membranes

As the embryo develops, it becomes enclosed within two protective membranes—the *chorion* and the *amnion*—that persist through to birth. Two other membranous sacs called the *yolk sac* and *allantois* are also observed during earlier phases, but these are transient, being absorbed or incorporated into developing embryonic tissues. The membranes together provide a range of activities including protection, nutrition, and waste disposal in the period until placentation has progressed sufficiently to assume some of those roles. Although these developments are concurrent, it is simpler to consider them separately.

Chorion

You will recall that the blastocyst has two outer layers of cells, the trophectoderm, which act to enable the blastocyst to invade the endometrial decidua. At around 2 weeks after fertilization, a third layer forms below the trophectoderm; these cells originated from the mesoderm layer of the embryo at gastrulation and have migrated outwards from it. Since this new layer is located outside the embryo proper, it is distinguished by the term *extraembryonic* mesoderm. It will have a critical role to play in development of the placenta; but for now, simply note that together these three layers will form the *chorion* around the embryo. As the embryo/fetus increases in size, the chorion bulges into the uterine cavity and will eventually grow to line the entire uterus, encapsulating the embryo within its internal, fluid-filled space.

The space within the chorion originated as the blastocoele cavity within the tiny blastocyst, but, with its new mesoderm-derived lining, it is now referred to as the *extraembryonic coelom*. We will meet this term again in relation to other coeloms (or cavities) inside the embryo. The extraembryonic coelom provides a source of nutrients and oxygen, derived from the decidua, during the very early stages of embryo development prior to placentation. It diminishes in volume as the space is taken up by the growing embryo/fetus. Placentation replaces its nutritive role, but the chorion continues to support the embryo, for example, by providing shock absorption when the mother is moving.

Amnion

The ectoderm layer of the bilaminar embryonic disc parts to form a small fluid-filled cavity within it. A thin layer of cells makes up the 'roof' of this *amniotic sac* (Fig. 3.7) and this layer is destined to form the *amniotic membrane*. As the cells begin to divide, the sac grows outwards and as it enlarges, it begins to extend down the sides of the developing embryo. The leading edges of the amnion eventually join to form a continuous layer that completely envelops the embryo, and hence the later fetus. The cavity inside it continues to fill with *amniotic fluid*.

Since the amnion has developed from the actual embryo, it is located inside the chorion, rather like one balloon inside another (Fig. 3.8). As the fetus grows, the amnion enlarges further and the chorionic fluid around it diminishes in volume as it is displaced by the growing amniotic volume. Eventually both the chorion and amnion extend to line the entire uterus and the two come into contact with each other; a thin layer of mucus

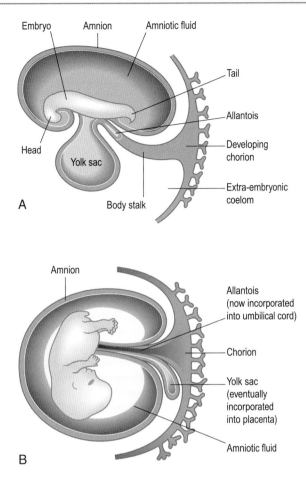

Fig. 3.8 The extraembryonic membranes. In (A) the embryo is almost enclosed by the outgrowing amnion. Placentation has only just commenced and the embryo is sustained by exchange with the extraembryonic fluid, facilitated by the extension into it of the yolk sac and allantois membranes. In (B) the embryo has become completely enclosed within the amnion. The functions of the yolk sac and allantois are increasingly replaced by the developing placenta; those membranes diminish and will eventually become incorporated into embryonic tissues. (Redrawn from Clancy J, McVicar A. *Physiology and Anatomy: A homeostatic approach*, 3rd ed, 2009, with permission from Hodder Education.)

prevents any frictional damage between the two membranes. In this way a dual membrane eventually lines the distended uterus, encapsulating the fetus which is now suspended in the amniotic fluid by its umbilical cord (see also Box 3.8).

Yolk Sac and Allantois

These sacs appear early in embryo development, before the full development of the amnion, and extend into the chorionic fluid. They have significant roles at this time by exchanging substances with the surrounding chorionic fluid, but neither sac is retained for long because the placenta eventually takes on those roles.

The *yolk sac* is formed from endoderm cells within the embryo as a fluid-filled cavity that distends outwards through the mesoderm and ectoderm, into the chorionic fluid. It exchanges nutrients and waste with the chorionic fluid in the period before the amnion has grown sufficiently to enclose the embryo. The externalized part of the yolk sac is eventually 'pinched off' and

BOX 3.8   Amniocentesis

Amniocentesis is the sampling of amniotic fluid and of the embryonic/fetal cells floating within it. Recall that both the chorionic and amniotic membranes grow outwards and eventually line the uterus, but that the fluid volume within the chorion is displaced by that inside the expanding amnion. Should clinicians wish to sample embryonic cells for karyotype screening, then the amniotic fluid is the most accessible material. Note, though, that access to it must be through both the chorion and amniotic membrane; this introduces a slight risk to the fetus and the pregnancy.

See also Box 3.7 regarding karyotyping at the earlier morula phase when the embryo itself has not formed.

subsequently degenerates; the rest is trapped within the embryo and grows to line a body cavity that has formed between the mesoderm and endoderm layers, inside the embryo—now called the *intraembryonic coelom*. As the embryo develops, this cavity will later provide the thoracic and abdominal cavities.

The *allantois* is an outgrowth from the yolk sac and has a role in gas exchange with the chorionic fluid, again prior to the amnion enclosing the embryo; it also provides urine storage. Externally, this sac rapidly becomes unnecessary when blood vessels within the *body stalk* (which connects the embryo to the developing placenta) enable more efficient exchange of respiratory gases; the allantois becomes incorporated into the stalk. Internally, the sac is incorporated into the developing urinary bladder.

Monozygotic Twinning and the Embryonic Membranes

Early splitting of the zygote within the first 2 days after fertilization produces two blastocysts which will each develop their own chorion and amnion, and may even have individual placentas (though these may fuse as they grow).

Later splitting (3–9 days after fertilization) is more complicated; the embryos may each have their own amnion, but the chorionic development that commenced with the blastocyst will have already advanced and so both embryos, with their amniotic membranes, will remain inside a single chorion. Such *monochorionic* twins will share the same placenta (the development of which involves the chorion, as described later in the chapter).

Even later splitting (9–12 days after fertilization) is rare, and often is not viable as it takes place after both the chorion and the amnion have formed. If viable, this late twinning may produce two embryos that share a single amnion, a single chorion, and a common placenta.

Placentation and the Umbilical Cord

The *placenta* initially develops from the chorion where it is in contact with the endometrial decidua. It is a complex organ responsible for the exchange of oxygen, nutrients and waste substances between the embryonic/fetal circulation and that of the mother. The significance of placentation is:

• A very large surface area is generated, allowing highly efficient exchanges with maternal blood that support the rapidly growing embryo.

• Maternal and fetal bloods are prevented from mingling. Remember that the embryo is genetically unique; this isolation of fetal cells from those of the mother is essential to prevent components of the maternal immune system rejecting the fetal tissue as non-self.

Formation of the placenta commences at the lacunar stage of blastocyst implantation, in which outgrowing layers of trophectoderm cells cause fluid-filled spaces (lacunae) to appear within the endometrial decidua. Recall that during this process, the trophectoderm is joined by a layer of extraembryonic mesoderm that has grown out from the developing embryo. These layers comprise the early chorion membrane; the next stage in placentation is for them to produce finger-like projections (*villi*) that extend into the lacunae. It is the vast number of villi that creates the massively increased surface area in the placenta. A feature of this process is that only the embryonic mesodermal cells can transform into blood vessels, so the mesodermal layer below the trophectoderm must push outwards to enable maximal exchange between maternal and embryonic blood.

There are three phases in the development of chorionic villi:

• The inner, extraembryonic mesoderm layer induces the overlying cytotrophoblast layer of the trophectoderm to form projections through the outer syncytium layer of the developing chorion. These projections are referred to as the *primary chorionic villi*, and they appear at the end of just 2 weeks post-fertilization.

• During the third week, the extraembryonic mesoderm layer itself pushes into the primary villi and projects from them as smaller *secondary chorionic villi*.

- Finally, some of the extraembryonic mesoderm cells within the secondary villi transform into blood vessels (capillary loops) which then project outwards from the secondary villi to produce even smaller projections, the *tertiary chorionic villi*.

Prior to this point, as noted earlier, lacunae (spaces) had formed in the nutritive layer of the uterine endometrium (the decidua) as a result of its digestion by the implanting embryo. The spaces were blocked, preventing the embryo coming into contact with maternal blood. Once the tertiary villi have formed, the lacunae are allowed to fill with maternal blood and so nutrient/waste exchange can commence between the maternal circulation and embryonic blood within the villi. The walls of the tertiary villi provide a physical barrier that continues to prevent direct contact between the two bloodstreams (see also Box 3.9).

The Fetoplacental Unit

The embryo/fetus is not a passive agent; it triggers, and even controls, numerous key processes to ensure pregnancy and its own subsequent development. For example, it has already been noted how the blastocyst secretes chemicals that are instrumental in its adherence to the uterine endometrium, and in transforming the endometrium at the site of implantation into a nutrient-rich decidua which helps to ensure the success of implantation.

Hormonal secretions from the embryo/fetus and placenta (referred to in this context as a *fetoplacental unit*) take this influence still further by acting on the mother's own physiology, triggering some of the adaptations required for her to support the pregnancy. In this way, the embryo/fetus actively contributes to its own development and sustainability. A prime example is the secretion of *human chorionic gonadotrophin* (*HCG*), firstly by the trophectoderm cells as the blastocyst implants in the decidua, and later by the chorion and placenta (both of which contain cells derived from the trophectoderm). This hormone is responsible for promoting the transformation of the discharged ovarian follicle (which released the secondary oocyte) into the *corpus luteum*, a tissue that secretes another hormone, progesterone. Progesterone, in turn, maintains the placenta and prompts further adaptations in the mother. The fact that HCG is secreted by embryonic rather than maternal tissue provides the basis for its use in pregnancy testing of maternal urine.

BOX 3.9   Placental (or Uteroplacental Vascular) Insufficiency

Uterine Blood Flow

Uterine blood flow is approximately 100 ml per minute in the non-pregnant state, equivalent to around 2% of cardiac output (at rest). At term, uterine blood flow may be as high as 700 ml per minute. To meet this demand, the mother has an increased blood volume; however, even with this, the uterus also receives a bigger proportion of the cardiac output—around 10%. Much of this increased blood supply supports the exchange of gases, water, nutrients and waste with the fetus.

Uterine blood vessels are highly dilated during pregnancy, meaning that placental blood flow is susceptible to inadequate maternal cardiac output and inadequate uterine arterial blood pressure (hence risk from hypovolaemia and, for example, general anaesthesia). Increased vascular resistance within the placenta also presents a critical risk to both the fetus (due to inadequate perfusion of the placenta) and the mother (due to an elevated total peripheral resistance and consequently hypertension). Hypertension is one of the key symptoms of *preeclampsia*.

Placental Insufficiency and Preeclampsia

Placental *insufficiency* refers to the occurrence of poor nutrient/gas exchange between the mother and her fetus. It is rare and usually arises as a consequence of inadequate development of the placenta such that maternal blood supply via the uterine artery cannot increase adequately as the fetus grows. Even more rarely, it might relate to disruption of the fetal blood supply to the placenta. The insufficiency conveys a serious risk of either inadequate fetal growth or maternal *preeclampsia*.

If preeclampsia occurs, it is most commonly observed after around 20 weeks of pregnancy. It is poorly understood but is characterized by increased maternal blood pressure and excess protein in the urine. It is associated with multi-organ problems and is a precursor of eclampsia, characterized by neurological fits that present a serious—even fatal—risk to the mother, but may also impact indirectly on the fetus.

A good overview of the risks, causes and complications of preeclampsia is presented on the UK National Health Service website:
https://www.nhs.uk/conditions/pre-eclampsia/causes/

The Umbilical Cord

Earlier, we saw how the mesodermal cells within the developing embryo also migrate out of the embryo as extraembryonic mesoderm, which extends outwards to become part of the chorion membrane and hence the placenta. It is also incorporated into the *body stalk* that connects the embryo to the chorion and is the precursor of the *umbilical cord* which joins the embryo to the developing placenta. That mesoderm transforms into capillaries which connect with blood vessels developing from mesoderm in the tertiary villi of the early placenta, and the circulatory system of the embryo, establishing a direct blood circulation between the embryo and the placenta. Eventually, the *umbilical cord* will contain two *umbilical arteries* that transfer blood from the embryo to the placenta, and an *umbilical vein* that returns blood to the embryo from the placenta, having exchanged gases and nutrients/waste with maternal blood.

MORPHOGENESIS (2–8 WEEKS AFTER FERTILIZATION)

The early folding of the embryonic disc laid down the fundamental structure of the body by putting in place the embryonic cell layers within a three-dimensional form, identifying the 'head' and 'tail' end of the baby, and the eventual locality of the thorax, abdomen, and left and right body sides. Further progress requires cells to *differentiate* (specialize) and take on the appropriate specialist functions. In this respect, *histogenesis* and *organogenesis* are terms that refer to the formation of tissues and organs, respectively, while *morphogenesis* (morph = shape) refers to the spatial organization that is necessary for their normal anatomical arrangement. Clearly, all three processes will generally occur together. Thus organ development requires:

- cells to differentiate into the four primary tissue types: connective tissue, muscle tissue, nervous tissue, and epithelial (lining) tissue. Within these, there are a variety of subtypes; for example, muscle tissue includes cardiac, smooth and skeletal muscle;
- the tissue types to be organized in such a way as to produce the functions required of the organ. For example, a cross section through the wall of the heart reveals an outer layer of connective tissue (epicardium), a middle layer of cardiac muscle (myocardium), and an inner layer of epithelial tissue (endocardium), together with coronary blood vessels, branches of nervous tissue and internal features such as heart valves;
- the organs to have a specific position and orientation within the body; again, this is exemplified by the location and overall structure of the four-chambered heart, including its relationship to major blood vessels;
- growth.

Such processes reflect the specific operation of particular genes, the timing of that operation, and their control within a genetic/epigenetic environment. It is beyond the scope of this book to discuss every process in depth, but the following sections provide two examples to illustrate intrinsic developmental processes (see also Box 3.10).

BOX 3.10   Stem Cells

All cells derive from the zygote, formed at fertilization of the ovum by a spermatozoon. All the trillions of future cells within the embryo, fetus, child and adult could therefore, in principle, be traced back to the zygote. This is because DNA (i.e., the genetic code) is conserved during cell division by mitosis and cells therefore maintain the same karyotype and genotypes. To a large extent this is true, but sporadic gene mutations, or those induced by environmental factors, will alter the genotypes of some individual cells throughout life. Fundamentally, though, the principle of DNA conservation means that the genetically-driven differentiation of specialized cells and tissues we observe in the embryo demonstrates what can be achieved by controlling the activation or deactivation of genes: this is why the genetic code is often referred to as a 'blueprint' for the body.

Stem cells are undifferentiated cells found in the early embryo and later embryo—and indeed in adults, though in much lower proportion. They are 'simple' in that they have little or no specialist function. However, 'switching' genes 'on' and 'off' in a given sequence and at a given time can cause them to develop characteristics of specialized cells—muscle cells, nerve cells, secretory cells, etc.

Differentiation of a cell requires numerous steps. In adults, most stem cells are already partially transformed, though they may not look like it. The further they are along this developmental 'road', the less flexible they become; simplistically, this means that a neural stem cell will only form functional nerve cells. Undifferentiated embryonic stem cells, some of which can be identified in adult tissues, are the least differentiated and have the capacity to be pluralistic; that is, to transform into one of a range of specialist cell types provided that the appropriate gene activation and deactivation patterns are generated.

All stem cells, therefore, are of potential value for stem cell therapy. It is a measure of how far genetic science has progressed that stem cells can now be extracted and genetic functioning manipulated to produce cells of a specific type for transplantation into a patient. The flexibility of embryonic stem cells in this respect makes them of particular value for harvesting from cord blood after birth.

Stages of Development of the Central Nervous System: An Example of Morphogenesis

The nervous system is the first organ system to begin to visibly differentiate. The primitive streak that appeared on the embryonic disc provides a focus for growth of the *notochord*, a rigid, cellular rod that stretches out along the length of the disc. This feature is not retained for long but has a role in initiating several developments. Formation of the nervous system, referred to as *neurulation*, begins when the notochord induces the overlying ectodermal cells to thicken and form a *neural plate* (Fig. 3.9). Around day 18, this plate develops a *neural groove* running lengthwise along the embryo; lateral folds then quickly close over the groove to produce the *neural tube*, which will become the brain and spinal cord. Some cells migrate to the outside of the tube to form the *neural crest*, which will produce tissues associated with the nervous system, for example, the meningeal membranes around the brain and spinal cord, and the Schwann cells that produce the insulating substance, myelin, around nerve cells. As the nervous system continues to develop, other cells transform into cells/tissues associated with the nervous system; for example, they become the cells of the adrenal medulla that secrete adrenaline, a hormone which acts in concert with the sympathetic nervous system and so remains functionally linked to neural tissue.

By 19 days after fertilization, the 'head' end of the neural tube has developed three expansions that will eventually become the forebrain, midbrain and hindbrain structures. The aggregation of nerve cells into *neural ganglia* at specific locations within the developing brain can now take place; for example, those of the

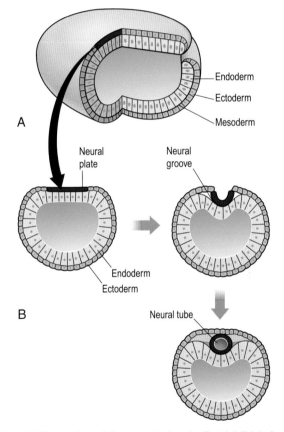

Fig. 3.9 Formation of the neural tube: the first (visible) sign of organ development in the embryo. (A) Simplistic view of the early embryo after folding of the embryonic cell layers (see also Fig. 3.7). For clarity, the mesoderm has been omitted. (B) The embryo in section, showing development of the neural tube from the embryonic ectoderm. (Redrawn from Clancy J, McVicar A. *Physiology and Anatomy: A Homeostatic Approach*, 3rd ed, 2009, with permission from Hodder Education.)

hypothalamus differentiate by the fifth week. Further along, the neural tube is transforming into the spinal cord; cells here differentiate either into *neurons* or into supportive cells. Some neurons that have migrated into central areas of the cord will make up the '*grey matter*' within the brain and spinal cord. Axons produced as outgrowths from some of these will eventually form connections with other neurons in the cord or developing brain, while other neurons will project away from the cord towards the developing viscera and muscles, directed by chemical attractants, and so form *peripheral nerves*. Eventually some of these—for example, the sensory neurons projecting from our toes to the midbrain—may become very long.

Thus histogenesis, organogenesis and morphogenesis combine to provide specialized cells, the spatial positioning of these cells in specialized tissues, and their

incorporation into the developing neural and associated organs, respectively.

Sex Differentiation

Sex differentiation, which takes place by the end of the eighth week, marks the final stage of embryo development. It is described here to provide an illustration of the way genes interact during development, and also the way in which functional changes as tissues/organs begin to operate can themselves be influential.

The tissues that will eventually form either male or female gonads develop simultaneously at the same site within the abdomen of the embryo, which at this point is sex-neutral but has bipotential in that it may become male or female depending upon the final differentiation of the gonadal tissue and its associated ducts, the *Wolffian* and *Müllerian* ducts (Fig. 3.10).

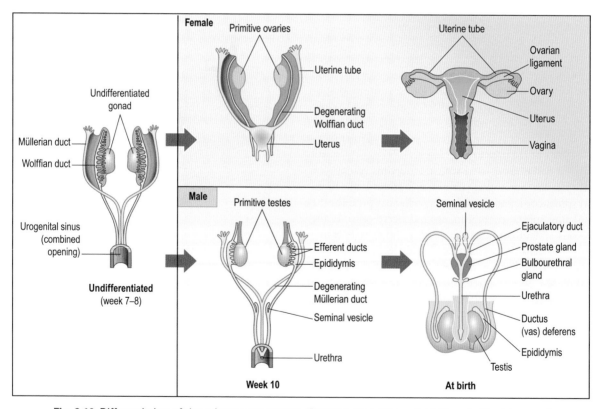

Fig. 3.10 Differentiation of the primary sex organs. (Redrawn from Clancy J, McVicar A. *Physiology and Anatomy: A Homeostatic Approach*, 3rd ed, 2009, with permission from Hodder Education.)

If a spermatozoon carrying a Y chromosome has fertilized the ovum (recall that males have an X and a Y chromosome, so the fertilizing spermatozoon will have one or the other), then male sex determination will be triggered in the embryo. Genes on the Y chromosome are activated for a short period of time and they in turn 'unmask' and stimulate other genes on the ovum-derived X chromosome; these genes promote differentiation of the nonspecific gonadal tissue into early testes. These begin to produce the male hormone testosterone but the glands also secrete another hormone called *Müllerian-inhibition substance (MIS)*:

- Testosterone promotes retention of the Wolffian ducts which will become the *vas deferens* and associated structures of the adult male reproductive tract, and external genitalia develop accordingly.
- MIS causes the Müllerian ducts to degenerate.

In contrast, if the ovum has been fertilized by an X chromosome–bearing spermatozoon, the absence of a Y chromosome in the embryo means that the critical testis-determining genes will not be present. Consequently, the early gonadal tissue will not produce testosterone and the male-promoting genes on the X-chromosome will remain masked; the gonads are thus 'programmed' to develop as ovaries and the embryo becomes female. Without testosterone, the Wolffian ducts regress and atrophy and, since no MIS is produced, the Müllerian ducts persist. These will develop into the *fallopian tubes* and *uterus* of the female tract.

Karyotype errors, for example XXY, XYY or XXX (i.e., an extra X chromosome in either male or female) shift the balance in sex differentiation (see Box 3.3). They do not alter the sex per se but may introduce exaggerated 'male' or 'female' characteristics, and/or affect fertility.

Genes and Morphogenesis

Over 80 years ago, Spemann and Mangold demonstrated that transplanting cells from specific points within a single newt embryo to another position on a recipient embryo could produce two (joined) newt embryos. In other words, both the cells of the recipient and the transplanted cells were capable of determining body axis, and of inducing precise morphogenesis in tissues adjacent to the transplant site.

There is likely to be more than one cluster of such cells, referred to as *organizers*, and they have since been identified in embryos of all animal groups—for example,

within the primitive streak that directs neurulation, discussed earlier. In these cells, gene 'families' such as *HOX* and *PAX* are activated and promote the production of proteins that stimulate differentiation in surrounding tissues by interacting with the genes and gene products of those cells. *HOX* genes are responsible for spatial orientation of cells and tissues along the head-tail axis of the embryo. *PAX* genes are *transcription factors*; they determine the activities of certain genes involved in cell specialization. Some genes have been shown to have a widespread involvement, for example the 'Hedgehog' gene and its subtypes cause the production of signalling proteins that influence cell developments and appear to have involvement in the morphogenesis of many organs, from intestines to the brain.

Collectively, the gene products that promote morphogenesis are known as *morphogens*. Among those best studied are the families of transcription factors (especially those produced by *HOX* and *PAX* genes) that interact with the DNA of cells to activate certain genes and hence govern how the cells look and function. Morphogens produced within a restricted area of tissue will spread away from that source; cells close to the source therefore are subjected to a high concentration whereas those a distance away receive a lower concentration. It is this concentration gradient that seems to influence how cells respond to the morphogen, including directions for migration or projection. The process is clearly very complex and highly coordinated. Readers are referred to technical reviews for more detail, for example Vuong-Brender et al. (2016).

Epigenetics

The complete sequencing of the human genome in 2004 (International Human Genome Sequencing Consortium, 2004) revealed a surprising finding: the human genome did not comprise the anticipated 100,000 genes or so, but rather around 20,000. A not insubstantial number—but still relatively small when compared with the vast range of proteins that the body synthesizes, and the complexity of cell regulation and differentiation. This consideration highlights that the great majority of DNA, which does not comprise actual genes, is unlikely to be 'evolutionary junk DNA' that was once thought to have accumulated in cells. Rather, those sections of DNA include repeated sequences of bases that could be replicate copies of genes or perhaps sections of DNA that influence the three-dimensional shape of the DNA molecule and thus control chromosome formation. Others influence gene expression, for example, by determining the level of DNA methylation (in which attachment of a methyl (CH3) molecule to a region of DNA acts to 'switch off' a gene by preventing protein synthesis).

The biochemical processes by which intracellular molecules regulate gene transcription (expression) during development are key to determining cell specialisation and functional requirements. Referred to as *epigenetics*, these mechanisms are a significant aspect of the interface by which environments may impact on development and on gene expression though life. The importance of the biochemical 'landscape' for development is that epigenetic mechanisms within cell nuclei seem to provide the means to control expression of the genetic code by timely activation of the embryo's genome. This is a big topic in modern cell biology; readers are referred to the review by O'Neill (2015) for more detailed information and reflections on epigenesis and embryo development. Because the epigenetic environment appears to have a significant role in progressing development, it is important to recognize that epigenetic influences on the genome might be reflected in errors of development such as dysplasia or congenital defects.

Dysplasia and Congenital Errors of Development

Dysplasia is a clinical term that refers to a failure of normal differentiation of tissue in the early embryo to an extent that anatomical and/or functional disorder occurs. *Congenital error* refers to dysplasia that arises from altered genes present within the zygote, that is, the embryonic cells are actually programmed to develop abnormally. Dysplasia might therefore be the consequence of:

- inherited genes;
- genetic change that has occurred *after* implantation of the embryo, occurring in the uterus either spontaneously or because of an extrinsic agent;
- the influence of an inappropriate biochemical environment in the uterus on the production or actions of morphogens.

The intrauterine environment is established before conception; it may involve inadvertent exposure of the woman to potentially harmful agents in her living environment or as a result of her lifestyle. External agents that induce developmental problems in the embryo/fetus are collectively referred to as *teratogens*. They have

to be introduced into the body; examples include toxins produced by certain bacteria, some prescribed drugs, and alcohol. Another cause of dysplasia might be that an important nutrient is missing; for example, a deficiency of folic acid may impact on the closure of the neural canal, producing *spina bifida*. In most instances, though, the cause for a particular dysplasia will be unknown, because so little is understood about how environmental factors impact on genes and how they interact. Increased understanding of morphogenesis will lead to better insights into the ways in which health behaviours influence fetal development.

The embryonic stage of development is particularly at risk of harm from extrinsic influences because all the organs are established during this period. In fact, as we have seen, the central nervous system begins to develop just 2 weeks after fertilization, and the heart very soon after; such early developments reflect the complexity of the central nervous system and the need to establish a blood circulation as soon as possible to facilitate growth. Morphogenesis is therefore most susceptible to adverse environmental exposures very early in the pregnancy and so maternal health behaviours are an important issue. Prior to implantation, the early embryo is exposed to the composition of the mother's uterine fluid, whereas at and around implantation, the composition of the decidua becomes instrumental. With placentation, the composition of the maternal blood and sufficiency of the placenta become key to continuing development.

However, a risk of dysplasia also continues into the fetal period (i.e., 9 weeks and more after fertilization; Fig. 3.11). All of the organs are established and in place (albeit perhaps in a rudimentary and nonfunctioning form) at this stage. The fetal period is characterized by growth and fine tuning of organogenesis, essential to provide *viability* at birth; for example, brain development continues with the formation of the cerebral cortex and its lobes at 12 to 14 weeks. Organ systems generally begin to function either more efficiently or perhaps even for the first time; for example, the kidneys commence urine production at around week 12. External body parts also begin to assume their final positions and body proportions change towards those seen at birth. Such developments continue to be genetically driven and so, as for early dysplasia, cells may still be sensitive to the environment provided by their mother.

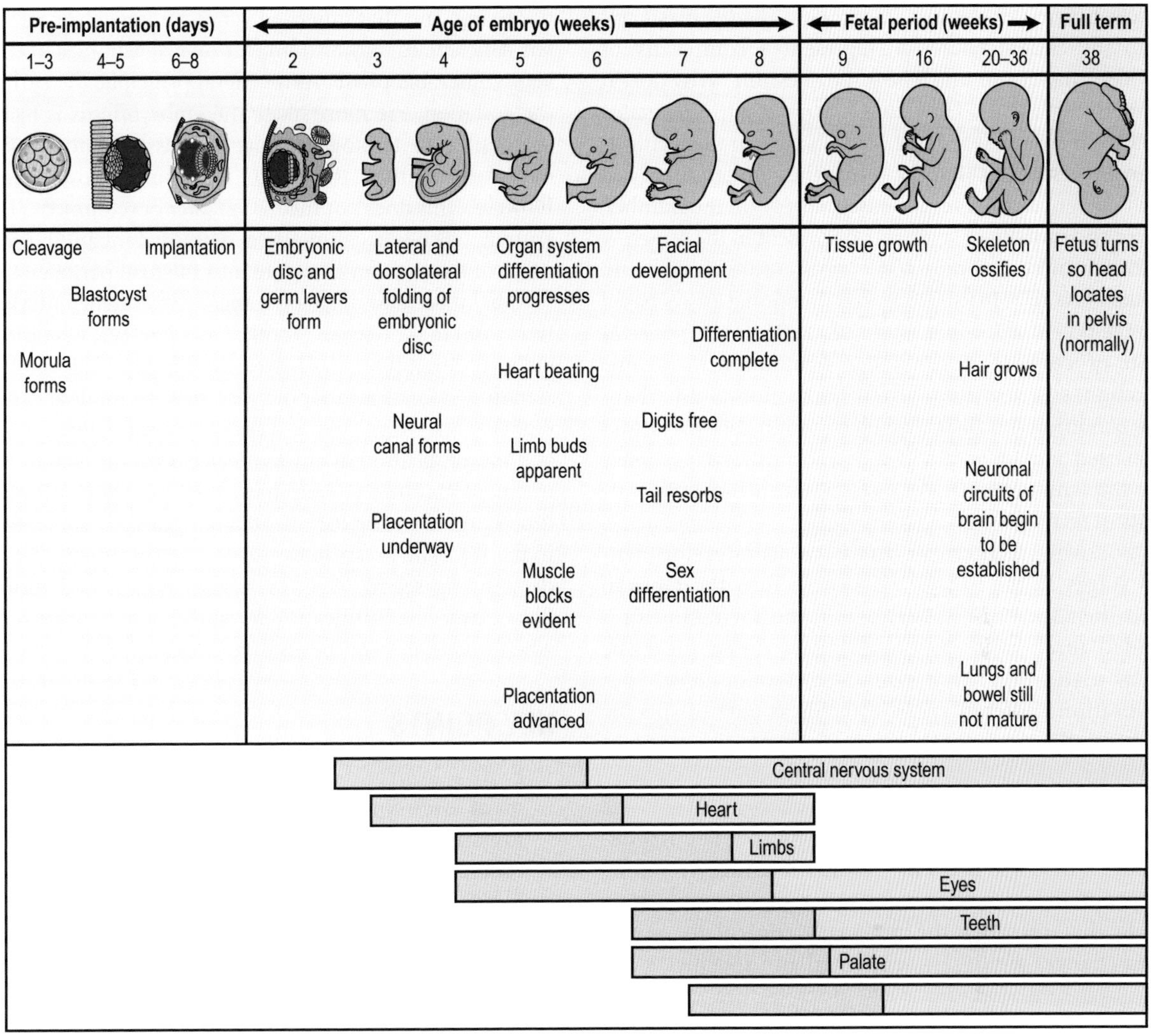

Pre-implantation (days)			◄———————— Age of embryo (weeks) ————————►							◄— Fetal period (weeks) —►			Full term
1–3	4–5	6–8	2	3	4	5	6	7	8	9	16	20–36		38

Pre-implantation			Age of embryo							Fetal period			Full term
Cleavage	Implantation		Embryonic disc and germ layers form	Lateral and dorsolateral folding of embryonic disc	Organ system differentiation progresses	Facial development				Tissue growth		Skeleton ossifies	Fetus turns so head locates in pelvis (normally)
	Blastocyst forms						Differentiation complete					Hair grows	
Morula forms				Neural canal forms	Limb buds apparent		Digits free						
							Tail resorbs					Neuronal circuits of brain begin to be established	
				Placentation underway									
					Muscle blocks evident		Sex differentiation						
												Lungs and bowel still not mature	
					Placentation advanced								

Fig. 3.11 **Chronology of embryonic/fetal development.** Horizontal bars at the bottom of the figure identify susceptibility to teratogenic agents – the darker the colour, the greater the developmental susceptibility. (Redrawn from Clancy J, McVicar A. *Physiology and Anatomy: A Homeostatic Approach*, 3rd ed, 2009, with permission from Hodder Education.)

SUMMARY

DNA becomes microscopically visible in a cell as chromosomes as the cell prepares to divide. The technique of chromosomal analysis, referred to as *karyotyping*, has been established since the 1970s but is becoming superseded by molecular genetic analysis, or *genotyping*, as a diagnostic tool. An understanding of genetics and the inheritance of genes provides insight into how errors in cell and tissue differentiation might arise in the embryo

or fetus. However, genetic processes in the embryo are only part of the story. Genes determine the form and specialist functions of cells throughout life, and these processes are also apparent during the production of sex cells, their interaction during fertilization and subsequent implantation of the blastocyst.

Production of the male and female sex cells, the survival of spermatozoa as they pass through the female tract, the chemical interactions that facilitate penetration of the oocyte by a single spermatozoon, the subsequent nuclear fusion events, and implantation of the blastocyst into the endometrium, all represent a complexity of process that not so much begs the question, 'Why does it sometimes fail?' as, 'How does it work at all?' Spermatozoa seem especially susceptible to failure in the fertilization process; the chemical events they undergo suggest that current fertility tests—based simply on the number, form and motility of spermatozoa present in the semen—will not necessarily provide an accurate assessment. Aitken (2006, 2018) suggests that functional assays based on the potential for movement of spermatozoa, penetration of cervical mucus, zona recognition, acrosome reaction, spermatozoon–ovum interaction and perhaps the conditions for interaction between the blastocyst and maternal endometrium (i.e., the conditions necessary for implantation) would represent much more accurate tests of fertility.

Following fertilization, there are clear developmental stages as the zygote transforms into the embryo and then the fetus. Gastrulation, the formation of a folded three-layer embryo that lays down the basic body plan, is a critical process in development. Specialisation (differentiation) of cells as part of specific tissues, the structural orientation of tissue types within a developing organ, cell migration to establish localisation of tissues and organs, and of course growth, must also proceed according to a defined developmental schema. This schema is underpinned by a 'program' of development inherent in our genetic code that provides the necessary control to ensure that changes are timely, sequential and specific.

Occurring alongside such processes are vital supportive aspects of pregnancy, including establishment of the chorion and amnion for protection and nutrition/excretion support prior to placental development, together with placentation and development of the umbilical cord to sustain the growing embryo/fetus.

Morphogens are vital to differentiation processes; genetic variation, a deficit of essential nutrients or the presence of substances that interfere with natural morphogen secretion/expression can have significant impacts on how cells, tissue and organs differentiate.

CONCLUSION

The focus in this chapter has been on inheritance and the anatomical development of the embryo, but it should be remembered that functional differentiation is also occurring, and that inherited genes, teratogens or nutrient deficiencies may also impact on cell activities in this very vulnerable phase. As a general principle, the earlier the gestation, the more likely the embryo/fetus is to be susceptible to teratogens; once the tissues and organs have formed, then the effects may not be so adverse. However, this does not mean that later developments are entirely safe because functional development and refinement of tissues continues late into the fetal period.

Our understanding of gene/environment interactions, and those between mother and embryo, that affect embryo development is increasing rapidly. That understanding is leading to potential new technologies for embryo screening and selection, genetic engineering, and the application of embryonic cells for medical treatments of children and adults. These are highly emotive topics and licensing for research is rigorously controlled in the UK. The pressure for further advancement of understanding seems likely to sustain ethical and moral debate as to the justification for such research, especially when undertaken in the embryo stages.

KEY POINTS

- Embryology is the study of an embryo's development after conception, characterized by the determination of its basic body plan and the subsequent differentiation of tissues and organs, directed by selective genetic activities.
- Our chromosomes occur as homologous pairs. Originating in the combination of chromosomes from our father and mother, the pairs represent a duplication; apart from the X and Y chromosomes, each chromosome has a homologous 'double', with the same genes present on each member of the pair. These 'pairs of genes', called 'alleles', provide a genotype that contributes to a given characteristic (physical or chemical), referred to as the phenotype.
- Genes enable our cells to produce proteins that often have highly specific actions. If the DNA structure of one member of an allele pair differs from the other, one member of the pair may assume dominance to the other 'recessive' copy. However, the distribution of chromosomes during gamete formation may result in the zygote having two copies of the recessive allele, in which case that allele may be expressed by its cells.
- A genetic mutation (change) occurs when the base sequence within an allele is altered; this may change

the size and/or shape of the protein which will be synthesized by the cell should that allele be expressed. The actual change may have no major consequence for cell function, but in some cases the effects of the new protein, or the absence of the normal one, on development and/or function can be profound.

- Chromosomes are either autosomal (22 pairs), contributing to most bodily functioning and the same in males and females, or sex chromosomes (1 pair, XX in females and XY in males), with primary functions related to sexual development and reproduction.
- Inheritance may be autosomal or sex-linked; sex-linked recessive disorders usually affect boys and result from mutations on the X chromosome, the Y chromosome containing very few genes and being unable to 'mask' the recessive alleles.
- Gastrulation—the formation of embryonic cell layers and folding of the embryo around 6 to 14 days after fertilization—lays down the fundamental structure of the body even at such an early age. Sex differentiation towards the end of the eighth week after fertilization signals the end of the embryonic period, and the start of the fetal period of growth and tissue maturation over the remaining months of the pregnancy.
- The term *dysplasia* describes a failure of normal differentiation of tissue in the early embryo, to an extent that an anatomical and/or functional disorder may occur. Dysplasia may result from inheriting abnormal genes (alleles), from the effects of extrinsic agents or teratogens on gene structure or expression, or from the lack of a nutrient essential for development.
- While the cause of dysplasia is often unknown, the embryo is particularly at risk of extrinsic influences because all organs are established during the first 8 weeks of development.
- A number of genetic technologies have been introduced within the past few decades. These technologies have generated moral and ethical debate concerning the manipulation of genes and are likely to continue to do so as new technologies and applications arise.

REFERENCES

Aitken, R.J., 2006. Sperm function tests and fertility. Int. J. Androl. 29 (1), 69–75

Aitken, R.J., 2018. Not every sperm is sacred; a perspective on male infertility. Mol. Hum. Reprod. 24 (6) 287–298.

Aplin, J.D., Ruane, P.T., 2017. Embryo–epithelium interactions during implantation at a glance. J. Cell. Sci. 130, 15–22.

Blackburn, S.T., 2018. Maternal, Fetal, & Neonatal Physiology: A Clinical Perspective, fifth ed. Elsevier, Missouri.

Collins, P., 2004. Dictionary of Medical Terms, 2004. fourth ed. London, Bloomsbury. Available from: www.collinsdictionary.com. Accessed March 2020.

Egbase, P.E., Al-Sharhan, M., & Grudzinskas, J.G., 2000. Influence of practice and length of uterus on implantation and clinical pregnancy rates in IVF and embryo transfer treatment cycles. Human Reproduction. 15(9): 1943–1946

International Human Genome Sequencing Consortium, 2004. Finishing the euchromatic sequence of the human genome. Nature 431 (7011), 931–945.

NHS, Health A–Z guide: Pre-eclampsia. Available from: https://www.nhs.uk/conditions/pre-eclampsia/causes/. Accessed Replece with March 27th 2020.

O'Neill, C., 2015. The epigenetics of embryo development. Anim. Front. 5 (1), 42–49.

Poolman, E.M., Galvani, A.P., 2007. Evaluating candidate agents of selective pressure for cystic fibrosis. Journal of the Royal Society Interface 4 (12), 91–98.

Rankin, J., 2017. Physiology in Childbearing: With Anatomy and Related Biosciences. 4th edition. Cambridge, Elsevier.

Rutherford, A., 2017. A Brief History of Everyone Who Ever Lived: The Stories in Our Genes. London, Weidenfeld & Nicholson.

Tosti, E., Ménézo, Y., 2016. Gamete activation: basic knowledge and clinical applications. Hum. Reprod. Update 22 (4), 420–439.

Van den Bergh, M., Emiliani, S., Biramane J., Vannin, A.S., Englert, Y., 1998. A first prospective study of the individual straight-line velocity of the spermatozoon and its influences on the fertilization rate after intracytoplasmic sperm injection. Hum. Reprod. 13 (11), 3103–3107.

Vuong-Brender, T.T.K., Yang, Z., Labouesse, M., 2016. C. elegans Embryonic Morphogenesis. Curr. Top. Dev. Biol. 116, 597–616.

4

Antenatal Screening and Testing: The Significance for the Health of the Newborn

Sharon McDonald and Sarah Fiadjoe

CHAPTER CONTENTS

INTRODUCTION

Much of the assessment that a midwife performs during the antenatal period, for example abdominal palpation or urinalysis, could be viewed as screening (NHS, 2018a). However, the term *antenatal screening* is largely associated with a complex range of biochemical and technological tests that are offered to women during pregnancy in order to identify preexisting conditions, diseases or anomalies in the fetus (see Chapter 11). In this chapter, we will concentrate on those screening tests included in the antenatal screening recommendations from the United Kingdom National Screening Committee (UK NSC), although it is recognized that their recommendations are not universally acknowledged (NSC, 2018; NICE, 2019a; WHO, 2016). The UK NSC has a responsibility to advise on, and support the implementation of, all aspects of antenatal and newborn screening programmes. This includes the introduction of any new screening programmes and monitoring the cost-effectiveness of continuing, modifying or withdrawing existing programmes (NSC, 2019; PHE, 2015a). You would be advised to read Chapter 3, which provides information relating to the fundamentals of genes and their inheritance as well as the stages of embryo development and the key features of specialisation and differentiation in the embryo. This will provide a greater understanding of the screening tests and their functions.

Communication, Information Sharing and Health Literacy

The introduction of increasingly sophisticated testing in the last decade or so means that information sharing in this area of care is more important than ever. Any communication around antenatal screening is complex, and women and their partners need time and space to really understand what they are being asked to consider. The General Medical Council is currently reviewing its consent guidelines and these will be available in late 2019, but the following principles, although now twenty years old, are still pertinent today.

> *'You must ensure that anyone considering whether to consent to screening can make a properly informed decision. …You should be careful to explain clearly: the purpose of the screening; the likelihood of positive/negative findings and possibility of false positive/negative results; the uncertainties and risks attached to the screening process; any significant medical, social or financial implications of screening for the particular condition or predisposition; follow up plans, including availability of counselling and support services'.*
>
> **General Medical Council (1999: 7)**

Parents-to-be need to be aware of what 'screening' for a condition actually means. They may mistake screening for diagnostic testing and so the starting point in any discussion should be to clarify this distinction (Box 4.1). This is important information, as an elementary understanding of *specificity* and *sensitivity* in relation to the tests performed on their baby is essential.

The terms specificity and sensitivity give rise to a *positive predictive value* and a *negative predictive value* which can result in the following in relation to antenatal screening: (Box 4.2).

Public Health England has produced a series of video animations that explain these principles, simplifying what is complex information to make it accessible to all. These can be found at https://www.gov.uk/guidance/nhs-population-screening-explained. Health literacy is described as the 'capacity to find, interpret and use information and health services to make effective decisions for health and wellbeing' (MoH, 2019). As health professionals, we have a responsibility to provide those in our care with clear and relevant health messages that

Box 4.1	Definition of Terms
What is screening?	The process of identifying the presence of a condition in an apparently healthy population.
What is a diagnostic test?	A test that determines or confirms the presence of the condition in an individual.
What is specificity?	Refers to the accuracy of the test in identifying people with the condition being screened for. A high specificity means that a high number of people are correctly identified.
What is sensitivity?	Refers to the ability of the test to correctly identify people who do not have the condition.

Adapted from New Zealand National Screening Unit (2019).

BOX 4.2	
True positive	The fetus has the condition and the test is positive.
False positive	The fetus does not have the condition but the test is positive.
True negative	The fetus does not have the condition and the test is negative.
False negative	The fetus has the condition but the test is negative.

empower them to make informed decisions. Other considerations in relation to decision-making are:

1. How does the concept of screening and each particular test relate to the cultural, spiritual and/or religious beliefs of the woman and her partner?
2. Are there potential emotional or psychological implications?
3. If the screening test is positive and a course of treatment or action is recommended, would the nature of the potential treatment be acceptable to the parents?

Hearing the results of a screening test may represent the first time a woman and her partner have considered the possibility of a 'less than perfect' baby (Healthtalk, 2017; ARC, 2019; National Childbirth Trust, 2019). It is therefore imperative that any discussion that takes place around screening is handled with sensitivity and without ambiguity (see Chapter 11).

Screening Programmes and Timelines

It is important to acknowledge that screening programmes do vary from country to country; although the primary focus here will be on the UK programme as an example, you a as a practitioner need to familiarize yourself with your own country's programme (i.e. New Zealand; National Screening Unit; pregnancy and Newborn screening https://www.nsu.govt.nz/pregnancy-newborn). Fig. 4.1 is an illustration of the United Kingdoms, antenatal and newborn screening programmes.

The early identification of any possible concerns offers the opportunity for women, their partners and the multidisciplinary team to discuss the options available to them. Fig. 4.1, The UK Screening Timeline, with optimum times for testing, is available online for women and health professionals (PHE, 2019a) and provides this information in a clear and understandable way. Another comprehensive resource for women and families is the Public Health England (PHE) publication *Screening Tests for You and Your Baby*, available online but given to all women antenatally in the United Kingdom (PHE, 2019b).

The UK NSC's current antenatal screening programmes are:
- Infectious disease screening
- Sickle cell and thalassaemia screening
- First and second trimester screening
- Fetal anomaly ultrasound

INFECTIOUS DISEASES SCREENING

Screening for infection in pregnancy enables early detection and treatment, which can significantly reduce the risk of vertical transmission from mother to child (PHE, 2018a).

The argument for offering routine testing for infectious diseases has a sound rationale which includes the need to minimize the risk to the fetus in the case of vertical transmission pathways, the need to treat the infection in the woman, and the need to protect the professionals involved in care or treatment. This routine testing can be viewed as diagnostic testing, in contrast to the screening programmes which, as discussed, predict the chance of a condition rather than making a direct diagnosis.

In the United Kingdom, systematic population screening for human immunodeficiency virus (HIV), hepatitis B (HBV), and syphilis is offered to all women in each pregnancy, irrespective of the stage of pregnancy when the woman presents for care (NHS, 2018b). The NHS Infectious Diseases in Pregnancy Screening (IDPS)

programme standards (PHE, 2018a) monitor the uptake of testing within maternity units. This enables a robust treatment plan to be offered, with the aim of optimizing the outcome for both the woman and her baby. This means that at a service level, consideration needs to be given to ensure that effective pathways are in place for women presenting late in pregnancy. This should be irrespective of the reason for their late presentation, which may be due to late booking, transfers into the area, concealed pregnancy or other reason. If no such pathway exists, additional care should be considered. The fact is that, unless we know for certain that women have been offered and have accepted screening, we cannot make assumptions.

HIV: What Is It and Why Do We Screen?

Screening for HIV in pregnancy identifies women with the infection in order to offer early treatment and appropriate care, and interventions to reduce the risk of mother-to-baby transmission (PHE, 2018a). HIV is a retrovirus that attacks and destroys CD4 cells, resulting in immunosuppression that may lead to acquired immunodeficiency syndrome (AIDS).

HIV is known to be transmitted through sexual contact, contact with contaminated blood products, and by vertical transmission during pregnancy, at birth or by breastfeeding (Avert, 2019).

Issues for Practice

The National Surveillance of HIV in Pregnancy and Childhood (NSHPC) in the United Kingdom reports that the risk of mother-to-child vertical transmission is now low (0.5%). This has resulted from optimal management, which includes antiretroviral therapy and appropriate obstetric and midwifery input. If left untreated, the risk increases to 25% (PHE, 2018a; Peters et al., 2018). If an HIV-infected woman is unsure of her HIV status, it is estimated that her baby has a 1 in 4 chance of infection. It is the usual practice within maternity units to share the care of confirmed HIV-positive women with a specialist multidisciplinary team. Both the British HIV Association (BHIVA) and the Children's HIV Association (CHIVA) stress that HIV-positive women and their families need specialist input in order to meet their defined needs. It is extremely important that the woman is fully aware of the possibility of a false negative result occurring if she is tested in the window period between infection and seroconversion. This needs to be carefully explained and it should

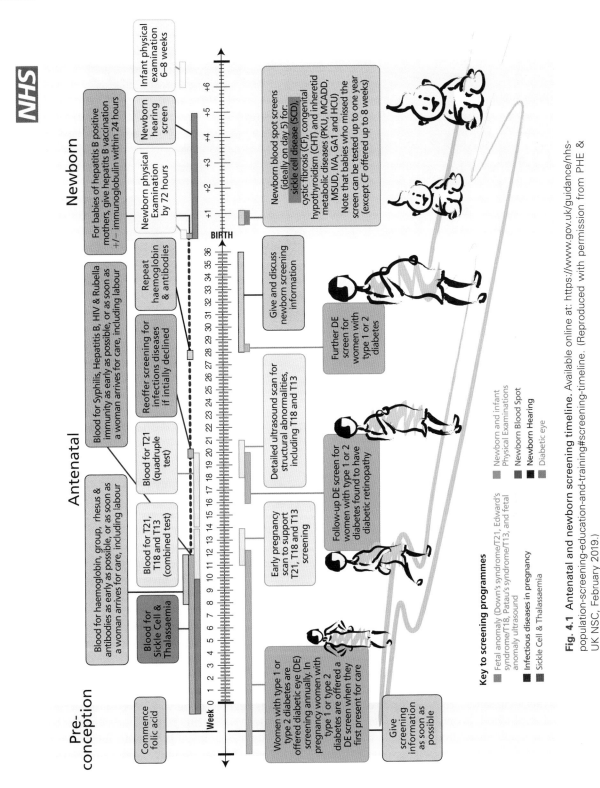

Fig. 4.1 Antenatal and newborn screening timeline. Available online at: https://www.gov.uk/guidance/nhs-population-screening-education-and-training#screening-timeline. (Reproduced with permission from PHE & UK NSC, February 2019.)

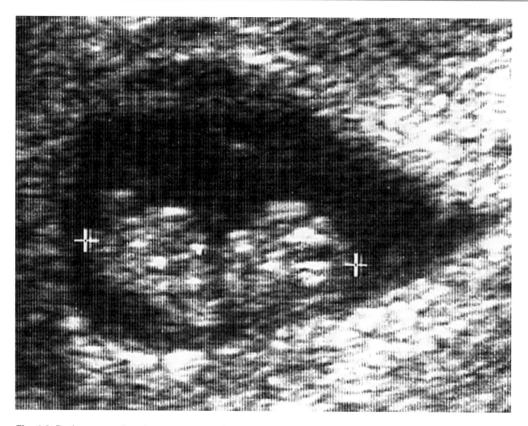

Fig. 4.2 Dating scan, showing crown-rump length of 24 mm, the mean for 8 weeks 6 days. (Reproduced from Smith NC and Smith APM, *Obstetric Ultrasound Made Easy* 2002, with permission from Elsevier Ltd.)

be made very clear that there remains a risk of acquiring HIV during pregnancy, if the woman or her partner participate in high-risk behaviour. All children registered as being born to HIV-infected women should be offered follow-up screening to establish infection status.

Hepatitis B (HBV): What Is It and Why Do We Screen?

Hepatitis B is an infectious disease of the liver caused by the hepatitis B virus, resulting in both acute and chronic infection. Chronic infectivity may result in cirrhosis and carcinoma of the liver, and up to 20% of chronic HBV carriers die from liver failure or hepatoma. HBV is a very infectious virus that is transmitted through all body fluids including saliva, semen, vaginal secretions, and contaminated blood. It can be transmitted by activities such as needle-sharing or by vertical transmission; mother to baby is the most common route globally (WHO, 2015a).

The aim of routine universal antenatal screening in pregnancy is to identify women who are infected by Hepatitis B or who are carriers, as their babies will be at risk of contracting HBV (NHS, 2018a; NICE, 2017; WHO, 2015a; WHO, 2015b). The screening test identifies the hepatitis B surface antigen (HBsAg) and has an accuracy of 99.9%. The presence of the hepatitis B e antigen (HBeAg) indicates high infectivity. Confirmed positive hepatitis B results require referral to gastroenterology and/or hepatology services (there may be some country-specific variation in referral pathways).

Issues for Practice

The hepatitis B vaccination programme for newborn babies is believed to be 95% effective if vaccination is completed (NICE, 2017). Vaccination involves an initial dose within 24 hours of birth and a further three doses at 1 month, 2 months and 12 months of age, with blood sampling to check for immunity (PHE, 2017a). It is important that health professionals caring for the baby are made aware this has been undertaken, to ensure the baby is protected by the vaccination programme and has immunity to hepatitis B.

Syphilis: What Is It and Why Do We Screen?

Syphilis is a sexually transmitted infection caused by a spirochaete, *Treponema pallidum*. If a pregnant woman has an untreated syphilis infection, the risk of losing her baby by miscarriage or stillbirth is approximately 50%. Even if the infection is treated, it has been reported that 15% of babies will either die or be delivered with congenital syphilis (transmitted either transplacentally or, rarely, via a lesion during breastfeeding). Babies who survive have been reported to suffer considerable morbidity, including nasofacial hypoplasia, blindness and deafness (PHE, 2018b).

Screening in pregnancy aims to identify women with an infection and offer treatment which will reduce the risk of the baby developing congenital syphilis. To prevent mother-to-fetus transmission, pregnant women should be offered screening for syphilis during the first trimester and again in the third trimester of pregnancy. Whilst syphilis is not prevalent in the United Kingdom, statistical evidence suggests that the global incidence is increasing, and it is identified as the second leading cause of stillbirth as a result of increased incidences of low birth weight, prematurity and newborn infection (PHE, 2018b; WHO, 2006). It therefore continues to be screened for in many other countries.

Issues for Practice

The screening test has an accuracy of more than 99%. Confirmed syphilis or equivocal results require urgent referral to genitourinary medicine (GUM) for antibiotic treatment and discussion regarding the risks to the baby. The treatment plan should then be negotiated with the woman and the multidisciplinary team, following guidelines established by the British Association for Sexual Health and HIV (BASHH, 2017). Benzathine penicillin is considered the most effective treatment. Contact tracing is also imperative to ensure that screening and treatment are offered to those who have had sexual contact with a woman who has been infected.

Rubella

Rubella (German measles) is an illness caused by the rubella virus; it presents with a characteristic rash and has an incubation period of between 14 and 21 days. No treatment is available during pregnancy for women found to be seronegative or found to be infected with the virus, because treatment may lead to the transmission of rubella. The virus can cause multiple problems for the baby including heart and eye defects and deafness.

Screening for rubella in pregnancy was discontinued in the United Kingdom (as in other countries) in 2016. This followed a review of the evidence (2003–2012) by the UK National Screening Committee which concluded that screening for rubella susceptibility during pregnancy did not meet the UK NSC criteria for a screening programme (PHE, 2018b). As a result of this decision, health professionals need to be vigilant and aware of the consequences for the fetus if primary rubella infection (German measles) occurs. During the first 12 weeks of pregnancy, the effects of rubella can be devastating. The risk of intrauterine transmission of rubella infection is greatest before 12 weeks but low after 16 weeks. In the first 8 to 10 weeks of pregnancy, infection results in severe fetal damage in up to 90% of cases. This risk is reduced to 20% between weeks 11 and 16, with a minimal risk up to 20 weeks and no risk after 20 weeks. Since the severity of congenital infection depends on the timing of maternal infection, it is understandable that this can be extremely worrying for the woman who is unaware of her immunity status. Women should be encouraged to check their immunity status with their GP prior to conception; if there are no records and the woman is already pregnant, she should seek to have the vaccination 6 weeks after the birth of her baby (NHS, 2018c). Other countries, such as New Zealand and Australia, continue to screen for rubella during pregnancy, but this is based on the premise that such screening aims to identify women who are nonimmune, so that they can be vaccinated after the birth to protect future pregnancies against rubella infection and its consequences (Australian DoH, 2019). We are witnessing a rise globally of the incidence of rubella.

SCREENING FOR SICKLE CELL AND THALASSAEMIA

- The haemoglobinopathies sickle cell and thalassaemia are both autosomal recessive inherited disorders of haemoglobin. The inheritance of two altered gene variants, one from each parent, results in an affected baby; inheritance of only one altered gene variant results in a healthy carrier.

- Sickle cell and thalassaemia screening is a genetic screening programme that identifies people who are genetic carriers for sickle cell, thalassaemia and other haemoglobinopathies (PHE, 2018b; PHE, 2018c).
- Worldwide, approximately 14–16 million people suffer from sickle cell disease; of these, an estimated 7% are pregnant women (Modell and Darlison, 2008).

Sickle Cell Disorders

Sickle cell affects the oxygen-carrying capacity of red blood cells. When the red blood cells of affected individuals are deoxygenated and under stress, they change to a sickle shape, preventing free passage through small capillaries. Then the cells form clusters and cause a blockage, which prevents oxygenation of the tissues. Sickle cell disorders originate from a variable set of conditions, but all present with chronic anaemia, jaundice and painful crisis, and can result in organ damage, infections and strokes.

Whilst it seems there is no reliable estimate of the total number of people living with Sickle Cell Disorders in the United Kingdom, there are approximately 310,000 healthy carriers, an estimated 12,000 people suffering with sickle cell disorders and a reported 350 affected pregnancies annually (PHE, 2018a, 2020). Sickle cell disorders can affect anyone from any population or ethnicity but are more common in people of African, African Caribbean, Middle Eastern, Mediterranean and South Asian (Indian sub-continent) ancestry (Modell & Darlison, 2008). It is thought that the presence of the sickle gene provides some resistance to malaria and this explains the genetic loading in populations where the incidence of malaria is high. Women from high-prevalence areas (High prevalence is defined as a fetal prevalence of sickle cell disorder greater than 1.5 per 10,000 pregnancies, PHE, 2020.) should be offered enhanced laboratory screening. Those units defined as low-prevalence trusts (fetal prevalence of sickle cell < 1.5 per 10,000 pregnancies) should offer screening to women using the family origin questionnaire (PHE, 2019) as well as a formal laboratory process of inspection of routine blood indices to screen for thalassaemia (PHE, 2018b).

Thalassaemia

It is estimated that 80–90 million (1.5%) of the world's population are carriers of beta-thalassaemia, and 5% are carriers of alpha-thalassaemia (Tidy and Bonsall, 2015).

The thalassaemias are an group of inherited blood disorders in which the body makes an abnormal form of haemoglobin. The disorder results in excessive destruction of red blood cells, causing anaemia. Thalassaemia occurs when there is an abnormality or mutation in one of the genes involved in haemoglobin production. There are different types, normally divided into alpha- and beta-thalassaemias. Beta-thalassaemia major is the most severe type and is commonly seen in the Mediterranean, Middle East and Asia, whereas severe alpha-thalassaemia is common in Southeast Asia and sickle cell anaemia predominates in Africa. Increased migration has seen haemoglobin disorders introduced into many areas throughout the world (Modell and Darlison, 2008).

Universal screening for thalassaemia was recommended by the World Health Organization in 1998 and the United Kingdom Thalassaemia Society (UKTS) in 2002. By 2008, much of Europe, Australasia, North America and parts of the Caribbean, Asia and India provided prenatal diagnosis and antenatal carrier screening as standard practice.

There are approximately 327,000 healthy carriers and more than 700 people with thalassaemia disorders in the United Kingdom; thalassaemia affects about 75 pregnancies per year, and approximately 25 babies will be born with thalassaemia major and 5 pregnancies will be affected with alpha-thalassaemia (Kai, 2006).

Alpha- and Beta-thalassaemia Major

Alpha-thalassaemia major is incompatible with extra-uterine life, whereas beta-thalassaemia major results in life-threatening anaemia and requires blood transfusions (usually every 4–6 weeks) and iron chelation therapy to prevent further illness.

Thalassaemia is currently screened on the red cell indices known more commonly as the full blood count (FBC) and this is the method of screening advocated by the Sickle Cell and Thalassaemia screening programme (PHE, 2018a).

Issues for Practice: Haemoglobinopathies

One of the important areas of concern is to raise the professionals' knowledge and understanding of the key aspects surrounding haemoglobinopathies. For counselling at-risk couples, the practitioner should have a good understanding of basic genetics, ethnicity and diversity factors, consanguinity and paternity issues. In response to these needs, a comprehensive training package is available to support professionals involved in antenatal and newborn screening (PHE, 2019b). In addition to this programme, professionals should make use of the family origin questionnaire as a tool for screening for haemoglobinopathies (PHE, 2019b).

Antenatal screening aims to detect carriers, provide genetic counselling if required, offer carrier couples the choice of prenatal diagnosis, and enable women to make reproductive choices. Ideally the process of screening, if required, should start at the first notification of pregnancy (between 8 and 10 weeks) to give the woman and her family some time to make decisions at an early gestation, and to complete any resulting action by the end of the 12th week of pregnancy. It has been argued that this approach is too late and that a prenatal diagnostic test would be much more beneficial and acceptable. It is reported that many parents feel unable to consider termination after 12 weeks' gestation and this evidence is linked to a reduced uptake of diagnostic testing with advancing gestation (ARC, 2019).

The most challenging problem faced by maternity units is how to ensure that women access services at an early stage so that timely screening, along with appropriate partner testing, can be offered. Partner testing gives rise to another complex debate about who tests the partner's blood and where his results are reported. Making decisions following antenatal diagnosis is difficult enough when the diagnosis is clear, but becomes even more complex when there is only an estimated risk of abnormality, or where the effects of the abnormality cannot be predicted; for example, if the woman has, or is a carrier of, a haemoglobinopathy, the baby's father should be offered screening so that if he is a carrier they can be offered diagnostic testing in pregnancy. If couples who are both healthy carriers decide to have children, there is a 1 in 4 chance with each pregnancy that the child will inherit the condition. Where both partners are carriers, or one is a carrier and the other has the disorder, or if the baby's father is not available, the couple/woman should be referred for further counselling to discuss the options available. This should include the offer of a diagnostic procedure, such as chorionic villus sampling (CVS). Services for CVS must be available for couples who may be likely to produce a child at risk of developing the condition. For those women who conceive by fertility treatment, their haemoglobinopathy status should be discussed and the appropriate pathway followed (PHE, 2018c). The

potential for stigma attached to the confirmation of carrier status should not be underestimated, particularly in close-knit communities or in some ethnic groups. It must also be acknowledged that screening may, on occasion, reveal unexpected results; for example, there may be issues relating to the paternity of the pregnancy. These concerns can be extremely disruptive and need to be dealt with professionally and with sensitivity. We should also remember that an error in labelling samples at collection, or not reporting that the pregnancy was a result of assisted conception, can also give an unexpected result that can raise issues of paternity/non-paternity.

There are many resources available to assist professionals in understanding these issues in more depth; many can be found online at Public Health England's website (PHE, 2019c; PHE, 2019d).

SCREENING FOR FETAL CHROMOSOME ABNORMALITIES

Almost universally, the recommended method of screening for fetal trisomy is *first-trimester combined screening*, where a number of factors such as maternal age, biochemistry (free beta-hCG and PAPP-A), and ultrasound measurement of fetal nuchal translucency (NT) are combined. The results of the screening calculation will indicate the chance of a woman having a baby with a trisomy (extra chromosome). The three common trisomies are trisomy 21 (Down syndrome), trisomy 18 (Edwards syndrome) and trisomy 13 (Patau syndrome). (NHS, 2019; New Zealand National Screening Unit, 2019). There is a cut-off value of 1:150 at term in the United Kingdom (although interestingly in New Zealand this is 1:300); women who are at increased chance of having an affected baby will be given their individual chance result. First and second trimester screening for twin pregnancy differs from that for singletons, and calculations of chance are determined by the chorionicity (dichorionic vs. monochorionic).

The universal introduction of maternal serum screening in the United Kingdom has been shown to decrease the birth prevalence of chromosomal abnormalities (PHE, 2018b). Some would argue that this decrease has come at an ethical cost in terms of an increase in the number of terminations for fetal anomaly (see Chapter 11).

Trisomy 21: Down Syndrome

Down syndrome (DS) occurs when an extra copy of chromosome 21 is passed on, usually during maternal meiosis (see Chapter 3). In the absence of prenatal diagnosis, the suggested birth prevalence is 1 in 800 births (PHE, 2015b). The age-related rates of Down syndrome are illustrated in Table 4.1.

It is well documented that chromosomal abnormalities like trisomy 21 are more likely to affect pregnancies in women of a higher maternal age (PHE, 2015b), but Down syndrome occurs across the spectrum of age groups, which is why universal DS screening should be offered to all women.

In the past, DS screening was offered on the basis of maternal age alone, and whilst the chance of older women having a baby with Down syndrome is higher, because women under 35 make up the majority of the child-bearing population, more babies with Down syndrome are born to younger women.

Trisomy 18 (Edwards Syndrome) and Trisomy 13 (Patau Syndrome)

Survival rates for babies with these trisomies are low, because the chromosome imbalances cause severe congenital abnormalities. Of those babies who survive to term, 10% may survive for the first year of life but rarely into adulthood. Babies born with Edwards syndrome (3 in 10,000 births) have an extra copy of chromosome 18 in all or some cells. Babies born with Patau syndrome (2 in 10,000 births) have an extra copy of chromosome 13 in all or some cells.

Second-trimester Screening: the Quadruple Test

The Fetal Anomaly Screening Programme standards recommend the *quadruple test* for second-trimester

TABLE 4.1 Maternal Age–related Risk of Having a Pregnancy Affected by Down Syndrome

Maternal age	Chance of baby having trisomy 21	Probability
20 years	1 in 1500	0.07%
30 years	1 in 900	0.1%
40 years	1 in 100	1%

Source Fetal Anomaly Screening Programme Handbook for ultrasound practitioners (PHE, 2015b).

screening if the window for first-trimester screening is missed for any reason (PHE, 2018b). The quadruple test combines maternal age with four biochemical markers (alpha-fetoprotein (AFP), human chorionic gonadotropin (hCG), oestriol-three (uE3) and inhibin-A, which can be measured from 14+2 weeks until 20 weeks of pregnancy. This assay has a lower detection rate and a higher screen positive rate than the first-trimester combined test; however, there is a need for a second-trimester screening test for women who book too late for first-trimester testing, or when an NT measurement cannot be obtained in the first trimester.

The evidence suggests there are advantages to screening earlier in pregnancy; early detection of any anomalies allows time for women and their partners to prepare and make psychological adjustments and to plan for the birth of the baby. Women need to be made aware of the options available to them. Health professionals should be respectful and nonjudgemental of whatever decisions women and their families make, and should ensure that women are offered whatever support they require to help them through the process (see Chapter 11).

Diagnostic Testing (Amniocentesis and CVS)

Amniocentesis, chorionic villus sampling (both invasive tests) and doppler velocimetry flow are not routinely offered to all women in pregnancy. Such testing is only indicated if there is a higher chance result or fetal chromosomal or biochemical defects are suspected (Ogilvie et al., 2014). All hospitals in the United Kingdom, and in most other high-income countries, now provide these diagnostic options.

CVS can be carried out from as early as 6 weeks in pregnancy and is used for analysis of the fetal karyotype, i.e., to define the number and visual appearance of the chromosomes in the cells of the fetus (see Chapter 3). This usually occurs from around 11 weeks following early screening, or sometimes at a woman's request if there is a history of an affected pregnancy . Amniocentesis is offered at a later gestation from 15 weeks onwards with 0.5–1% chance of miscarriage (RCOG, 2017, 2020; Ogilvie & Akobkar, 2014).

Noninvasive Prenatal Testing (NIPT)

The most recent addition to the antenatal screening portfolio—and perhaps the most controversial—is noninvasive prenatal testing (or screening; NIPT or NIPS) which can be carried out only 10 weeks into a pregnancy, and possibly even earlier (PHE, 2017b). The

TABLE 4.2   National Standards: Thresholds for Performance

This standard provides assurance that screening is offered to everyone who is eligible and each individual who chooses to accept screening has a conclusive screening result.

Screening Strategy	THRESHOLDS	
	Acceptable	Achievable
T21	Standardized DR 85%	
	Standardized SPR 1.8%–2.5%	Standardized SPR 1.9%–2.4%
T18/T13/T21/T18/T13	Standardized DR 80%	
	Standardized SPR 0.1%–0.2%	Standardized SPR 0.13%–0.17%
	Standardized DR 80%	
	Standardized SPR 1.8%–2.5%	Standardized SPR 1.9%–2.4%
Quadruple (T21)	Standardized DR 80%	
	Standardized SPR 2.5%–3.5%	Standardized SPR 2.7%–3.3%

*The Detection Rate (DR) and Screen Positive Rate (SPR) for the quadruple test relate to singleton pregnancies only.
Source: PHE (2019), https://www.gov.uk/government/publications/fetal-anomaly-screening-programme-standards/standards-valid-from-1-april-2018#standard-1-fetal-ano.

technique is able to detect small fragments of DNA known as cell-free DNA (cfDNA) in the mother's serum following a simple blood test. The majority of these fragments will be from the mother but a small proportion (described as the *fetal fraction*) will be from the fetus. By examining the cfDNA in the fetal fraction, it is possible to identify whether the fetus has the standard number of chromosomes (46) or has an aneuploidy (abnormal number of chromosomes). False positive rates for cfDNA are estimated to be 0.1% for each trisomy, compared with conventional first-trimester screening which has a 3%–5% false positive rate (ARC, 2019).

In spite of the significant increase in accuracy of previous screening methods, the test is not 100% accurate. The sensitivity and specificity of the test are not perfect and it can sometimes produce a false positive or false negative result; for this reason, it remains classified as a screening rather than a diagnostic test. It cannot currently analyze all chromosomes, and therefore it cannot replace CVS or amniocentesis; a screen positive will result in a referral for invasive diagnostic testing. However, it is reported that the introduction of the test has led to a reduction in the number of referrals because of its greater accuracy in the detection of trisomies. It also reduces the risk of miscarriage carried by the invasive procedures of CVS and amniocentesis. NIPT cannot identify structural and non-genetic

abnormalities and these are still better excluded by ultrasound (MoH, 2019). It should be noted that NIPT is less likely to provide an informative result in obese women, because they often have insufficient fetal fraction, increasing the likelihood of false negative results (Zozzarro-Smith et al., 2014).

There are some ethical concerns about the future development of NIPT in relation to the potential number of conditions that such testing may eventually be able to identify and the ramifications of such discovery. There has been some criticism that the introduction of NIPT has been industry-driven and little room has been left for engagement in ethical debate (Vanstone et al., 2018). The Royal Australian and New Zealand College of Obstetricians and Gynaecologists (RANZCOG) comment that the direct-to-consumer marketing of such screening is problematic because support for decision-making via pre-test and post-test counselling is not always available (RANZCOG, 2015).

In 2016 the UK NSC recommended that NIPT become part of the NHS FASP programme. Its introduction for 'all pregnant women whose chance of having a baby with Down, Edwards or Patau syndromes is greater than 1 in 150' (PHE, 2017b) started gradually in 2018. It is anticipated that the test will become part of the universal package of care provided by the NHS; however, it is currently only provided for this pre-screened group of pregnant women accessing maternity care. In other countries—New Zealand, for example—the test is not part of the publicly funded screening programme and at the time of publication it remains a user-pays, non-scheduled test. This means that essentially a two-tier model of screening exists for those who can afford it and those who cannot (MoH, 2019).

FETAL ANOMALY SCREENING: ULTRASOUND SCANS

In many ways, the application of ultrasound in obstetrics revolutionized the management of pregnancy and its potential complications. Routine ultrasound scans are used widely in many settings in antenatal care, and have been for many decades. Scans are popular with women and their families; a moving image of the baby may make the pregnancy seem more real, and women have come to expect it. From clinical experience, most women do not decline scans in pregnancy. This may imply that scans are an accepted part of routine antenatal care, or it may be because the role of ultrasound in antenatal screening is not fully understood. Clinicians agree that ultrasound scans should be used with caution in pregnancy because the long-term implications are not truly known; even though low-frequency ultrasound has not been shown to be unsafe in pregnancy, its use should be kept to a minimum and scans should only be performed for a justified clinical indication or based on sound evidence (NHS Screening Programme, 2015; PHE, 2015b; RCOG, 2000). However, Wagner (2019) identified that 'although we now have sufficient scientific data to be able to say that routine prenatal ultrasound scanning has no effectiveness and may very well carry risks, it would be naive to think that routine use will not continue'. Whilst two scans are offered routinely in pregnancy and form part of the UK National Antenatal Screening Programme, an increasing number of scans are offered universally as a result of, for example, earlier dating scans due to NIPT and the increasing number of customized growth scans (RCOG, 2000). For most women the first scan usually takes place between 10 and 14 weeks and includes a blood sample taken to test for trisomy 21 and/or trisomies 13 and 18, with a second scan for fetal anomalies between 18+0 and 20+6 weeks. The timing of the scans allows for further diagnostic tests if required, and ensures women have time to consider any decisions about continuing their pregnancy. The British Medical Ultrasound Society (British Medical Ultrasound Society,

https://www.bmus.org/) state that the primary aim of a dating scan is to establish gestational age, viability, the number of fetuses and chorionicity if more than one fetus is detected. Additionally, maternal pelvic and/or uterine or fetal abnormalities may also be identified.

The 18- to 20-week scan screens for anomalies associated with morbidity or disability, or that would benefit from intrauterine or extrauterine interventions. The identification of a major fetal abnormality could be viewed as a means of offering choices to a woman and her partner regarding their pregnancy and birth. The FASP sets a standard for 11 structural conditions to be screened for (with a 50% chance that the conditions may not be detected on the scan), including anencephaly, cleft lip, exomphalos, serious cardiac anomalies and bilateral renal agenesis (PHE, 2018b; PHE, 2015b). Detection rates will depend upon the severity of the anomaly, the training and experience of the person performing the scan, and the quality of the ultrasound machine used. Structures within organizations will also have an impact; for example, whether they encourage high-quality ultrasound scans, how much time they allocate for individual scans, the intensity of staff workload, and the provision of staff support and training.

Accurate determination of the expected date of birth (EDB) is a critical piece of information for both clinicians and clients; an accurate gestational age guides the optimal time for most screening tests in pregnancy, and the information has profound personal, social and medical implications for a woman. Historically, a normal pregnancy gestation has been calculated based on Naegele's rule, taking the first day of the last menstrual period (LMP) and adding 9 months and 7 days, based on a regular 28-day menstrual cycle. This method makes a normal gestation period 280 days from conception to birth. Several studies have been conducted to examine reliability of LMP versus ultrasound to date pregnancy. An inaccurate EDB may expose women to inappropriate interventions during their pregnancy, such as early induction of labour (PHE, 2015b).

A dating scan is shown in Fig. 4.2, in which the crown–rump length is being measured. This measurement, based on BMUS guidelines, is recommended for dating pregnancies from 6 weeks up to 13 weeks' gestation; after 13+1 and up to 25+6, the pregnancy should be dated based on head circumference and femur length (PHE, 2015b).

An increased NT can indicate the presence of chromosomal abnormalities like trisomy 21, and is sometimes associated with cardiac anomalies. Care must be taken to ensure that women understand the possible implications of, and have consented to, this specific type of scan. Unusual findings at a routine dating scan can result in ethical and moral dilemmas for women, their partners and also sonographers. The appearance of an increased NT has the potential to set the wheels of the screening programme in motion, without either explicit explanation or consent. The onus is therefore on the sonographer, midwife, GP or obstetrician to engage patience and time explaining the possible implications to women and their partners. It is important that both professionals and women are aware of the limitations of ultrasound examinations, as this may have an impact on the reported anguish and dissatisfaction experienced by some women when potential chromosomal or structural abnormalities have not been identified antenatally. Women should be provided with accurate information, both written and verbal, prior to the scan, so that informed choices can be made. Efforts should be made to ensure women understand that scan findings cannot guarantee a 'perfect baby'.

CONCLUSION

We hope we have given you a comprehensive overview of the range of antenatal screening tests available to women, and explored some of the issues women and professionals face. It is imperative that informed consent is obtained prior to any examination or procedure of clinical significance (GMC, 2018). All the screening programmes rely on early access to the midwife so that information and choices can be offered. There is great

potential and clearly documented advantages to offering screening early in pregnancy; therefore, midwives need to rise to the challenge of seeing women as early as possible. There is strong evidence to support midwives being more involved in pre-conception care, as this would be the best time to discuss and even offer some of the screening tests.

Never assume that a woman has consented to screening tests by default, simply by attending for a blood test or scan in pregnancy. Women need to understand what they are consenting to and the possible consequences and implications of all the tests discussed. Midwives need to be mindful that women may be engaged in wishful thinking, based on the anticipation of a positive outcome. In an ideal world, all professionals should be nonjudgemental and have complete respect and understanding for the choices and decisions that women and their families make (NICE, 2019; ARC, 2019).

The standard practice for communicating results to parents following high-chance results or suspicion of abnormalities is to offer a face-to-face appointment to discuss the results and the options that are available, in addition to providing support. The UK NSC and Antenatal Results and Choices (ARC) provide training to support sonographers, midwives and general practitioners in ways to communicate effectively when the outcomes are not quite what the parents may be expecting; the issue of communication is addressed further in Chapters 11, 12 and 15). Public Health England has also produced a number of training resources to support health professionals in their initial training and continuing professional development (PHE, 2019d).

PARENTS' STORY

Cayne's Story

My name is Anna, and I am a hospital-based midwife. My son Jay is the eldest of my four children, and Jamie is his partner of 4 years. Aiden, their first child, was 2 years old when Jamie became pregnant for the second time. They have given me permission to share their story about their baby Cayne.

On the day of Jamie's anatomy scan, I received a call from Jay. I thought he was calling to tell me the sex of the baby as they had been so excited about knowing. He said they were having another boy, which they were really

happy about, and that everything looked good, but that the baby had a wee gap in the front of his mouth. I instantly knew it was a cleft, having cared for parents welcoming babies with clefts into the world, and that we would be in for a challenging journey. Jay and Jamie were initially overwhelmed with the news. Jamie questioned if it was her fault, whether she had done something wrong in the pregnancy to cause it. However, they also knew from the outset that they loved their wee boy very much. A week or so after the anatomy scan, we went to the hospital to have a

Continued

Cayne's Story

meeting with a fetal and maternal medicine consultant. Another more detailed scan of the baby's face was performed, and it was very easy to see that the cleft was on the right side and was fairly large. The consultant offered Jamie an amniocentesis. It was such a big decision to make at such short notice, but Jamie and Jay decided they did not want to risk miscarriage for the small chance of a genetic abnormality being diagnosed. The consultant had said that Cayne didn't have any other markers that would indicate the presence of a syndrome, such as a structural heart defect or limb abnormalities.

A meeting was organized with the specialist cleft team a few weeks later. This team supports all the children and families in our region. They analyse the specific needs of the baby related to the cleft. The team consists of orthodontists, maxillofacial surgeons, dentists, nurses, speech and language therapists, and plastic surgeons. We met with seven different specialists over a 2-hour period, which was overwhelming, and trying to absorb all the information they were sharing with us was challenging. Jay and Jamie said that having me there to help them remember everything was really helpful. The first year sounded very daunting with two surgeries a few months apart and I felt so much compassion for what my family would have to cope with in the short and long term.

Jamie's pregnancy progressed normally and she continued to receive regular midwifery care from her wonderful continuity midwife. After all the meetings with specialists, we had to wait until the baby was born to see what would happen with regard to issues such as feeding, or whether he would need to be admitted to NICU. The plan was for Jamie to labour and birth in hospital so that specialist help was on hand, although NICU staff were not required to attend the birth. Jamie's waters broke at 37+6 weeks and she went straight into labour. I was blessed to be invited to the birth and Cayne was born after 4 hours of established labour and a one-push second stage! His Apgar scores were 7 at 1 minute and 7 at 5. He was in good condition at birth but at about 3 minutes of age, it was identified that he needed CPAP; there were signs of respiratory distress with oxygen levels around 55% and no sign of improvement with CPAP. He was taken to NICU for breathing support, where they struggled to find a way to maintain his oxygen saturations due to the cleft complicating how they could ventilate him. It was a very emotional and stressful time for Jay and Jamie. They found it disturbing seeing Cayne in the incubator with monitors, alarms, wires and tubes. Jamie found it really hard that everyone else had handled him while she had to

stay in the birthing room for a while before she could visit him. She was shocked by both the rapid birth and at how fast Cayne had been whisked away to NICU. Both Jay and Jamie were nervous about how they would feel seeing him for the first time, and it was made harder by the fact that he was in the neonatal unit.

Cayne was in NICU for 20 days, initially for respiratory support and then for help with feeding. Jay learned how to insert a nasogastric tube and we learned how to tube-feed. We also learned how to feed him with a special bottle and Jamie worked hard at expressing her breast milk. Unfortunately, she needed surgery for some abscesses under her arm the day after Cayne was born and then went on to develop pneumonia. It seemed so unfair that she had become so unwell after everything else. The logistics of having a baby in hospital and a toddler at home, with no transport, were very challenging and exhausting. I don't think they could have managed without my support.

Getting Cayne home was a huge milestone, but sadly within a week he had to go back into hospital for bronchiolitis caused by RSV. He ended up in ICU as he needed extensive breathing support, which was once again complicated by the cleft; the anatomy of his cleft meant that it was very difficult to get a seal on the oxygen mask. He was sedated as when he moved, the seal on the mask was compromised. He was in hospital for 8 days and although it was hard, Jay and Jamie enjoyed connecting with other parents in NICU, feeling a sense of shared experience. They have been in contact with Cleft New Zealand, a foundation to support families of children born with clefts.

We recognize that this is only the start of a long journey. Cayne will have his first operation to repair the cleft at around 3 months of age. At the moment he has tape over his lips to try to keep them from growing further apart. The surgery will bring the lips together and then at about 5 months the repair of his palate will commence. He also has a small ventricular septal defect (VSD), but this is expected to close spontaneously.

Having a baby with a cleft has been hard but Jay and Jamie are blessed in having a strong relationship and are able to support and care for each other. They feel that my support has been invaluable to them and although it has been hard, it's also been wonderful to be a granny to my lovely grandsons. The couple had incredible support from their midwife. The childcare centre that Aiden attends was able to extend his hours while Cayne was in hospital, which was so helpful. The cleft team have been so supportive and have worked together to manage Cayne's specific needs and to support Jay and Jamie.

KEY POINTS

- Women must be encouraged to access midwifery services early so they can be offered screening choices as early in pregnancy as possible.
- Early discussion of screening tests allows women informed choices.
- Women should have nondirective, clear information about all screening tests available in pregnancy and their consequences.
- Informed consent should always be gained prior to any scan examination and screening test.

REFERENCES

Antenatal Results and Choices (ARC), 2019. Helping parents and professionals through antenatal screening. Available from: https://www.arc-uk.org/. Accessed February 2019.

Australian Government Department of Health Pregnancy Care Guidelines. 37—Rubella. https://www.health.gov.au/resources/pregnancy-care-guidelines/part-f-routine-maternal-health-tests/rubella. Accessed March 2020.

Avert Information on HIV, 2019. Global information and education on HIV and AIDS Information on HIV. Available from: https://www.avert.org/public-hub. Accessed February 2019.

British Association for Sexual Health and HIV (BASHH), 2017. Available from: https://www.bashh.org/guidelines. Accessed February 2019.

General Medical Council (GMC), 2018. General Medical Council decision making and consent supporting patient choices about health care. Draft Guidance. https://www.gmc-uk.org/-/media/gmc-site-images/ethical-guidance/related-pdf-items/consent-draft-guidance/consent-draft-guidance.pdf?la=en&hash=E85F0DD8C7033541BF51F1C619EF992B1A45A188.

Healthtalk, 2017. Ending a pregnancy for fetal abnormality. Available from: http://www.healthtalk.org/peoples-experiences/pregnancy-children/antenatal-screening/topics. Accessed February 2019.

Kai, J., 2006. Pegasus for Front Line Professional—Handbook. University of Nottingham, Version 1.5.3, Cambridge, Pegasus Press.

Ministry of Health (MoH), 2019. National Screening Unit. Available from: https://www.nsu.govt.nz/health-professionals/antenatal-screening-down-syndrome-and-other-conditions/procedures-guidelines-2. Accessed April 2019.

Modell, B., Darlison, M., 2008. World Health Organization Global Epidemiology of Haemoglobin Disorders and Derived Service Indicators Bulletin of the World Health Organisation. Available from: https://www.who.int/bulletin/volumes/86/6/06-036673/en/. Accessed January 2019.

National Childbirth Trust (NCT), 2019. Antenatal Screening and Testing Information. Available from: https://www.nct.org.uk/pregnancy/tests-scans-and-antenatal-checks/antenatal-screening-and-testing-information. Accessed February 2019.

NHS Screening Programme, Fetal anomaly screening programme. https://assets.publishing.service.gov.uk/government/uploads/system/uploads/attachment_data/file/443865/FASP_ultrasound_handbook_July_2015_090715.pdf.

National Institute for Clinical Excellence (NICE), 2019. Antenatal care for Uncomplicated Pregnancies (CG62). Available from: https://www.nice.org.uk/guidance/cg62/chapter/Woman-centred-care. 2019. Accessed February 2019.

National Institute for Health and Care Excellence (NICE), 2017. Hepatitis B (Chronic): Diagnosis and Management: Clinical Guideline 165. Available from: https://www.nice.org.uk/guidance/cg165. Accessed February 2019.

National Screening Committee (NSC), 2019. Available from: https://www.gov.uk/government/groups/uk-national-screening-committee-uk-nsc. Accessed January 2019.

National Screening Committee (NSC), 2018. Available from: https://www.gov.uk/government/groups/uk-national-screening-committee-uk-nsc. Accessed March 2019.

New Zealand National Screening Unit, 2019. https://www.nsu.govt.nz/pregnancy-newborn-screening/antenatal-screening-down-syndrome-and-other-conditions/about-test

NHS, 2008. Antenatal and Newborn Screening Programme. Available from: https://www.gov.uk/topic/population-screening-programmes. Accessed February 2019.

NHS, 2018a. Antenatal Checks and Tests. Available from: https://www.nhs.uk/conditions/pregnancy-and-baby/antenatal-care-checks-tests/. Accessed February 2018a. Accessed March 2019.

NHS, 2018b. Your Pregnancy and Baby Guide. Available from: https://www.nhs.uk/conditions/pregnancy-and-baby/screening-blood-test-infectious-diseases-pregnant/. Accessed February 2019.

NHS, 2018c. Vaccinations. Available from: https://www.nhs.uk/conditions/vaccinations/mmr-vaccine-when-needed/. Accessed February 2019.

NHS, 2019. https://www.nhs.uk/conditions/pregnancy-and-baby/screening-amniocentesis-downs-syndrome/

Ogilvie, C., Akolekar, R., 2014. Pregnancy loss following amniocentesis or CVS sampling—time for a reassessment of risk. J. Clin. Med. 3 (3), 741–746. Available from: https://www.ncbi.nlm.nih.gov/pmc/articles/PMC4449654/. Accessed February 2019.

Peters, H., Thorne, C., Tookey, P.A., Byrne, L., 2018. National audit of perinatal HIV infections in the UK, 2006–2013: what lessons can be learnt? HIV Medicine published by John

Wiley & Sons Ltd on behalf of British HIV Association. HIV Med. 19, 280–289. Available from: https://onlinelibrary.wiley.com/doi/epdf/10.1111/hiv.12577. Accessed February 2019.

Public Health England (PHE), 2015a. Criteria for Appraising the Viability, Effectiveness and Appropriateness of a Screening Programme. Available from: https://www.gov.uk/government/publications/evidence-review-criteria-national-screening-programmes/criteria-for-appraising-the-viability-effectiveness-and-appropriateness-of-a-screening-programme#the-test. Accessed February 2019.

Public Health England (PHE), 2015b. Fetal Anomaly Screening Programme Handbook for Ultrasound Practitioners. Available from: https://assets.publishing.service.gov.uk/government/uploads/system/uploads/attachment_data/file/443865/FASP_ultrasound_handbook_July_2015_090715.pdf. Accessed February 2019.

Public Health England (PHE), 2017a. DH Immunisation Against Infectious Disease. Hepatitis B: the Green Book, Chapter 18 London. Available from: https://www.gov.uk/government/collections/immunisation-against-infectious-disease-the-green-book. Accessed February 2019.

Public Health England (PHE), 2017b. Introducing Non-Invasive Prenatal Testing to Antenatal Screening—Progress so Far. Available from: https://phescreening.blog.gov.uk/2017/03/24/introducing-non-invasive-prenatal-testing-to-antenatal-screening-progress-so-far/. Accessed June 2019.

Public Health England (PHE), 2018a. Infectious Diseases in Pregnancy Screening Programme Standards. Available from: https://www.gov.uk/government/publications/infectious-diseases-in-pregnancy-screening-programme-standards. Accessed March 2019.

Public Health England (PHE), 2018b. Fetal Anomaly Screening Programme (FASP) Standards. Available from: https://www.gov.uk/government/publications/fetal-anomaly-screening-programme-standards. Accessed March 2019.

Public Health England (PHE), 2018c. Understanding haemoglobinopathies. Available from: https://www.gov.uk/government/publications/handbook-for-sickle-cell-and-thalassaemia-screening/understanding-haemoglobinopathies. Accessed March 2019.

Public Health England (PHE), 2019a. Antenatal and Newborn Screening Timeline. Available from: https://www.gov.uk/guidance/nhs-population-screening-education-and-training#screening-timeline. Accessed February 2019.

Public Health England (PHE), 2019b. Screening Tests for you and our Baby. Available from: https://assets.publishing.service.gov.uk/government/uploads/system/uploads/attachment_data/file/800673/Screening_tests_for_you_and_your_baby.pdf. Accessed June 2019.

Public Health England (PHE), 2019c. Sickle Cell and Thalassaemia Screening: Education and Training. Available from: https://www.gov.uk/guidance/sickle-cell-and-thalassaemia-screening-education-and-training. Accessed February 2019.

Public Health England (PHE), 2019d. NHS Population Screening: Education and Training. Available from: https://www.gov.uk/guidance/nhs-population-screening-education-and-training#annbresource. Accessed February 2019.

Public Health England (PHE), 2019e. Antenatal and Newborn Screening e-Learning Module. Available from: https://portal.e-lfh.org.uk/Component/Details/446948. Accessed March 2020.

Public Health England (PHE), 2019f. Family Origin Questionnaire. Available from: https://assets.publishing.service.gov.uk/government/uploads/system/uploads/attachment_data/file/780349/SCT19_FOQ_updated_February_2019.pdf. Accessed February 2019.

Public Health England (PHE), Immunisation Against Infectious Disease (The Green Book). 2014. Available from: https://www.gov.uk/government/collections/immunisation-against-infectious-disease-the-green-book. Accessed February 2019.

Public Health England, 2020. NHS Sickle Cell and Thalassaemia Screening Programme 2017-2018 Data Report. https://assets.publishing.service.gov.uk/government/uploads/system/uploads/attachment_data/file/870090/Sickle_cell_and_thalassaemia_screening_annual_data_report_1_April_2017_to_31_March_2018.pdf.

Royal Australian and New Zealand College of Obstetricians and Gynaecologists (RANZCOG), 2015. DNA-Based Noninvasive Prenatal Testing for Fetal Aneuploidy. Available from: https://www.ranzcog.edu.au/news/DNA-based-Noninvasive-Prenatal-Testing-for-Fetal-A. Accessed April 2019.

Royal College of Obstetricians & Gynaecologists (RCOG), 2000. Ultrasound Screening for Fetal Abnormalities. RCOG, London. Available from: http://itpack31.itarget.com.br/uploads/cuf/arquivos/Ultrasound_Screening-GUIDELINE-ROYAL_COLLEGE.pdf. Accessed March 2019.

Royal College of Obstetricians & Gynaecologists (RCOG), 2013. Small-for-Gestational-Age Fetus, Investigation and Management (Green-top Guideline No. 31). Available from: https://www.rcog.org.uk/en/guidelines-research-services/guidelines/gtg31/. Accessed June 2019.

Royal College of Obstetricians & Gynaecologists (RCOG), 2017. Amniocentesis and Chorionic Villus Sampling: Guideline No. 8. RCOG Press, London. Available from: https://www.rcog.org.uk/guidelines.

Tidy, C., Bonsall, D., 2015. Thalassemia. Available from: https://patient.info/doctor/thalassaemia-pro. Accessed June 2019.

Vanstone, M., Cernat, A., Nisker, J., Schwartz, L., 2018. Women's perspectives on the ethical implications of non-invasive prenatal testing: a qualitative analysis to inform health policy decisions. BMC Med. Ethics 19 (1), 27. doi:10.1186/s12910-018-0267-4.

Wagner, M., 2019. Ultrasound More Harm Than Good? Birth International. Available from: https://birthinternational.com/article/pregnancy/ultrasound-more-harm-than-good/. Accessed June 2019.

World Health Organization, 2006. WHO Publication Prevention of Mother-to-Child Transmission of Syphilis (100). Available from: http://www.who.int/reproductivehealth/publications/maternal_perinatal_health/prevention_mtct_syphilis.pdf. Accessed February 2019.

World Health Organization, 2015a. WHO Guidelines (98), HIV Testing. Available from: http://www.who.int/hiv/pub/guidelines/hiv-testing-services/en/. Accessed March 2019.

World Health Organization, 2015b. Guideline on When to Start Antiretroviral Therapy and on Pre-Exposure Prophylaxis for HIV (99). Available from: http://www.who.int/hiv/pub/guidelines/earlyrelease-arv/en/. Accessed March 2019.

World Health Organization, 2016. WHO Recommendations on Antenatal Care for a Positive Pregnancy Experience (52). Available from: https://apps.who.int/iris/bitstream/handle/10665/250796/9789241549912-eng.pdf;jsessionid=37089D90824309B11A8FD4636E0C16B8?sequence=1. Accessed March 2020.

Zozzaro-Smith, P., Gray, L.M., Bacak, S.J., Thornburg, L.L., 2014. Limitations of aneuploidy and anomaly detection in the obese patient. J. Clin. Med. 3 (3), 795–808. doi:10.3390/jcm3030795. Accessed March 2019.

Useful websites

www.antenataltesting.info
ARC Antenatal Results and Choices is a national charity that provides information to expectant and bereaved parents throughout and after the antenatal screening and testing process, www.arc-uk.org
www.cafamily.org.uk
www.cpdscreening.phe.org.uk/sct-externaltraining
British HIV Association (BHIVA), https://www.bhiva.org/
British Medical Ultrasound Society, https://www.bmus.org/
Children's HIV Association (CHIVA), https://www.chiva.org.uk/

5

Influences on the Health of the Newborn, Before and During Pregnancy

Lorna Davies

CHAPTER CONTENTS

Everyone needs to understand that improving the condition of the fetus will have personal, social and economic benefits. The time has come to realize that, in a sense, it is not just women who are pregnant but it is the family and the whole of society.

Nathanielsz et al. (2003)

The primary purpose of this chapter is to consider the effect on the fetus and newborn of influences during the antenatal period. Some of these influences may continue to shape health and well-being into childhood and way beyond. The secondary purpose is to consider how we identify such factors in our discussions with women in order to tailor and optimize care for them and their babies.

In an age of advanced scientific knowledge and rapidly evolving technology, we may feel that we have a reasonable appreciation of the factors that influence the development and growth of the fetus during gestation. For example, we recognize from numerous research studies that cigarette smoking during pregnancy increases the risk of spontaneous miscarriage (Pineles et al., 2014). We are aware that certain medications can have teratogenic effects on the fetus. We know that infections can cross the placenta and cause irreversible negative effects on the unborn baby, and that some foods contain substances that can cause early fetal demise. As well as the obvious physical factors that may affect the fetus and newborn child, there are more subtle, nebulous aspects of our complex lives that can affect the growth and development of a baby. For example, what effect does the mother being in an abusive relationship have on the growth and development of her fetus? How does putting a pregnancy on hold emotionally following the discovery of a potential chromosomal anomaly affect the outcome after birth?

In recent decades, we have become aware that there may be a causal relationship between early life experience and later risk of disease. We are now aware, for example, that there is almost certainly a link between low birth weight and chronic disease in later life—notably ischaemic heart disease (Barker, 1992; Belbasis et al., 2016), obesity and diabetes (Jornayvaz et al., 2016). Other studies have shown that lower birth weight is associated with higher blood pressure in childhood (Chen, Srinivasan and Yao, 2012). This possible 'programming' of disease during 'critical windows' in fetal life has been attributed to the mechanism of oxidative stress and is a theory that has gained a strong following in the scientific world (Ávila et al., 2015; Rodríguez-Rodríguez et al., 2018).

EPIGENETICS

As touched upon in the discussion of embryology in Chapter 3, our understanding of influences on both the short- and long-term health and well-being of the baby is growing exponentially as scientists move further into the territories of epigenetics, brain architecture and development. The development of the field of epigenetics has added a whole new layer of complexity to the study of fetal and perinatal health. Epigenetics refers to the external modifications to DNA that enable genes to switch 'on' and 'off'. These changes do not alter the DNA sequence, but they do influence the way in which cells interpret genes. Any external stimulus that can be identified by the body has the potential to cause epigenetic modification (Simmons, 2008). For example, there is evidence that physical exercise causes changes in the pattern of epigenetic marks in muscle and fatty tissues (Rönn et al., 2013). Another factor is exposure to trauma, perhaps resulting from family violence during childhood, which appears to affect DNA methylation patterns (Suderman et al., 2014). The question of epigenetic inheritance has stimulated considerable interest and debate in recent years. However, although our understanding of this area is increasing exponentially, it is still not exactly clear which exposures influence epigenetic markers, or what the precise mechanisms and effects are. The notion of intergenerational impacts on health is a compelling theory, and there is evidence to suggest that what we do in our lives may be detected within gene expression for generations to come (Simmons, 2008). This is an important consideration that applies to paternity as well as maternity. So, although the emphasis in this chapter is primarily on the part that the mother plays in fetal development, the health and well-being of the father are also key determinants (Day et al., 2016). Prior to conception, if a man is nutritionally deficient, exposed to environmental pollutants, smokes, drinks alcohol and/or takes recreational drugs, he could inadvertently be compromising the health status of his future offspring. After conception, he may influence the future health of his child by, amongst other things, transferring infection to his partner, continuing to smoke or creating stress in his partner's life (Cefalo and Moos, 1995). What we are not so sure about currently is the interplay between maternal and paternal influences with regard to epigenetics; this missing link could further our understanding of this

important influence on health and well-being in uterine life and beyond. (Day et al., 2016) By taking gene expression into account, we can begin to appreciate the importance of a broader perspective when we work with women and their families.

It would be impossible within this chapter to cover the enormous range of potential factors and to discuss all their implications for midwifery practice, but Fig. 5.1 illustrates the vast number of factors and the interconnections between them. We will focus on a small number of individual areas that represent the much broader range of influences. Other sources of impact are addressed elsewhere in the book.

THE SIGNIFICANCE OF HISTORY-TAKING

The growth and healthy development of the baby is governed not only by hereditary factors, but by the mother's health and nutritional status, reproductive history, socioeconomic and demographic status, and psychological, emotional and spiritual well-being.

An important part of antenatal care which impacts on neonatal health is acquiring a history that is as comprehensive as possible in order to identify factors that may impact on fetal and newborn health. If we consider the unique characteristics of each pregnancy, we can see from the factors illustrated in Fig. 5.1, and their interconnectivity, that the list is potentially limitless.

PRECONCEPTION CARE

Healthy women have a greater chance of becoming pregnant, having a healthy pregnancy and giving birth to a healthy baby, and the same could be said for healthy fathers. In an ideal world, pregnancy would not occur until the factors that may serve to enhance or confound the health and well-being of any baby had been considered. Parents-to-be planning a pregnancy would have ready access to preconception care in order to optimize the health and well-being outcomes for both mother and baby (Dean et al., 2014). Maternal (and consequently fetal and newborn) health is influenced by a range of determinants of health that include social circumstances, preexisting medical conditions, mental health, sexual health, nutrition, immune status, environmental contaminant exposure, and substance use. In order to mitigate any risks related to these factors, the preconception health of the woman/couple should be

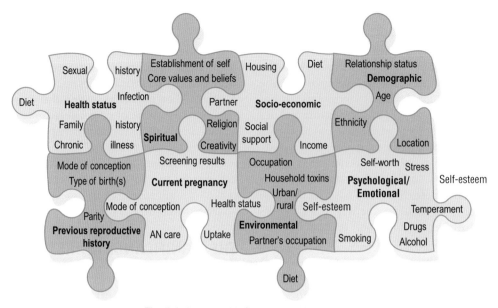

Fig. 5.1 Antenatal Influences. *AN,* antenatal

assessed and therapy or counselling around any identified factors should be considered.

However, in spite of the increasing evidence supporting the value and importance of preconception planning, this aspect of care remains a low-profile service in many health care systems. There are a number of reasons why this may be the case. It is estimated that only 45% of pregnancies are actually planned (Wellings et al., 2013), which means that broader targeting may be required. The funding of a service for preconception care is not clear cut, because it is viewed as the responsibility of many in the system (e.g., GPs, health visitors, midwives, NGOs) rather than being a clearly identified pathway. In 2017 a situation analysis study carried out in Scotland, canvassing the views of both non–health professionals and health professionals, identified that a lack of awareness of preconception health was hampering attempts to introduce preconception programmes of care (Goodfellow et al., 2017). Public Health England (PHE) has recently launched an initiative (Jesurasa, 2018) proposing that preconception care should be considered a cornerstone of primary care. The document indicates that preconception advice should be provided as a life-course health initiative with an opportunistic element at key points in the reproductive life course of women, although there is less of a focus on men. The document suggests that this should be achieved via a multidisciplinary effort including midwives, health visitors, public health nurses and general practitioners. This initiative supports the goals of the Maternity Transformation Programme that aims to ensure safer births; it therefore has specific significance for midwives who, as primary care workers with a focus on health promotion and health education, are well positioned to take a key role in this development. What is particularly heartening about the document is its focus on equitable access and the principle of 'proportionate universalisms', which means that although the initiative is aimed at providing a service for all, more resources can be targeted for those with clearly defined needs. Those needs could be related to socioeconomic factors, preexisting medical conditions, previous childbirth outcomes, or other factors. Addressing them in this way may help to reduce inequality and improve outcomes for higher-need client groups whilst meeting the needs of all.

FACTORS THAT MAY INFLUENCE FETAL HEALTH

The following section will explore some of the factors that are already perceived as either covert or manifest threats to the health and well-being of the baby. It is important to stress at this juncture that, although the risk factors are categorized for ease of study, the reality is, as we know, never so unambiguous. The many elements that may contribute to the outcome are often enmeshed and difficult to extricate, which makes researching some of these areas quite problematic from both a methodological and analytical perspective.

Environmental Toxins

Although there is an abundance of information available on the effects of smoking, drinking alcohol and using drugs, there would appear to be a dearth of accessible information about environmental pollutants and their effects on embryonic and fetal development. Researchers claim there are many confounding variables which make it difficult to determine categorically what the effects on the unborn child of exposure to substances such as heavy metals, ionizing radiation and organic solvents may be.

Over 85,000 synthetic chemicals are currently utilized commercially, and approximately 1000 new chemicals are introduced annually. Only a percentage of these potential environmental toxins have been adequately tested to determine their effect on humans; in fact, comprehensive data exist for only about 25% (EPA, 2017).

Studies carried out in a number of different countries indicate that environmental toxins play an active role in the increasing rate of low birth weight babies (Miranda, 2009). A study in Germany (Karmaus and Wolf, 1995) identified that occupational exposure to wood preservatives among pregnant workers was linked to low birth weight.

A recently published US study that analyzed data for 500,000 women between 1997 and 2011 in an agricultural region of California found that the number of birth abnormalities increased by 5% to 9% in women exposed to high levels of pesticides (Larsen et al., 2017). An increased risk of birth defects has also been noted in female flower workers in Kenya (Saina et al., 2017) and Brazil (Cremonese, 2014). These international studies represent just a very small sample of the escalating literature on environmental toxins; in our globalized world, they have significance wherever we are situated, because products from one country can very easily turn up on the other side of the world.

Several studies and systematic reviews have found a correlation between low birth weight (LBW), birth defects and drinking water contamination (Infante-Rivard, 2004; Aschengrau, 2009). In a systematic review

of 16 studies, Bove et al. (2002) identified that not only was LBW more likely where drinking water contamination was present, but that neural tube defects, oral clefts, cardiac defects and choanal atresia were also more prevalent; they suggested these findings warranted follow-up studies as a matter of urgency.

The presence of environmental endocrine-disrupting chemicals (EDCs), particularly in drinking water, has been a matter of concern to some in the scientific community for some time. These chemicals are external compounds that can interfere with the synthesis, secretion, action and elimination of hormones that occur naturally within the body, and thus they are able to modify the operation of the hormonal system on the body's organs. Oestrogen, progesterone, androgens, bisphenol A and bichlorinated bisphenol are all examples of EDCs that are found in drinking water, albeit at generally low levels (Burkhardt-Holm, 2010). Although many manufacturers have removed bisphenol A from their products (often as a result of legislation), the replacements may carry similar risks to babies (Worland, 2015). Endocrine disruptors are believed by some researchers to be linked with many diseases and disorders, including cancers, obesity, prematurity, autism, allergies and pubertal development disorders. It is theorized that EDCs attach to endogenous hormone receptors within the body and either mimic the hormones that occur naturally within the body or prevent them from binding to the receptor. Although the risk is not proven, the precautionary principle should apply (Burkhardt-Holm, 2010). It is claimed that using a water filter may help to eliminate some of the risks associated with EDCs, as might limiting the number of chemicals in the household wherever possible (Touraud et al., 2011).

Before and during pregnancy, a woman and her partner may have to consider occupational exposure to potential teratogens that may be found in the workplace. Table 5.1 highlights some of the areas where steps should be taken to ensure that the woman and her unborn baby are not placed at unnecessary risk. Under COSHH regulations (Control of Substances Hazardous to Health Regulations, 2002), employers must carry out a proper risk assessment to identify potential hazards to pregnant workers. Each individual workplace should be evaluated and steps taken to minimize or eliminate exposure. For example, in the aviation industry, where concerns about ionizing radiation from galactic cosmic rays on the pregnancies of personnel were expressed,

TABLE 5.1   Occupational Exposure to Reprotoxic Agents

Agent	Industry or Occupational Group	Reported Effects of Female Exposure	Reported Effects of Male Exposure
Organic solvents in general	Painting, degreasing, shoemaking, printing, dry cleaning, metal industry and several other fields of industry	Reduced fertility, menstrual disorders, fetal loss, birth defects, preterm birth, neurobehavioural effects, childhood leukaemia	Delayed conception, reduced semen quality, fetal loss, birth defects
Benzene	Petrochemical industry, laboratory personnel	Fetal loss, reduced fertility, low birth weight	
Carbon disulphide	Viscose rayon industry	Menstrual disorders	Decreased libido and potency
Some ethylene glycol ethers and their acetates	Electronics industry, silk screen printing, photography and dyeing, shipyard painting, metal casting, chemical industry, other industries	Reduced fertility, fetal loss, birth defects, menstrual disorders	Reduced semen quality
Tetrachloroethylene	Dry cleaning, degreasing	Reduced fertility, fetal loss	
Toluene	Shoe industry, painting, laboratory work	Reduced fertility, fetal loss	
Metals			
Lead	Battery industry, lead smelting, foundries, pottery industry, ammunition industry and some other metal industries	Reduced fertility, fetal loss, preterm birth, low birth weight, birth defects, impaired cognitive development	Reduced semen quality, reduced fertility, fetal loss, birth defects
Inorganic mercury	Lamp industry, chloralkali industry, dental personnel	Reduced fertility, menstrual disorders, fetal loss	Fetal loss
Pesticides[a]	Agriculture, gardening, greenhouse work	Reduced fertility, fetal loss, birth defects, preterm birth, reduced fetal growth, neurodevelopmental effects, childhood leukaemia	Reduced sperm quality, reduced fertility, fetal loss, birth defects, childhood cancer
Pharmaceuticals			
Anaesthetic gases	Operating rooms, delivery wards, dental offices	Fetal loss, reduced birth weight, preterm birth, birth defects, reduced fertility	
Nitrous oxide	Operating rooms, delivery wards, dental offices	Fetal loss, reduced birth weight, reduced fertility	
Antineoplastic agents	Hospitals, pharmaceutical industry	Menstrual dysfunction, reduced fertility, fetal loss, premature birth, low birth weight, birth defects	
Carbon monoxide	Iron and steel foundries, welding, food industry, car repair, service stations	Preterm birth, intrauterine death	

[a]Examples of pesticides with adverse effects in men include dibromochloropropane (DBCP), 2,4-dichlorophenoxyacetic acid (2,4-D), ethylene dibromide, chlordecone, carbaryl, alachlor, atrazine and diazinon.

many aviation authorities have issued a radiation exposure level for pregnant cabin staff (ICRP, 2016).

Unlike the threats of tobacco, alcohol and recreational drugs, a pregnant woman will probably find it impossible to avoid exposure to all environmental toxins, particularly within the food chain and water supply, or as an occupational hazard. Alone, most of these exposure levels are unlikely to cause harm to the unborn baby, but the fact remains that we do not know what the so-called 'safe' levels are for many substances, and the effect of multiple exposures is unknown. For example, if a woman is eating foods with a high pesticide residue, living near a waste dump and working with solvents in her job, then her baby is statistically at greater risk of developing a congenital abnormality.

It is therefore critically important to take a good booking history in order to help the woman identify some of the risks she may not previously have considered. She may, for example, be able to change her duties temporarily within her workplace, limit the amount of fish she consumes, invest in a water filter, purchase organic produce, or consider moving, at least temporarily, to an area further away from the landfill waste site in her present vicinity. This is not about scaring your clients, but about creating awareness and giving them options with regard to minimizing any potential risk to their unborn baby.

Stress

Pregnancy is a time of considerable stress for many women. It could be said that there are many additional stressors for women during this time. The so-called minor problems of pregnancy can create major crises for some women, while making decisions about which antenatal screening tests to have may create anxiety for others (Chapter 4). Intimate partner violence has been noted in 3% to 15% of pregnancies (Devries et al., 2010), and one can imagine the levels of stress that this must trigger.

Although the data relating to psychological stress and birth outcomes are not always easy to interpret, an increasing number of studies support the argument that high levels of stress may have a detrimental effect on the well-being of the baby.

The biochemical effects of stress include hypercortisolism and an imbalance of the hypothalamic–pituitary–adrenal axis which may contribute to congenital defects, preterm birth and low birth weight at term (Randall, 2015). Women who experience preterm birth have significantly higher plasma corticotropin-releasing hormone (CRH) levels than those in control groups, regardless of their gestation (Sandman, Davis and Glynn, 2012). CRH is produced by the brain and the placenta and is also the first hormone our brains produce when we are faced with stress. Placental activation of the maternal pituitary–adrenal axis manifests in the same way as the classic endocrine response to stress (Hobel et al., 1999). When exposure to cortisol becomes prolonged and persistent it can lead to chronic stress, which affects memory, impairs cognition, decreases thyroid function, and has implications for cardiovascular health (O'Connor et al., 2013).

Psychosocial stress during pregnancy can also increase inflammatory markers and alters cytokine production across pregnancy (Coussons-Read et al., 2007). Cytokines, produced by immune cells, coordinate and initiate defence functions in the body. This suggests that stress in the antenatal period may alter maternal physiology, and specifically immune function, in a way that can result in pregnancy complications such as pre-eclampsia and premature labour.

It is recognized that high levels of stress and anxiety may result in depression. Brummelte et al. (2006) suggested that women may be more susceptible to depression during pregnancy because the fluctuating levels of hormones, including corticosterone, create a state of hypercortisolism which is associated with depression. In New Zealand, a research study was carried out using a sample group of 550 women and children. The women were all identified as having been subjected to high levels of stress during the antenatal period. All of the children were born at full term, yet half of them were small for gestational age. The children were tested cognitively at the age of 3½ years; the researchers identified that maternal stress and lack of social support during pregnancy were significantly associated with lower intelligence test scores (Slykerman et al., 2005).

Approximately 10% to 15% of pregnant women are said to suffer from antenatal depression. This is a similar rate to that for depression in the postnatal period. It is believed that depression rates for women are higher during pregnancy than at any other time. (O'Keane and Marsh, 2007). In 2018, a UK longitudinal study provided evidence that young women birthing today are far more likely to have perinatal depression than were their mother's generation (Pearson et al., 2018). However, the literature around the prevalence of depression in pregnant as opposed to non-pregnant women would seem to be less than equivocal. Another study demonstrated that awakening salivary cortisol levels are naturally higher in pregnant than non-pregnant women, which may suggest that they are programmed to cope with stress more effectively in pregnancy (Weerth and Buitelaar, 2005). It may be that women do have a biochemical compensatory mechanism to enable them to cope with the additional demands of pregnancy, but if the balance is tipped—as sometimes happens with the increasing demands of pregnancy—then the effects could be injurious for the future well-being of the child. For example, the findings of the Avon Longitudinal Study of Parents and Children suggest a correlation between exposure to antenatal depression and offspring depression at age 18, particularly in female children (Quarini et al., 2016). Whether there is an increased incidence or not, the fact remains that, in most studies, depression during pregnancy is the strongest predictor of postnatal depression (Faisal-Cury and Menezes, 2012). The effects of postnatal depression on child development are well documented and include behavioural adjustment problems and poor cognitive and language development (Murray, Halligan and Cooper, 2010).

The symptoms of antenatal depression may also take their toll on the well-being of the fetus. Depressed pregnant women may eat and sleep less well, and are more likely to smoke and drink alcohol (Tong, 2016). They are also less likely to seek antenatal care. The symptoms of depression during pregnancy are similar to those at other times of life, but they are sometimes masked by the ongoing changes that occur during pregnancy, such as tiredness and changing body image (Schetter and Tanner, 2012).

One of the key roles of the midwife is that of health educator; the antenatal period offers an unparalleled opportunity to provide women and their families with information that may help them at other points in their lives, including education about stress management and depression. Antenatal social and education groups may help to develop support networks for the woman and her partner. As peer group members, they may also be aided in identifying and normalizing some of the changes occurring in their lives by the recognition that they are not alone. Mindfulness has been found to have

positive benefits for some women during pregnancy by restoring central nervous system equilibrium and providing tools for coping with anxiety and depression (Duncan et al., 2017). It can also help women to create a closer attachment with their babies, as can using relaxation techniques, visualizing, talking to, and perhaps listening to music with, their babies (Marsh-Prelesnik and Davies, 2007).

Although the importance of identifying depression in the antenatal period is increasingly recognized, there may be a need for broader use of screening tools in antenatal care (Kingston et al., 2017). However, identifying depression is worthless without timely, accessible and user-friendly treatment facilities. We also need to ensure that, as midwives, we are aware of best practices (both nonpharmacological and pharmacological) for helping the woman to deal with depression during pregnancy.

Current changes in antenatal provision have, in some areas, led to a decrease in antenatal visits and a reduction in the number of antenatal classes. Such action could isolate women even further, thereby increasing their chances of becoming depressed and not being identified. This means that midwives may need to become more creative in the ways in which they deliver their services, targeting those women identified as having the greatest need.

Nutrition

Evidence increasingly suggests that one of the most significant gifts a woman can provide for her baby is a nutritionally dense uterine environment during pregnancy. Nutrition has been held up as the cornerstone in determining pregnancy outcomes as well as the health and well-being of the baby (Gluckman et al., 2015). Suboptimal maternal nutrition during pregnancy has been linked with a number of adverse outcomes, including low birth weight (<2500 g), preterm birth and intrauterine growth restriction.

Impaired fetal growth has been associated with negative short- and long-term outcomes, such as increased perinatal morbidity and mortality, infant mortality and childhood morbidity. As we have already established, children who experience restricted growth in utero are also more likely to show poor cognitive development and neurological impairment. Additionally, particular nutrient deficiencies have been linked to many congenital anomalies and birth defects.

It would seem, however, that the current dietary practices of pregnant women do not necessarily conform with current health recommendations (Bookari, Yeatman and Williamson, 2017). One possible example of this is the frequently cited increasing rates of obesity (Opray et al., 2015). Obesity appears to be associated with an increased risk of many of the adverse pregnancy outcomes identified earlier; the recording of body mass index (BMI) has subsequently become an increasingly significant feature within antenatal care in the past few years (Davies and Deery, 2014). The physiological changes of pregnancy that are designed to increase maternal energetic efficiency and liberate fetal substrates are not as effective when obesity is present, and may lead to conditions such as preeclampsia and gestational diabetes in the woman and hyperinsulinism in the newborn (Cedergren, 2004).

However, the current focus on obesity may detract attention from the fact that women of normal weight (or who are underweight) may have a diet deficient in the nutrients that are essential for optimal fetal development. In the much cited fetal origins theory, Barker (1992) hypothesizes that permanent metabolic and endocrine changes occur as a result of adaptation to undernutrition in fetal life and that this can result from any form of malnutrition. This phenomenon is referred to as 'the thrifty phenotype' (Hales and Barker, 2001). In situations where nutrients are scarce, these changes would ensure survival; however, where nutrition is plentiful, they predispose the child to health problems in later life. The well-documented Dutch Famine Study Cohort offered scientists the unique opportunity to measure the effects of famine on human health in a modern, developed and literate country, albeit one subjected to the ravages of war. The study showed that pregnant women exposed to famine produced offspring who were more susceptible to diabetes, obesity, cardiovascular disease, microalbuminuria and other health problems (Roseboom et al., 2001). The study provides an illustration of the theory of epigenetic influences, whereby epigenetic events, modified inter alia by diet, carry the potential for an intergenerational effect.

Could our current epidemics of similar types of ill health be the result of epigenetic activity caused by malnutrition? Type II diabetes, until recently unheard of in children under 16, is now steadily increasing; there may now be up to 7000 cases in the United Kingdom (Diabetes UK, 2018). Obese children and adolescents are also more likely to have higher levels of cholesterol, triglycerides, lipoproteins and low-density lipoproteins, and low levels of high-density lipoproteins. This pattern correlates strongly with heart disease in later life. They are also more likely to develop hypertension and osteoarthritis (Gluckman et al., 2015).

The nutritional literature offered to pregnant women places an emphasis on 'risk' foods that they should leave out of their diet—soft cheeses, raw egg products, swordfish, etc.—rather than what they should be putting in. It is important that women are aware of the foodstuffs (listed in Table 5.2) that should be avoided where possible during pregnancy, but a heavy emphasis on food safety can leave women feeling less than safe and somewhat confused (Paterson, Hay-Smith and Treharne, 2016). It is equally important, if not more so, that they are aware of those constituents of diet that will encourage the growth of a healthy baby. The antenatal period offers an ideal opportunity for the woman and her family to focus on dietary and lifestyle adaptations as part of a life-based knowledge and skills approach. However, it does require a proactive and positive approach to food and nutrition, which might call for increased attention to nutritional literacy in healthcare education and professional development (Davies and Deery, 2014).

The dietary recommendations for pregnant women are not dissimilar to those for adults generally; a healthy, well-balanced diet should enable the baby to receive most of its needs with minimal supplementation (Williamson, 2006). However, there are a few notable exceptions which should be briefly addressed. The physiological changes that take place during pregnancy will usually compensate for the woman's increased need for iron, without the need for iron supplementation. A 2019 review of 49 studies in 29 countries over a 22-year period suggests that approximately 40–60% of European women have low to depleted iron reserves 60% (Milman 2019). This increases the chances of preterm birth and low birth weight (Scholl, 2011).

A number of women will therefore require iron supplementation during pregnancy. Interestingly, there does not appear to be any global or even local consensus regarding the most accurate way of obtaining information relating to the pregnant woman's iron status (Calje and Skinner, 2017). A wide variety of biochemical indicators—including haemoglobin (Hb), serum ferritin (SF) and serum transferrin receptor (sTfR)—are

TABLE 5.2   Foods Women Are Advised to Avoid During Pregnancy

Food	Reason	Effect
Swordfish Shark Marlin	High methylmercury levels	Neurological effects
Tuna (limit to 1 or 2 times a week)	High methylmercury levels	Neurological effects
Soft cheeses Pate Ready-to-eat meats Unpasteurized milk/products	Listeria	Miscarriage Preterm birth Stillbirth or perinatal death
Raw egg products	Listeria	Miscarriage
Undercooked meat & poultry	*Escherichia coli* *Campylobacter* *Salmonella*	Preterm birth Stillbirth or perinatal death
Unwashed raw vegetables	Toxoplasmosis	Vision & hearing loss Impaired cognitive development Seizures
Liver	Overconsumption of vitamin A	Birth defects
Hummus/tahini	*Salmonella*	Fetal infection Perinatal death
Raw sushi or ceviche	*Vibrionaceae a* Salmonella Protozoan species	Neurological defects
Honey	Has been associated with botulism	

used to assess the iron status, but the most effective way of obtaining the information remains elusive (Madhavan Nair et al., 2004).

Women are routinely advised to complement their diet with a folic acid supplement during the periconception period, up to and including the 12th week of pregnancy, as it is well documented that this can reduce the incidence of neural tube defects (NTDs) (De-Regil et al., 2015). However, a Cochrane review in 2013 suggested that some of the other claims related to higher levels of folic acid supplementation in pregnancy, such as increased birth weight, higher placental weight and prolonged gestation, did not stand up to scrutiny (Lassi et al., 2013). The recommended dosage of folic acid varies by country; for example, in the United Kingdom the dose is 400 μg per day, while in New Zealand it is 800 μg daily.

Vitamin D is the most recent addition to the list of supplements advised during pregnancy. NICE recommends that women should take 10 μg of Vitamin D daily throughout pregnancy and whilst breastfeeding. However, a Cochrane review advised that the evidence for Vitamin D supplementation as a universal recommendation remains unclear. Although Vitamin D may decrease the risk of preeclampsia, it may increase the risk of preterm birth. (Palacios et al., 2019).

It would seem that the importance of nutrition in pregnancy has never been given the full attention it deserves; studies in different countries have identified that midwives have less than adequate knowledge of nutrition, or lack the confidence to provide such information for women (Arrish, Yeatman and Williamson, 2014). It has also been identified that nutrition could be given a more prominent profile in the professional development requirements of both GPs and health visitors (Van Teijlingen et al., 1998). This is something the health sector needs to take on board in order to improve perinatal and life course outcomes.

Pregnancy is a time when women are more open to change, and nonjudgemental support at this time could reduce or even prevent complications related to diet (Cheyney and Moreno-Black, 2012). By changing habits and behaviours around food and eating, women could improve the health outcomes for their baby as well as benefiting their own health. Health professionals therefore need to communicate the benefits of good nutrition, and inform women how they can best provide a nutritionally rich environment for their baby and themselves during pregnancy.

Alcohol

Some years ago an advertising campaign in New Zealand used the copy headline 'It's not what we're drinking, it's how we're drinking'. This sobering reminder is something that may have even greater significance for women considering conceiving or who are already pregnant. Many countries have taken the abstinence line, advocating that 'no level is safe' in relation to the use of alcohol in pregnancy. The consumption of alcohol during pregnancy is inconsistent between countries, possibly because of different cultural and social attitudes around drinking alcohol. This can create challenges when it comes to obtaining an accurate picture of what, when and how much alcohol women imbibe during the childbearing period, because locally generated data do not always give enough information for broader conjecture. Findings can also be quite variable between studies, which is likely to reflect differences in study methodologies, but which again leaves a less than clear slate on which to draw conclusions.

It has been mooted that women are not always candid about what and when they are drinking. As a result, they may choose not to disclose what is really happening for them, leading to a less than accurate appraisal of the situation (Callinan and Ferris, 2014). Furthermore, it has been argued that the evidence for abstinence during pregnancy is not particularly strong; there are studies demonstrating that low to moderate consumption of alcohol in pregnancy has little effect on the executive function of the children at the age of 5 (McCarthy et al., 2013). This argument is not invalid, but could lead to confusion in the targeted group when, for example, the headline of the Harvard Health Publishing website states 'Drinking a little alcohol in pregnancy may be ok' (Lewine, 2018) Finally, from a global perspective, campaigning around this public health area has come under fire as being less than well planned or evidence based (France et al., 2013).

As a result of these factors, it would seem that although many women are aware that alcohol use decreases their chance of having a healthy baby, many have limited knowledge about more specific aspects, such as the nature of the conditions that babies can present with (Peadon et al., 2010; Parackal et al., 2006).

Teratogenic Effects of Alcohol

Alcohol is a well-known teratogen that may continue to affect the fetus beyond the early embryonic stages of development. It crosses the barrier of the placenta, producing equivalent concentrations in fetal circulation. The brain and central nervous system of the unborn child are especially sensitive to alcohol exposure in the antenatal period, and the resulting effects may cause a disorder that falls under the umbrella of fetal alcohol spectrum disorder (FASD).

Fetal alcohol spectrum disorder. Fetal alcohol spectrum disorder may affect 3% to 5% of mainstream school-aged children, with many remaining undiagnosed (May, 2014). The main characteristics of the disorder are listed in Table 5.3, although it should be noted that there is no typical FASD profile (Gibbard, 2009); the individual presentation and the degree of severity experienced may vary from infant to infant.

FASD is a nondiagnostic term that includes fetal alcohol syndrome and other FASDs (Box 5.1), and those

---

TABLE 5.3 Main Characteristics of Fetal Alcohol Spectrum Disorder

- Facial anomalies, which include: small eye openings; flat, thin upper lip; little or no philtrum; reduction in ear length; flattened midface
  Three of the facial features should be present for consideration of FASD. (May, 2014)
- Growth retardation in at least one of the following respects:
  - low birth weight
  - weight loss which is not due to poor nutrition
  - low weight-height ratio
- Central nervous system abnormalities in at least one of the following areas:
  - small head size at birth
  - structural abnormalities in the brain
  - poor fine motor skills, poor eye–hand coordination, hearing loss not related to injury or illness or poor gait when walking

BOX 5.1 **Varying Presentations of FASD**

Partial fetal alcohol syndrome (pFAS)	These children will not necessarily have the three facial features required for diagnosis.
Alcohol-related neurodevelopmental disorder (ARND)	These children have none of the facial features, but present with cognitive and behavioural issues relating to damage to their central nervous system.
Alcohol-related birth defects (ARBD) (this term is rarely used now)	Defects of the skeletal system or major organs but not the behavioural or cognitive issues seen in people with FAS.

Adapted from MoH, 2015.

children who may be affected by fetal alcohol exposure but may not have a diagnosis because they do not quite meet the clinical criteria of having been exposed to alcohol in utero. This is because the diagnostic criteria for these disorders are not clinically consistent, and clinicians would have to prove that a person was exposed to alcohol in the womb to give them a diagnosis of any disorder other than FASD (Göransson et al., 2004).

We may assume that these problems will only present in the babies of women who have serious issues with alcohol and who consequently are drinking excessively throughout their pregnancy. However, although most studies of FASD pinpoint the long-term heavy use of alcohol as the cause of problems for the child, it has been suggested that there is a 2- or 3-day 'critical period' a few weeks after conception when the developing fetus is especially vulnerable to alcohol effects (Siegelman and Rider, 2014). It is possible, though not proven, that even one drinking session of five or six drinks early in the pregnancy could be enough to cause neurobehavioural effects. (MoH, 2004).

As previously discussed, it is difficult to obtain data illuminating how widespread the problem of alcohol use in pregnancy actually is. Women are often reluctant to share this sort of information with anyone, including health professionals, for fear of being subjected to social disapproval and judgemental attitudes. The approach of the midwife or other health professional is therefore very important in establishing whether there is a problem with alcohol and, if so, how serious a threat it presents to the fetus.

Disclosure is far more likely when a good relationship is established with the woman. Göransson et al. (2004) found that poor communication between primary care, social services and other agencies can lead to the woman not being identified as having a problem in the antenatal period. The study concluded that midwives had a tendency to deal with the problem themselves and were in fact convinced that most women gave up drinking during pregnancy. A woman's reluctance to disclose may be based on a fear of having her baby removed by the authorities, or of being stigmatized in some way. Anecdotally at least, these findings would appear to still have a strong relevance; a recent study from the United States suggests that policies relating to alcohol in pregnancy are leading to women spurning any attempts to provide help, fearing draconian consequences such as the threat of imprisonment or of having their baby taken from them (Stone, 2015). We may need a more effective way of identifying pregnant women with dependency problems, but we equally need to be able to offer them appropriate support and referral if necessary.

The Canadian Pediatric Society suggests that prevention efforts should target women both before they become pregnant and during their childbearing years. It also recognizes the importance of including the partners, families, and the community of such women, stressing that all efforts need to be family-centred and culturally sensitive, so that they are able to contextualize the significance of alcohol in pregnancy. Its recommendation is that communication needs to be comprehensive, and that women should draw on all services appropriate to their often complex social, economic and emotional needs (Schröter, 2010).

The information that midwives and other carers provide must be consistent, evidence-informed and contemporaneous; there is almost certainly a need for further ongoing professional development in this area. Such education should aim to provide counselling skills that motivate, and support lifestyle change for, at-risk women.

CONCLUSION

Becoming pregnant and growing a baby are complex physiological processes. There are numerous factors that affect the embryo and fetus in utero, and it would be impossible to tell any woman that 'these are *your* definitive risk factors and this is what you must aim to eliminate or avoid during pregnancy'. In this chapter, we have chiefly explored matters that could be termed as psychosocial. If we had included existing medical conditions, for example, or cultural issues, the complexity of the subject would have been further compounded. How can we extrapolate one potential risk factor without looking at the bigger picture? Life is complicated and the influences that shape us into individual beings are so hugely varied that, although generalizations can be made, nothing can ever be assumed.

The interrelated factors and events that represent the physical, social, emotional, psychological and spiritual elements of our lives mean there will always be things that appear to defy logic. Why did Sarah, a health-conscious vegetarian of optimal weight who ran marathons before becoming pregnant, give birth to a baby with a marked congenital condition? Or why did Bethana, a 17-year-old with a heart murmur, who has dabbled with a variety of different drugs and binge-drinks at weekends, give birth to a baby who appears to be physically perfect?

What we can do is to advise women, where possible, to seek out advice preconception, as this may encourage healthy lifestyle changes. We can aim to provide up-to-date, evidence-based information on the relative risks of the identifiable factors in a woman's life, bearing in mind the potential for epigenetic significance. This may help to at least minimize exposure to any potential threat. Midwives and other health professionals also have a responsibility to acquaint themselves with resources in their community that are able to offer further specialized support for some of the identified areas of influence.

However, the most significant action on the part of the practitioner would be to accept the notion that this *is* a complex, multifaceted and interconnected area, and that by compartmentalizing we may be offering illusory solutions. Adopting a broader and more holistic approach to practice may enable us to be more responsive to the specific context of the individual woman and, in so doing, support her in producing a baby who is able to enjoy an optimal state of health from the outset.

KEY POINTS

- There are many aspects of our complicated lives that may affect the growth and development of a baby.
- The health and well-being of the father is a key determinant in the outcomes of neonatal health.

- An important part of antenatal care which impacts on neonatal health is the acquisition of a comprehensive history from the mother.
- We should be advising women, where possible, to seek out advice before they conceive, as this may encourage healthy lifestyle changes.
- Midwives and other health professionals have a responsibility to acquaint themselves with resources available in their community.
- Adopting a broader and more holistic approach to practice may enable us to be more responsive to the specific context of the individual woman.

REFERENCES

Arrish, J., Yeatman, H., Williamson, M., 2014. Midwives and nutrition education during pregnancy: a literature review. Women Birth 27 (1), 2–8.

Aschengrau, A., Weinberg, J.M., Janulewicz, P.A., Gallagher, L.S., Winter, M.R., Vieira, V.M., et al., 2009. Prenatal exposure to tetrachloroethylene-contaminated drinking water and the risk of congenital anomalies: a retrospective cohort study. Environmental Heal. 1, 8–44. doi:10.1186/1476-069X-8-44.

Ávila, J.G., Echeverr, I., de Plata C.A., Castillo, A., 2015. Impact of oxidative stress during pregnancy on fetal epigenetic patterns and early origin of vascular diseases. Nutr. Rev. 73 (1), 12–21. doi:10.1093/nutrit/nuu001.

Barker, D.J.P. (Ed.), 1992. Fetal and Infant Origins of Adult Disease. London, BMJ Books.

Belbasis, L., Savvidou, M.D., Kanu, C., Evangelou, E., Tzoulaki, I., 2016. Birth weight in relation to health and disease in later life: an umbrella review of systematic reviews and meta-analyses. BMC Med. 14 (1), 147. doi:10.1186/s12916-016-0692-5.

Bookari, K., Yeatman, H., Williamson, M., 2017. Informing nutrition care in the antenatal period: pregnant women's experiences and need for support. Biomed Res. Int. 2017, 4856527. Available from: https://www.hindawi.com/journals/bmri/2017/4856527/cta/.

Bove, F., Shim, Y., Zeitz, P., 2002. Drinking water contaminants and adverse pregnancy outcomes: a review. Environ. Health Perspect. 110 (Suppl. 1), 61–74.

Brummelte, S., Pawluski, J.L., Galea, L.A., 2006. High post-partum levels of corticosterone given to dams influence postnatal hippocampal cell proliferation and behavior of offspring: a model of post-partum stress and possible depression. Horm. Behav. 50, 370–382.

Burkhardt-Holm, P., 2010. Endocrine disruptors and water quality: a state-of-the-art review. Int. J. Water. Resour. Dev. 26, 477–493. doi:10.1080/07900627.2010.489298.

Calje, E., Skinner, J., 2017. The challenge of defining and treating anemia and iron deficiency in pregnancy: a study of New Zealand midwives' management of iron status in pregnancy and the postpartum period. Birth. 44, 181–190. doi:10.1111/birt.12282.

Callinan, S., Ferris, J., 2014. Trends in alcohol consumption during pregnancy in Australia. Int. J. Alcohol Drug Res. 3 (1), 17–24.

Cedergren, M.I., 2004. Maternal morbid obesity and the risk of adverse pregnancy outcome. Obstet. Gynecol. 103, 219–224.

Cefalo, R.C., Moos, M.K., 1995. Preconceptional Health Promotion: A Practical Guide, second ed. London; Mosby.

Chen, W., Srinivasan, S.R., Yao, L., Li, S., Dasmahapatra, P., Fernandez, C., et al., 2012. Low birth weight is associated with higher blood pressure variability from childhood to young adulthood: the Bogalusa Heart Study. Am. J. Epidemiol. 176 (Suppl. 7), S99–S105.

Cheyney, M., Moreno-Black, G., 2010. Nutritional counselling in midwifery and obstetric practice. Ecol. Food. Nutr. 49, 1–29.

Control of Substances Hazardous to Health Regulations (COSHH), 2002. Health and Safety Executive. Available from: https://www.hse.gov.uk/coshh/. Accessed 13 January 2020.

Coussons-Read, M.E., Okun, M.L., Nettles, C.D., 2007. Psychosocial stress increases inflammatory markers and alters cytokine production across pregnancy. Brain. Behav. Immun. 21 (3), 343–350.

Cremonese, C., Freire, C., De Camargo, A.M., De Lima, J.S., Koifman, S., Meyer, A., 2014. Pesticide consumption, central nervous system and cardiovascular congenital malformations in the South and Southeast region of Brazil. Int. J. Occup. Med. Env. 27 (3), 474–486.

Davies, L., Deery, R., 2014. Conversations about food. In: Davies, L., Deery, R., (Eds.), Nutrition in Pregnancy and Childbirth; Food for Thought. London, Routledge.

Day, J., Savani, S., Krempley, B.D., Nguyen, M., Kitlinska, J.B., 2016. Influence of paternal preconception exposures on their offspring: through epigenetics to phenotype. Am. J. Stem. Cells. 5 (1), 11–18. Available from: www.AJSC.us/ISSN:2160-4150/AJSC0030217.

Dean, S.V., Lassi, Z.S., Imam, A.M., Bhutta, Z.A., 2014. Preconception care: closing the gap in the continuum of care to accelerate improvements in maternal, newborn and child health. Reprod. Health. 11 (Suppl. 3), S1.

De-Regil, L.M., Peña-Rosas, J.P., Fernandez-Gaxioloa, A.C., Rayco-Solon, P., 2015. Effects and safety of periconceptional oral folate supplementation for preventing birth defects. *The Cochrane Database of Systematic Reviews* (12): CD007950. doi:10.1002/14651858.

De-Regil, L.M., Palacios, C., Lombardo, L.K., Peña-Rosas, J.P., 2016. Vitamin D supplementation for women during pregnancy. Cochrane Database Syst Rev, (1), CD008873. doi:10.1002/14651858.CD008873.pub3.

Devries, K.M., Kishor, S., Johnson, H., Stöckl, H., Bacchus, L.J., Garcia-Moreno, C., et al., 2010. Intimate partner violence during pregnancy: analysis of prevalence data from 19 countries. Reprod. Health. Matters 18 (36), 158–170.

Diabetes UK, 2018. Nearly 7,000 children and young adults with Type 2 diabetes. Available from: https://www.diabetes.org.uk/about-us/news/children-young-adults-type-2-rise. Accessed 23 January 2019

Duncan, L.G., Cohn, M.A., Chao, M.T., Cook, J.G., Riccobono, J., Bardacke, N., 2017. Benefits of preparing for childbirth with mindfulness training: a randomized controlled trial with active comparison. BMC Pregnancy Childbirth 17, 140. doi:10.1186/s12884-017-1319-3.

EPA, 2017. Regulatory Information by Topic. Toxic Substances. Available from: https://www.epa.gov/regulatory-information-topic/regulatory-information-topic-toxic-substances. Accessed February 2019.

Faisal-Cury, A., Menezes, P.R., 2012. Antenatal depression strongly predicts postnatal depression in primary health care. Braz. J. Psychiatry. 34, 446–450.

France, K.E., 2011. Creating persuasive messages to promote abstinence from alcohol during pregnancy. PhD thesis Edith Cowan University. Available from: https://ro.ecu.edu.au/cgi/viewcontent.cgi?referer=https://www.google.co.nz/&httpsredir=1&article=1414&context=theses. Accessed April 2019.

Gibbard, B. 2009. Extent and impact on child development. In E. Jonsson, L Dennett, G Littlejohn (eds). Fetal Alcohol Spectrum Disorder (FASD): Across the lifespan. Alberta, Canada: Institute of Health Economics.

Gluckman, P., Hanson, M., Seng, C.Y., Bardsley, A., 2015. Nutrition and Lifestyle for Pregnancy and Breastfeeding. Oxford University Press, Oxford.

Goodfellow, A., Frank, J., McAteer, J., Rankin, J., 2017. Improving preconception health and care: a situation analysis. BMC Health Serv. Res. 17, 595. doi:10.1186/s12913-017-2544-1.

Göransson, M., Faxelid, E., Heilig, M., 2004. Beliefs and reality: detection and prevention of high alcohol consumption in Swedish antenatal clinics. Acta Obstetricia et Gynecologica Scandinavica, 83: 796–800. doi:10.1111/j.0001-6349.2004.00461.x.

Hales, C.N., Barker, D.J., 2001. The thrifty phenotype hypothesis. Br. Med. Bull. 60, 5–20.

Hobel, C.J., Dunkel-Schetter, C., Roesch, S.C., Castro, L.C., Arora, C.P., 1999. Maternal plasma corticotropin-releasing hormone associated with stress at 20 weeks' gestation in pregnancies ending in preterm delivery. Am. J. Obstet. Gynecol. 180 (1 Pt 3), S257–S263.

ICRP Publication 132, 2016. Radiological protection from cosmic radiation in aviation. ANN. ICRP 45 (1), 1–48.

Infante-Rivard, C., 2004. Drinking water contaminants, gene polymorphisms, and fetal growth, Environ. Health. Perspect. 112 (11), 1213–1216.

Jesurasa, A., 2018. Making the Case for Preconception Care. Public Health England. Available from: https://assets. publishing.service.gov.uk/government/uploads/system/ uploads/attachment_data/file/729018/Making_the_case_ for_preconception_care.pdf. Accessed January, 2020.

Jornayvaz, F.R., Vollenweider, P., Bochud, M., Mooser, V., Waeber, G., Marques-Vidal, P., 2016. Low birth weight leads to obesity, diabetes and increased leptin levels in adults: the CoLaus study. Cardiovasc. Diabetol. 15, 73. doi:10.1186/s12933-016-0389-2. Accessed January 2019.

Kalkhoran, S., Glantz, S.A., 2016. E-cigarettes and smoking cessation in real-world and clinical settings: a systematic review and meta-analysis. Lancet Respir Med. 4 (2), 116–128. doi:10.1016/S2213-2600(15)00521-4.

Karmaus, W., Wolf, N., 1995. Reduced birthweight and length in the offspring of females exposed to PCDFs, PCP, and lindane. Environ. Health. Persp. 103 (12), 1120–1125.

Kingston, D., Austin, M.P., Veldhuyzen van Zanten, S., Harvalik, P., Giallo R., McDonald, S.D., et al., 2017. Pregnant women's views on the feasibility and acceptability of web-based mental health E-screening versus paper-based screening: a randomized controlled trial. J. Med. Internet. Res. 19 (4), e88. doi:10.2196/jmir.6866.

Larsen, A.E., Gaines, S.D., Deschênes, O., 2017. Agricultural pesticide use and adverse birth outcomes in the San Joaquin valley of California. Nat. Commun. 8, 302.

Lassi, Z.S., Salam, R.A., Haider, B.A., Bhutta, Z.A., 2013. Folic acid supplementation during pregnancy for maternal health and pregnancy outcomes. Cochrane Database Syst. Rev. (3), CD006896. doi:10.1002/14651858.CD006896.pub2.

Lewine, H., 2018, Drinking a little alcohol early in pregnancy may be OK. Harvard Health Publishing. https://www. health.harvard.edu/blog/study-no-connection-between-drinking-alcohol-early-in-pregnancy-and-birth-problems-201309106667

Madhavan Nair, K., Bhaskaram, P., Balakrishna, N., Ravinder, P., Sesikeran, B., et al., 2004. Response of hemoglobin, serum ferritin, and serum transferrin receptor during iron supplementation in pregnancy: a prospective study. Nutrition. 20 (10), 896–899.

Marsh-Prelesnik, J., Davies, L., 2007. The rhythm of life. In: Davies, L. (Ed.), The Art and Soul of Midwifery. Elsevier, Edinburgh.

May, P.A., Baete, A., Russo, J., Elliott, A.J. et al., 2014. Prevalence and characteristics of fetal alcohol spectrum disorders. Pediatrics 134(5), 855–866. doi: 10.1542/peds.2013-3319.

McCarthy, F.P., O'Keeffe, L.M., Khashan, A.S., North, R.A., Poston, L., McCowan, L.M., et al., 2013. Association between maternal alcohol consumption in early pregnancy and pregnancy outcomes. Obstet. Gynecol. 122 (4), 830–837. doi:10.1097/AOG.0b013e3182a6b226.

McCubbin, A., Fallin-Bennett, A., Barnett, J., Ashford, K., 2017. Perceptions and use of electronic cigarettes in pregnancy. Health Educ. Res. 32 (1), 22–32.

Milman, N.T., 2019. Dietary iron intake in women of reproductive age in Europe: A review of 49 studies from 29 countries in the period 1993–2015. Journal of Nutrition and Metabolism 2019, Article ID 7631306, https://doi. org/10.1155/2019/7631306.

Ministry of Health (MoH), 2015. Taking Action on Fetal Alcohol Spectrum Disorder (FASD): A Discussion Document. Ministry of Health, Wellington.

Miranda, M.L., Maxson, P., Edwards, S., 2009. Environmental contributions to disparities in pregnancy outcomes. Epidemiol. Rev. (1), 67–83.

Mund, M., Louwen, F., Klingelhoefer, D., Gerber, A., 2013. Smoking and pregnancy—a review on the first major environmental risk factor of the unborn. Int. J. Environ. Res. Public Health 10, 6485–6499. doi:10.3390/ ijerph10126485.

Murray, L., Halligan, S., Cooper, P., 2010. Effects of postnatal depression on mother–infant interactions and child development. In: Bremner, J.G., Wachs T.D. (Eds.), The Wiley-Blackwell Handbook of Infant Development. Wiley-Blackwell, Chichester.

Nathanielsz, P.W., Berghorn, K.A., Derks. J.B., et al., 2003. Life before birth: effects of cortisol on future cardiovascular and metabolic function. Acta. Paediatr. Scand. 92 (7), 766–772.

NHS, 2018. Statistics on women's smoking status at time of delivery- England 2nd Quarter 2017-18. Available from: https://digital.nhs.uk/data-and-information/publications/ statistical/statistics-on-women-s-smoking-status-at-time-of-delivery-england/statistics-on-womens-smoking-status-at-time-of-delivery-england-quarter-2-july2018-to-september-2018/part-2. Accessed March 1, 2019.

O'Connor, T.G., Bergman, K., Sarkar, P., Glover, V., 2013. Prenatal cortisol exposure predicts infant cortisol response to acute stress. Dev. Psychobiol. 55 (2), 145–155. doi:10.1002/dev.21007.

O'Keane, V., Marsh, M.S., 2007. Depression during pregnancy. BMJ. 334 (7601), 1003-1035.

Opray, N., Grivell, R.M., Deussen, A.R., Dodd, J.M., 2015. Directed preconception health programs and interventions for improving pregnancy outcomes for women who are overweight or obese. Cochrane Database Syst Rev (7), CD010932. doi:10.1002/14651858.CD010932. pub2.

Palacios, C., Kostiuk, L.K., Peña-Rosas, J.P., 2019. Vitamin D supplementation for women during pregnancy. Cochrane Database of Systematic Reviews 2019, Issue 7. Art. No.: CD008873. DOI: 10.1002/14651858.CD008873.pub4.

Parackal, S., Parackal, M., Ferguson, E., et al., 2006. Awareness of the effects of alcohol use during pregnancy among New Zealand women of childbearing age. A report submitted to the Alcohol Advisory Council and Ministry of Health. University of Otago. https://www.alcohol.org.nz/sites/default/files/documents/Hazards%20of%20alcohol%20use%20while%20pregnant.pdf.

Paterson, H., Hay-Smith, E.J.C., Treharne, G.J., 2016. Womens experiences of changes in eating during pregnancy: a qualitative study in Dunedin. New Zealand. Aust. N. Z. J. Ment. Health Nurs. (52), 5–11.

Peadon, E., Payne, J., Henley, N., D'Antoine, H., Bartu, A., O'Leary, C., 2010. Women's knowledge and attitudes regarding alcohol consumption in pregnancy: a national survey. BMC Public Health 10, 510.

Pearson, R.M., Carnegie, R.E., Cree, C., Rollings, C., Rena-Jones, L., Evans, J., et al., 2018. Prevalence of prenatal depression symptoms among 2 generations of pregnant mothers: the avon longitudinal study of parents and children. JAMA. Netw. Open. 1 (3), e180725. doi:10.1001/jamanetworkopen.2018.0725.

Pineles, B.L., Park, E., Samet, J.M., 2014. Systematic review and meta-analysis of miscarriage and maternal exposure to tobacco smoke during pregnancy. Am. J. Epidemiol. 179 (7), 807–823.

Quarini, C., Pearson, R.M., Stein, A., Ramchandani, P.G., Lewis, G., Evans, J., 2016. Are female children more vulnerable to the long-term effects of maternal depression during pregnancy? J. Affect. Disord. 189, 329–335.

Randall, M., 2015. The Physiology of Stress: Cortisol and the Hypothalamic-Pituitary-Adrenal Axis. DUJS Online. Available from: http://dujs.dartmouth.edu/fall-2010/the-physiology-of-stress-cortisol-and-the-hypothalamic-pituitary-adrenal-axis. Accessed March 2019.

Rodríguez-Rodríguez, P., Ramiro-Cortijo, D., Reyes-Hernández, C.G., López de Pablo, A.L., González, M.C., Arribas, S.M., 2018. Implication of oxidative stress in fetal programming of cardiovascular disease. Front. Physiol. 9, 602. doi:10.3389/fphys.2018.00602.

Rönn, T., Volkov, P., Davegårdh, C., Dayeh, T., Hall, E., Olsson, A.H., et al., 2013. A six months exercise intervention influences the genome-wide DNA methylation pattern in human adipose tissue. PLOS Genet. 9 (6), e1003572. doi:10.1371/journal.pgen.1003572.

Roseboom, T.J., van der Meulen, J.H., Ravelli, A.C., Osmond, C., Barker, D.J., Bleker, O.P., 2001. Effects of prenatal exposure to the Dutch famine on adult disease in later life: an overview. Twin. Res. 4 (5), 293–298.

Saina, E.J., Kennedy, N., Odima, N., Otara, A.M., 2017. Levels of awareness on safety and health in use of agro-chemicals among large scale flower farm workers in Uasin Gishu County. Kenya. Res. Humanit. Soc. Sci. 7 (13) 14.

Sandman, C.A., Davis, E.P., Glynn L.M., 2012. Psychobiological Stress and Preterm Birth, Preterm Birth—Mother and Child. In: Morrison, D.J. (Ed.), InTech. Accessed March 1, 2019. Available from: http://www.intechopen.com/books/preterm-birth-mother-and-child/psychobiological-stress-and-preterm-birth.

Schetter, D.C., Tanner, L., 2012. Anxiety, depression and stress in pregnancy: implications for mothers, children, research, and practice. Curr. Opin. Psychiatry 25 (2), 141–148.

Scholl, T.O., 2011. Maternal iron status: relation to fetal growth, length of gestation, and iron endowment of the neonate. Nutr. Rev. 69, S23–S29.

Schröter, H., 2010. Fetal alcohol spectrum disorder: diagnostic update. Paediatr Child Health. 15 (7), 455–456.

Shahtahmasebi, S. 2003. The correlates of teenage smoking: some problems with interpreting the evidence. Int J Adolesc Med Health. 15(4), 3073–320.

Skogerbø, Å., Kesmodel, U.S., Wimberley, T., Støvring, H., Bertrand, J., Landrø, N.I., et al., 2012. The effects of low to moderate alcohol consumption and binge drinking in early pregnancy on executive function in 5-year-old children. BJOG: Int J. Obstet. Gynaecol. 119, 1201–1210. doi:10.1111/j.1471-0528.2012.03397.x.

Siegelman, C., Rider, E.A., 2014. Life-Span Human Development. Wadsworth Cengage Learning, Boston MA.

Sinead, M.C., Cameron, S.T., 2015. Social issues of teenage pregnancy. Obstet. Gynaecol. Reprod. Med. 25 (9), 243–248.

Simmons, D., 2008. Epigenetic Influences and Disease. Nature Educ. 1 (1), 6.

Slykerman, R.F., Thompson, J.M., Pryor, J.E., Becroft, D.M., Robinson, E., Clark, P.M., et al., 2005. Maternal stress, social support and pre-school children's intelligence. Early. Hum. Dev. 81, 815–821.

Stewart, D.E., Robertson, C., Robertson, E., et al. 2003. Postpartum depression: literature review of risk factors and interventions Toronto Public Health: University Health Network Women's Health Program. Accessed March 2019. Available from: https://www.who.int/mental_health/prevention/suicide/lit_review_postpartum_depression.pdf.

Stone, R., 2015. Pregnant women and substance use: fear, stigma, and barriers to care. Health Justice. 3:2. https://www.ncbi.nlm.nih.gov/pmc/articles/PMC5151516/.

Subbaraman, M.S., Roberts, S.C.M., 2019. Costs associated with policies regarding alcohol use during pregnancy: results from 1972-2015 vital statistics. PLoS ONE 14 (5), e0215670. doi:10.1371/journal.pone.0215670.

Suderman, M., Borghol, N., Pappas, J.J., Pinto Pereira, S.M., Pembrey, M., Hertzman, C., et al., 2014. Childhood abuse is associated with methylation of multiple loci in adult DNA, BMC Med. Genomics. 7, 13. doi:10.1186/1755-8794-7-13.

Tong, V.T., Farr, S.L., Bombard, J., D °Angelo, D., Ko, J.Y., England, L.J., 2016. Smoking before and during pregnancy among women reporting depression or anxiety. Obstet. Gynecol. 128 (3), 562–570.

Touraud E., Roig B, Sumpter J.P., Coetsier, C., 2011. Drug residues and endocrine disruptors in drinking water: Risk for humans? Int. J. Hyg. Environ. Health. 214, 437–441.

Van Teijlingen, E.R., Wilson, B., Barry, N., 1998. Effectiveness of interventions to promote healthy eating in pregnant women and women of childbearing – a review. Health Education Authority (HEA), London

Warren, C.W., Lea, V., Lee, J., Jones, N.R., Asma, S., McKenna M., 2009. Change in tobacco use among 13–15 year olds between 1999 and 2008: findings from the global youth tobacco survey. Glob. Health Promot. 16, 38–90.

Weerth, C., Buitelaar, J.K., 2005. Cortisol awakening response in pregnant women. Psychoneuroendocrinology 30, 902–907.

Wellings, K., Jones, K.G., Mercer, C.H., Tanton, C., Clifton, S., Datta, J., et al., 2013. The prevalence of unplanned pregnancy and associated factors in Britain: findings from the third National Survey of Sexual Attitudes and Lifestyles (Natsal-3). Lancet 382 (9907), 1807–1816.

Williamson, C.S., 2006. Nutrition in pregnancy. Nutri. Bul.31 (1), 28–59.

Whittington, J.R., Simmons, P.M., Phillips, A.M., Gammill, S.K., Cen, R., Magann, E.F., et al., 2018. The use of electronic cigarettes in pregnancy: a review of the literature. Obstet. Gynecol. Surv. 73 (9), 544–549. doi:10.1097/OGX.0000000000000595.

Worland, J., 2015. Why 'BPA Free' may be meaningless. Time Magazine. Available from: http://time.com/3742871/bpa-free-health/.

Zacharasiewicz, A., 2016. Maternal smoking in pregnancy and its influence on childhood asthma. ERJ Open Res. 2 (3), 00042-2016. doi:10.1183/23120541.00042-2016.

6

Maternal and Newborn Transition: Adjustment to Extrauterine Life

Lorna Davies and Julie Richards

CHAPTER CONTENTS

INTRODUCTION

For a moment, imagine you are attending a birth. As the baby makes its way from the supportive sanctuary of the intrauterine world, imagine what they might need in order to maximize the ease of transition to the extrauterine environment they are about to encounter.

From the evidence we now have, it is probable that the baby would ask to be born into a warm environment with as little sensory stimulation as possible, with no bright lights or loud noises to startle. In ideal circumstances, the baby would remain with its mother and would be able to enjoy immediate skin-to-skin contact. The baby would spend this early period making eye contact with its mother, listening to the familiar tones of her voice, gaining a recognition of her own unique scent. After about 45 minutes or so, the baby would negotiate a way to its mother's breast by wriggling up her abdomen, activating an ancient knowledge of survival by touching, smelling, licking and usually latching on to the breast for the first feed (Buckley, 2015). Following this, a few hours' sleep might be required to recover from the hard work of being born.

This process demands little physical action on the part of the midwife, who will be able to observe quietly and assess both mother and baby as they commence their 'babymoon'; she may be watching expectantly for the arrival of the placenta. Without active intervention, she will ensure the baby is making the anticipated responses, is alert, and has good colour and tone. She is confident that the baby is warm enough because the room feels warm. She has placed a warm dry towel over the baby, and the mother is providing an optimal thermoregulatory environment by providing skin-to-skin contact. There is no sense of urgency. The initial physical examination of the newborn, and other tasks such as weighing the baby, can be undertaken at a later stage. For the time being, the most important thing is that mother and baby are able to initiate this important stage in the process of attachment. If left well alone, everything else will follow the 'species-specific sequence of events' that the human race has evolved over many millennia (Bergman, 2005).

Within this biological econiche, the baby is able to make certain crucial physiological adaptations in order to initiate breathing and maintain regular respirations. This optimal habitat will also facilitate effective thermoregulation and regulation of metabolic processes, allow the baby access to adequate nutrition, and to eliminate waste and ward off infection.

Clearly, the midwife must have a sound knowledge and understanding of the physiological processes in order to facilitate a safe transition. She will need to be able to use appropriate assessment and to intervene where necessary if, for example, resuscitation measures are needed (Chapter 7). This paradigm, however, is not predicated on a belief that safety and sanctity are mutually exclusive concepts. On the contrary, if there is nothing to make it unsafe, and the sanctity of the birth and the hours following it are honoured, then for the vast majority of the time, safety will accompany sanctity.

By respecting this sanctity and by having a comprehensive understanding of the complex physiology, the attending midwife will play an important and 'actively passive' role in fortifying the mother–baby dyad.

AN INTEGRATED APPROACH: THE MOTHER–BABY DYAD

The first hour after birth sees a carefully synchronized series of physiological events that enable stabilization in both mother and baby, as well as furthering the process of attachment that has hopefully already started in pregnancy. For this reason, the hour after birth is referred to by some as the golden hour (Lerner and Moscati, 2001). The immediate 3- to 4-hour postpartum period following the birth of the placenta has popularly been embraced as the fourth stage of labour (Kaur, Kaur and Saha, 2014) although others have referred to the first few months as the fourth trimester (Karp, 2003). The concept of a fourth trimester, be it 1 hour, several hours or even several months, implies a continuum which bridges the internal and external worlds of the newborn. It is a recognition that the baby does have to undertake profound physiological changes in order to initiate a life independent of its mother—but equally that the dependence of the baby on its mother does not cease immediately with the first breath and the birth of the placenta. The mother continues to meet the needs of her baby as she did when the baby was encased within the membranes and amniotic fluid. Her body will continue to provide the baby with nourishment, as the breast replaces the placenta in this role, and will provide an environment to assist the baby in making the required metabolic adaptations by keeping it warm, ensuring a more regular breathing rate and stable heart rate, and by increasing oxygenation saturation (Hunt, 2008).

We acknowledge that, at first glance at least, this ideal may not be possible for every mother and baby. Among many other reasons, it may be that the mother has had a caesarean birth, given birth to a sick or preterm baby, or that she feels a sense of ambivalence after a long and arduous labour. However, we must always consider what value the ideal transitional environment has to offer, and the significance of the state of sanctity, which should ideally always be observed. Then, as caregivers, we may be better able to understand the huge significance of this time, and find creative ways of ensuring that the baby, in less than optimal circumstances, is given as much opportunity as possible to reap the benefits of a physiologically sound start in life.

NEONATAL ENERGY TRIANGLE

If the baby is unable to make the necessary physiological adaptations because of illness or prematurity, then a variety of interventions may be employed. These may include assisted ventilation, placing the baby in an incubator, monitoring blood glucose levels and introducing supplementary feeds. However, these interventions are sometimes introduced without a sound rationale, or are required because of iatrogenic effects. Some of the practices that we carry out as professionals do not necessarily aid in facilitating ideal conditions during this crucial time of changeover; some may even actively hinder a successful transition. The irony is that the innate survival mechanisms of the newborn ensure that the baby will usually overcome the hurdles we may unintentionally create—in spite of, not because of, the things we do 'to' and 'for' them in the first few minutes and hours of life.

Practices such as early cord clamping (which, although decreasing in prevalence, still occurs) and unnecessary separation of mother and baby may, as we will see, contribute to a less than optimal start in life.

Aylott (2006) talks about the *neonatal energy triangle*. This provides a logical yet integrated overview of the three physiological needs that must be met in order for the newborn baby to transition successfully from fetal to extrauterine life, and of the three most common difficulties encountered: hypothermia, hypoxia and hypoglycaemia.

These three conditions can be categorized as independent from one another, but they are equally interrelated as events that can threaten to disturb the successful transition of the newborn (Aylott, 2006).

The glycaemic status of the newborn, its thermoregulatory mechanism, and efficient respiratory functioning are vital physiological functions that are inextricably interrelated. Body temperature, blood glucose levels and oxygen concentrations adapt according to the requirements of the body during a normal state of health. 'Adequate amounts of oxygen and glucose are essential for normal cellular metabolism, and a neuro-thermal state is required for the successful functioning of the enzymatic systems that regulate cellular function' (Aylott, 2006).

If we simply consider these three physiological processes as discrete occurrences in an attempt to make them easier to understand, we may inadvertently subject the baby to unnecessary interventions. Conversely, the result may be an oversimplification, leading to a lack of recognition when problems do occur and a subsequent failure to offer appropriate intervention. These functions are closely interrelated and vital, as an integrated unit, to the successful transition from uterine to extrauterine life.

In order to understand fully why many routine practices may influence neonatal health, both advertently and inadvertently, it is necessary to revisit the physiology of the newborn, and then to relate that to practice.

CARDIORESPIRATORY TRANSITION

In spontaneous physiological birth, the baby's transition from fetus to newborn is designed to be gentle and supportive. The maintenance of the placental circulation via a pulsating umbilical cord provides circulatory and respiratory support, enabling the newborn to gradually achieve the significant physiological changes required at birth (Mercer and Skovgaard, 2002).

Over the last decade, research on the timing of cord clamping has confirmed physiological benefits for the newborn of deferring the process. These benefits relate to the transfer of oxygenated blood from the placenta to the newborn through the maintenance of a patent umbilical cord (McDonald et al., 2013). The physiological changes that occur during the transition from intrauterine to extrauterine life will be discussed from this perspective.

Fetal Circulation

During intrauterine life, the fetus is distinctly separate from, yet completely supported by, the mother's physiological processes. Blood, flowing through an effectively functioning placenta and umbilical cord, provides the transport medium for oxygen and nutrients to support growth and development, and permits the elimination of waste products via the maternal circulation. The presence of fetal haemoglobin supports the fetus to extract oxygen effectively from the maternal circulation across the placenta. Fetal blood contains mostly fetal haemoglobin (HbF) which has a higher affinity for oxygen than neonatal or adult haemoglobin and is at a higher concentration (180–200 g/l, compared with adult levels of 140–175 g/l). The higher oxygen affinity of HbF supports the binding of more oxygen from the maternal circulation; the higher concentration supports fetal perfusion (McEwan, 2017). Fetal haemoglobin also enables oxygenation of the fetus at a lower oxygen saturation than that of the neonate. Oxygen saturation values vary from 85% in blood received directly from the placenta via the umbilical vein through to 35% as the blood returns to the placenta via the abdominal inferior vena cava and umbilical arteries (Kiserud and Acharya, 2004). High-oxygen blood is blended and shunted to the organs of greatest need, with the coronary arteries and brain receiving the highest saturations (Singh and Tissot, 2018).

Prior to birth, the fetal cardiovascular system (Fig. 6.1) is a complex parallel process facilitated by various structures and shunts, whereas following birth, it becomes a sequential series of steps (Singh and Tissot, 2018). There are three fetal haemodynamic structures within the fetal circulation: the ductus venosus, foramen ovale and ductus arteriosus. These structures assist in distributing oxygenated blood from the maternal circulation around

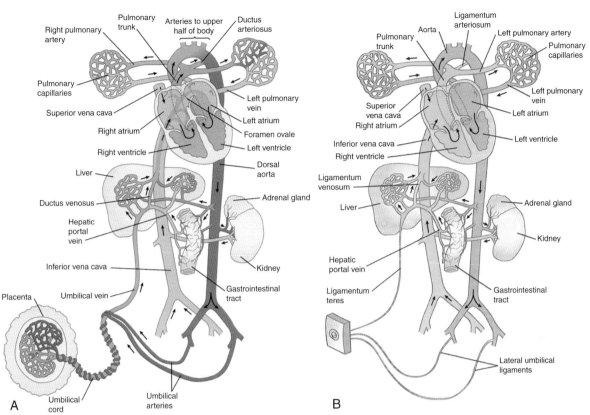

Fig. 6.1 Fetal Circulation.

the fetal body, creating a unique and flexible system to support intrauterine life and also preparing the fetus for extrauterine life (Kiserud and Acharya, 2004).

The *ductus venosus* connects the umbilical vein to the inferior vena cava (IVC) prior to entering the heart, shunting well-oxygenated umbilical blood away from the liver towards the right atrium (Kiserud and Acharya, 2004). Within the IVC, the well-oxygenated blood has a higher kinetic energy than the less oxygenated blood returning from the lower body. This results in the well-oxygenated blood forcing open the *foramen ovale*, a vertical opening between the two atria, and entering the left atrium, thus avoiding the pulmonary circulation. This same blood is then pumped into the aorta, where it is prioritized to the brain and heart. The less oxygenated blood coming from the IVC is directed to the right atrium, then the right ventricle, and flows into the pulmonary artery. The *ductus arteriosus*, a wide muscular vessel, creates a connection between the pulmonary artery and the aorta, redirecting 90% of this less oxygenated blood to the aorta, with only 10% entering the

pulmonary circulation. Prostaglandin and nitric oxide maintain the patency of the ductus arteriosus, which is particularly vulnerable to prostaglandin antagonists in the third trimester (Singh and Tissot, 2018; Kiserud and Acharya, 2004).

In utero, one-third of the blood of a full-term fetus and one-half that of a preterm fetus is in the placenta for gas exchange with the maternal circulation. The total fetoplacental blood volume is estimated to be between 105 and 115 ml/kg (Linderkamp, 1982; Yao, Moinian and Lind, 1969). The placenta requires 40% to 50% of the fetal cardiac output per minute, with the lungs requiring only 10% (Singh and Tissot, 2018; Mercer and Erickson-Owens, 2012). The haemodynamic structures in the fetal circulation redirect blood away from the lungs because cardiac output requirements are minimal during fetal life.

At term, the fetal lungs contain approximately 30 ml/kg of fluid. This fluid is produced by the lung epithelium and supports tissue growth and development (Hooper et al., 2010), as well as maintaining high resistance to blood flow, known as vascular resistance. In contrast, the placenta is a low-resistance system, maintaining low systemic vascular resistance (SVR) and ease of blood flow in the fetus (Kluckow and Hooper, 2015).

Haemodynamic Transition

In the moments immediately following birth, the cardiac output to the lungs must increase from 10% to between 45% and 55%, to perfuse the pulmonary vascular bed. In order to achieve this and maintain perfusion of the other organs, the newborn requires a transfusion of the blood within the placenta. This is achieved with an intact and unclamped umbilical cord, and ensures a blood volume containing red blood cells and stem cells is transferred. If the cord is clamped immediately, thereby eliminating access to the extra blood volume, the required blood will be redistributed from other areas of the newborn's circulation, making these organs vulnerable to underperfusion (Mercer and Erickson-Owens, 2012).

The intermittent high-pressure contractions around the time of birth and during the third stage of labour significantly increase the blood flow from placenta to baby (Katheria et al., 2017). Once the baby is born, the intact umbilical cord continues to provide blood volume for the significantly increased requirements of the pulmonary circulation (Kluckow and Hooper, 2015).

Lung aeration from respiration rapidly reduces pulmonary vascular resistance at birth, further increasing the pulmonary blood flow. This enables the newborn to switch its source of oxygenation and venous return from umbilical blood flow to the pulmonary circulation (Kluckow and Hooper, 2015). The blood flowing through the intact cord over the next 5 minutes (Farrar et al., 2010) continues to provide blood volume and oxygen to support a gentler transition to extrauterine life (Mercer and Skovgaard, 2002).

To further explain the haemodynamics: in the fetal circulation, oxygenated blood from the umbilical vein is prioritized to the left ventricle via the foramen ovale to firstly oxygenate the heart and brain (Singh and Tissot, 2018). If the umbilical cord is clamped soon after birth, the blood volume to the left ventricle is significantly reduced, decreasing cardiac output and resulting in fluctuating arterial pressure. The cerebral blood flow is most vulnerable during this time. Once respirations commence, pulmonary vascular resistance decreases significantly and pulmonary blood flow increases, providing the venous return to the left ventricle. This

reinstates cardiac output, but with less than ideal blood volume. If commencement of respiration is delayed, the newborn will become hypoxic as well as experiencing low cardiac output. During this time, the newborn is particularly vulnerable to hypoxic brain injury (Kluckow and Hooper, 2015).

It was previously thought that the umbilical arteries, which return blood to the placenta, constrict within a minute of birth, maintaining blood volume within the newborn, and that the umbilical vein remains open until the cord is white and flaccid (Mercer and Skovgaard, 2002). A 2015 study by Boere et al. challenged this belief, identifying that both umbilical and venous blood flow can be bidirectional and are more complex than first believed. The authors noted that breathing influenced venous blood flow, which only became continuous when breathing was established. Arterial blood flow was pulsatile and completed prior to cord pulsations ceasing. They concluded that placental transfusion was based on physiology and emphasized the importance of breathing being established before the cord was clamped (Boere et al., 2015).

Pulmonary Transition

The fetal lungs are prepared for breathing by the in utero presence of lung fluid, fetal breathing movements and the production of surfactant. Lung fluid volume supports lung compliance and is equivalent to the functional residual capacity (FRC) once respiration is established. Surfactant production increases from 32 weeks; surfactant acts as an interface between air and liquid through a monolayer lining, reducing the surface tension. Fetal breathing movements commence as early as 10 weeks, increasing with gestation and regulating lung fluid and the stretching of lung tissue. Fetal breathing movements decrease in frequency immediately before labour (Blackburn, 2007).

For breathing to occur at birth, the lungs are required to rapidly change their function from a 'wet' organ to a 'dry' organ for effective gas exchange. This change is assisted by a reduction in lung fluid in the days before labour and an increase in fetal glucocorticoids and thyroid hormones that readies the sodium absorption mechanism in the lung epithelium. The stress of labour raises fetal adrenaline levels, which triggers the sodium absorption mechanism, drawing fluid from the lungs through to the interstitial space (Vali et al., 2015). Recent animal studies demonstrate that most lung fluid absorption occurs with inspiration (van Vonderen et al., 2014), driving fluid from the airways to the adjacent lung tissue for absorption by the lymphatic and pulmonary circulations (Kluckow and Hooper, 2015). The 'vaginal squeeze' as the baby is born expels some upper respiratory tract fluid, although it is now recognized that progressive flexion of the fetus as labour progresses, rather than chest compression, is more likely to assist this (van Vonderen et al., 2014).

Multiple factors stimulate breathing at birth; these include cold, touch, recoil of the chest, changes in blood oxygen and carbon dioxide levels, and cord clamping (Blackburn, 2007).

The specific mechanisms responsible for the commencement of continuous breathing are not completely understood (Hillman, 2013; van Vonderen et al., 2014). Increased oxygenation immediately after birth appears to stimulate respiration, whereas hypoxia appears to weaken or remove respiratory drive. This is also evident in utero, where hypoxia inhibits breathing movements (van Vonderen et al., 2014). The baby becomes responsive to hypoxia and hypercapnia, similar to an adult, in the first hours following birth (Blackburn, 2007).

The newborn respiratory rate is irregular and ranges from 30 to 60 breaths per minute. The first breaths are deeper and longer, with short inspiration and longer expiration (Vali et al., 2015). The long expiration contributes to the FRC, which has been identified in animal studies to be mostly established over the first five breaths. Breath holding, crying and grunting, also known as expiratory braking, help to maintain FRC and prevent liquid moving back into the airways (van Vonderen et al., 2014). FRC creates an alveolar reservoir which contributes to the stabilisation of oxygen tension (PaO_2) and prevents lung collapse (Blackburn, 2007).

At birth, the oxygen saturation (SpO_2) of newborn blood reflects the physiologically lower oxygen saturation of fetal blood and will take several minutes to rise to normal extrauterine levels with the establishment of regular breathing. Oxygen saturation is a more accurate indication of effective physiological transition than colour assessment, due to its greater objectivity. Dawson et al. (2010) assessed the oxygen saturations at birth of infants who required no supplementary oxygen, reporting that the median length of time for a term newborn to reach ≥90% oxygen saturation was 8 minutes. Infants who were preterm or born by caesarean delivery took longer to reach this level (Dawson et al., 2010).

Maintaining placental blood flow with an intact umbilical cord enables the newborn to complete hemodynamic and respiratory transition with greater ease. There is now consensus from the multiple physiological studies that occurred in the last century (and more recent practice-based studies) that deferring cord clamping to enable placental transfusion supports the well-being of both full-term and preterm babies (McDonald et al., 2013; Rabe et al., 2012). The exact sequence of events for pulmonary transition with a patent umbilical cord is yet to be defined. Mercer and Skovgaard (2002) provide evidence that pulmonary blood flow, augmented by contractions, aids the opening of alveoli, which enables respiration, whereas Kluckow and Hooper (2015) cite alternative evidence demonstrating that lung ventilation lowers pulmonary vascular resistance, which increases pulmonary blood flow. Both sources of evidence are from animal studies because the invasive nature of the studies would make it unethical to undertake them on human newborns. Kluckow and Hooper refer to clamping the umbilical cord after lung ventilation has occurred as 'physiologically based cord clamping' instead of deferred or delayed cord clamping. There is now evidence to challenge the theory that placental transfusion can be guaranteed by timing alone (Boere et al., 2015).

Structural Cardiovascular Changes Following Birth

Following birth, intrauterine cardiovascular structures—the ductus venosus, foramen ovale and ductus arteriosus—become modified to support the newborn's extrauterine function. Perfusion of the lung vasculature and the removal of lung fluid reduces the pulmonary vascular resistance, and constriction of the umbilical blood flow increases systemic vascular resistance. These processes facilitate closure of these three structures (McEwan, 2017).

In utero, the ductus venosus shunted a significant proportion of the oxygenated blood from the umbilical vein to the inferior vena cava, bypassing the liver. This structure, and the umbilical vein, become closed relative to the umbilical blood flow or when the cord is clamped (Singh and Tissot, 2018).

The foramen ovale, a valvular opening between the two atria, remains patent in fetal circulation due to the flow of high–kinetic energy blood from the umbilical vein and a right atrial pressure higher than that of the left atrium. Following removal of the umbilical blood flow, increased lung perfusion at birth and establishment of respiration, the pressures in the two atria equalize, causing the foramen ovale valve to close (Singh and Tissot, 2018). This closure is functional and a patent foramen ovale may persist until pressures within the heart stabilize over the next 24 to 48 hours. Anatomical closure occurs by 2½ years of age (Blackburn, 2007).

In utero, the ductus arteriosus shunts the majority of the blood entering the pulmonary artery to the descending aorta, maintaining minimal blood flow to the lungs. Following birth, as PaO_2 rises with respiration and increased pulmonary blood flow, the ductus arteriosus, which is sensitive to oxygen, begins to constrict; this constriction maintains effective blood flow through the pulmonary circulation. Removal of the placenta also reduces the circulation of prostaglandins, further supporting closure (Singh and Tissot, 2018). Functional closure of the ductus arteriosus begins following birth and is complete in the majority of babies by 96 hours, with permanent anatomic closure by 2 to 3 months (Blackburn, 2007). The changes in these structures in the transition from fetus to newborn are summarized in Table 6.1.

Influences on Extrauterine Transfusion

Several practices during maternity care influence the amount of blood that is transferred from the placenta to the baby following birth; most of these relate to active management of the third stage of labour. These practices were frequently introduced without robust evidence to identify their effect on either mother or baby (Vali et al., 2015).

Timing of Cord Clamping

The point at which the cord is clamped, in relation to birth, can significantly affect the volume of blood transferred to the baby. Active management of the third stage of labour became common practice in the mid-20th century, with the aim of reducing postpartum haemorrhage. Immediate cord clamping, preventing any transfer of blood from the placenta to the baby after birth, was the first step in the procedure (McDonald et al., 2013). Farrar et al. (2010) undertook a study to estimate the amount of placental blood transfused to the baby following birth. They weighed 26 babies, with the cord intact, commencing immediately after birth. By

TABLE 6.1	Fetal and Neonatal Circulation	
System	**Fetal**	**Neonatal**
Pulmonary blood vessels	Receive 10% of cardiac output Minimal perfusion and constricted blood vessels with high vascular resistance Lungs contain fluid	Receive 40%–55% of cardiac output Increased blood volume, increasing perfusion, vasodilation of vessels and reducing vascular resistance Distended capillaries support alveoli structure and air entry Lung fluid absorbed into capillary circulation
Systemic blood vessels	Dilated with low resistance One-third of blood volume circulating through the placenta while two-thirds is in the term fetus Oxygen saturation 35%–85%	Increased systemic blood volume and blood pressure with completion of placental transfusion Increasing oxygen saturation
Ductus venosus	Connects umbilical vein to inferior vena cava Shunts well-oxygenated blood away from liver towards heart	Closure occurs with cord clamping
Ductus arteriosus	Wide muscular vessel connecting the pulmonary artery to the descending aorta Shunts up to 40% of cardiac output, bypassing the lungs	Blood flow through ductus arteriosus reduced due to increased left arterial pressure Closure triggered by increasing blood oxygen levels and decreasing prostaglandins
Foramen ovale	Opening between the left and right atrium to evenly distribute the flow of blood Enables highly oxygenated blood to pass directly into left atrium	Establishment of the pulmonary circulation and increased vascular resistance causes increased pressure in left atrium and closes the one-way valve

Adapted from London et al., 2003.

TABLE 6.2 **Effects of Placental Transfusion Following Birth on Human Neonatal Organ Systems**
Cardiovascular
Increased cardiac output
Increased blood pressure
Reduced bradycardia
Increased oxygen saturation
Pulmonary
Increased pulmonary blood flow
Increased lung fluid absorption
Central Nervous System
Increased cerebral blood flow
Reduced intracranial haemorrhage
Improved neurodevelopmental outcome
Haematological
Increased circulating blood volume
Increased red cell mass
Increased plasma volume
Increased stem cells

Adapted from Niermeyer and Velaphi, 2013.

converting weight to volume, they estimated that between 24 and 32 ml/kg of blood was transferred from the placenta, within 2 minutes for most babies but up to 5 minutes in some cases. This equated to between 30% and 40% more blood volume (83–110 ml mean volume) than if the cord had been clamped immediately. Although this was a small prospective observational study, it supports the findings of a much earlier randomized control trial (Yao et al., 1969); that study, of 111 newborns, measured an increase in blood volume of 19% by 1 minute and 32% by 3 minutes, with minimal change after this period. This study also measured a 60% increase in red blood cell volume in the newborn as a result of the placental transfusion.

Resuscitation

In most hospital environments, a need to resuscitate the baby has become a reason to clamp and cut the cord and transfer to the Resuscitaire, despite the documented benefits of the baby establishing respirations before cord clamping (Tissot and Singh, 2018; Kluckow and Hooper, 2015). Practitioners are now being encouraged to consider how they can resuscitate the respiratory-depressed newborn with the cord intact (Niermeyer and Velaphi,

2013; Hutchon, 2014; see also Chapter 7). An alternative way to obtain a rapid placental transfusion for the baby is umbilical cord milking or stripping. Current evidence suggests this technique provides similar benefits to delayed cord clamping without any apparent harm (Katheria et al., 2017; Mercer and Erickson-Owens, 2012) although the practice is yet to be widely adopted.

Position and Gravity

The position of the baby following birth, influenced by gravity, can affect the rate and volume of placental transfusion. Yao and Lind (1969) demonstrated that gravity impacts on the transfusion volume and rate, with babies held more than 10 cm above the introitus having smaller transfusions and those held more than 10 cm below the introitus having faster transfusions. If babies were held within 10 cm above or below the introitus, there was no difference compared to being at the introitus. Mercer and Erickson-Owens (2012) tell us that a baby placed on the maternal chest will require 5 minutes for a full placental transfusion because of its elevation above the introitus.

Use of Uterotonics

Uterotonic drugs do not appear to increase the volume of placental transfer to the baby. A 1968 study (Yao, Hirvensalo and Lind, 1968) divided women into two groups; after birthing their babies, one group was given intravenous methylergometrine at birth, and the other group after the cord was clamped. Placental transfusion in the group given methylergometrine at birth was essentially completed by 1 minute, compared with 3 minutes for the non-methylergometrine group. The volume of blood transferred was the same for both groups. In a smaller study by Farrar et al. (2010), intramuscular or intravenous oxytocin was administered to all women having either a vaginal birth or a caesarean delivery, before or after cord clamping. This study showed no difference in either the volume of placental transfusion between vaginal births and caesarean births, or the rate of transfer with oxytocin use compared with no oxytocin use. The authors note that the use of oxytocin, which is now commonly used in place of ergot alkaloid, may have influenced the different outcome with regard to rate of transfusion.

Stem Cell Collection

Stem cells are the body's early unspecialized cells, its ultimate repair system and one of nature's gifts to maintain well-being through life (Lawton, 2015). Fetal blood contains large numbers of stem cells. The important characteristic of a stem cell is its ability to self-renew multiple times while remaining unchanged, and its potential to differentiate into other types of cells in the body. Stem cells collected from the first stages of embryo development are termed totipotent or omnipotent, meaning they are completely unspecialized; they are the only cell type that can become any other cell, including placental cells. The stem cells in cord blood at birth are pluripotent (can develop into all cell types in the body) and multipotent (can develop into more than one cell type). At birth, haematopoiesis (the production of blood cells from stem cells) transfers from the liver to the bone marrow where the cells become more specialized, losing their pluripotent ability (Tolosa et al., 2010). The blood of preterm babies has a higher concentration of stem cells because of their immaturity (Mercer and Erickson-Owens, 2012).

It is the unique pluripotent ability of the stem cells in cord blood that has led to cord blood collection and banking. During our relatively short history of active management of the third stage of labour, umbilical cord blood has been generally considered a waste product and routinely discarded within the placenta (Armitage et al., 2006). This has been the rationale for the collection and efficient use of precious unused stem cells. Stem cells from cord blood have treated a variety of disorders including haematological, immunological, metabolic and oncological disorders, with a lower incidence of immune rejection because of their immaturity. Animal studies have also demonstrated that umbilical cord blood given to rats alleviates the neurological symptoms of cerebral palsy (Tolosa et al., 2010). It is important to acknowledge that most stem cell treatments are unlikely to be autologous (i.e., donor and recipient are the same person) because the disease process being treated would also be inherent within the stem cells. The probability of a donor having an autologous stem cell transplant in their life ranges from 1:400 to 1:200,000 (Sullivan, 2008).

Both Tolosa et al. (2010) and Lawton et al. (2015) acknowledge that if physiology were to be as unimpeded in human birth as it is with other mammals, the baby would receive a full complement of stem cells via the placental transfusion, as well as receiving the blood volume to support haemodynamic transition. It is recognized that the newborn's organs are not yet fully developed at birth; most newborn disease processes originate from development or immaturity. Tolosa (2010) suggests that a loss of stem cells could impact on newborn disease as well as diseases associated with aging.

Cord blood collection for storage and later use obtains between 50 and 200 ml of blood, with amounts less than 40 ml being discarded (Waller-Wise, 2011). Cord blood banks recognize that parents may want to delay umbilical cord clamping for their baby's benefit at birth; this significantly reduces the amount of cord blood collected after 60 seconds following birth and may result in the cord blood being discarded. A study by Ciubotariu et al. (2018) found that up to 46% of cord blood collections did not reach the required volume for banking when cord clamping was deferred for more than 1 minute.

There appears no doubt that stem cell transplants will support the health of many unwell people thanks to their unique ability to repair and renew almost any tissue. What is important, though, is that the current health of the newborn is not compromised to treat a potential illness in the future.

Benefits of Delayed or Deferred Cord Clamping

Numerous randomized controlled trials have now been undertaken to determine the effects of delaying cord clamping at birth compared with immediate cord clamping, and have demonstrated multiple benefits for both full-term and preterm babies (McDonald et al., 2013; Rabe et al., 2012). These benefits will be explored here in the context of both term and preterm babies.

Support of Physiological Transition

We have already seen the way in which the increased blood volume aids physiological transition at birth. The average blood volume transferred during placental transfusion is 30 ml/kg, leading to a transfer of around 105 ml in a 3500-g baby. On average, this represents 30% of the fetal–placental blood volume (Mercer and Erickson-Owens, 2012). Niermeyer and Velaphi (2013) describe how most organ systems in the body benefit from placental transfusion. These are identified in Table 6.1.

In the preterm baby (i.e., one born before 37 weeks), the overall effect is more profound; in one study, delayed cord clamping of 60 seconds or more resulted in a 32% reduced risk of mortality during the hospital stay (Fogarty, 2018). In another study, delayed cord clamping was also associated with a reduction in the risk of intraventricular haemorrhage, necrotizing enterocolitis and the need for blood transfusion (Rabe et al., 2012).

Increased Oxygenation and Decrease in Anaemia

Fetal blood has a higher haemoglobin count than adult blood; placental transfusion will increase the red blood cell volume by up to 60% when compared with immediate cord clamping (Yao et al., 1969). The increased red cell volume enhances oxygen carrying capacity during extrauterine transition and positively affects oxygen saturations (Fogarty, 2018). Placental transfusion contributes up to a further 75 mg of iron, which is extracted from the red blood cells after birth and stored as ferritin until required; this quantity of stored iron will meet growth and development requirements for 3 to 4 months longer than that which would follow immediate cord clamping (Mercer and Erickson-Owens, 2012). This is particularly significant for babies born to anaemic mothers, because the maternal transfer of iron during pregnancy will be reduced relative to their iron stores (van Rheenen and Brabin, 2004). Mercer and Erickson-Owens (2012) discussed a range of studies that identified iron deficiency in infancy as having long-term detrimental effects including social and emotional behaviour problems, decreased cognitive ability and poor school performance.

Increased Brain Myelin Content

Myelin-producing cells require iron for maturation and function. A recent trial by Mercer et al. (2018) identified increased brain myelin in babies who had delayed cord clamping compared with those who had immediate cord clamping. Newborns were randomized to immediate cord clamping (less than 20 seconds) or delayed cord clamping (5 minutes). Cord milking five times was used as a proxy for delayed cord clamping when required. At 4 months, infants in the delayed clamping group had significantly higher ferritin levels that correlated with increased myelin content in brain areas associated with motor, visual and sensory processing.

Risks of Delayed Cord Clamping

Opposition to delayed cord clamping has focused on the increased blood volume and red blood cell transfer, with concern that they may cause polycythaemia and hyperbilirubinaemia respectively (Saigal and Usher, 1977) and a generalized belief that the baby would become 'overtransfused'. Understanding of the benefits

of placental transfusion for the newborn, in particular those born prematurely, has been enhanced in recent years with our increased understanding of physiology. Over the last 20 years, multiple research trials have searched for any detrimental effects from delayed cord clamping. In one such study, there was an increase in the number of late clamped term babies requiring phototherapy for jaundice (4.36% compared with 2.74% for early clamped babies), although there was no increase in the presence of clinical jaundice (McDonald et al., 2013). Another study showed that for preterm infants, peak bilirubin levels were higher in the delayed cord clamping group, although there was no increase in the need for phototherapy (Rabe et al., 2012). Overall, any detrimental effects are considered minimal by comparison with the benefits of delayed cord clamping, although this will need to be weighed against the availability of resources for managing potential problems.

Clotting Mechanisms

A further potential benefit of delayed cord clamping is the impact on the baby's clotting factors. For many years, midwives have debated the need to give vitamin K to a newborn baby, and have questioned its effect on a finely balanced haematological system (see Chapter 15). The cord blood contains the full complement of clotting factors required at birth; it would seem logical that reducing the transfer of blood at birth by prematurely clamping the cord will reduce the amount of clotting factors. Bonnar et al. (1971) investigated the blood coagulation systems of both mother and baby immediately after birth and suggested that the process of normal birth activates the mother's and the baby's clotting and fibrinolytic systems. They also identified high levels of fibrinolytic activity in the baby, which may suggest a mechanism to ensure placental blood flow is maintained until complete.

Lotus Birth

In a physiologically managed birth, the cord is tied or clamped and cut following the delivery of the placenta. If the woman and her partner choose a lotus birth, they request that the cord is not cut but is left naturally to dry and separate at the umbilicus of the baby (Buckley, 2005). The placenta can be drained, dried, salted and wrapped and tucked in beside the baby.

This process supports placental transfusion in its purest form, because only the baby decides when the process is complete; this point will be individual to each baby, based on its physical condition at birth. The cord dries to a sinew by 48 hours, and separation at the umbilicus then occurs, usually between 3 and 10 days (Buckley, 2005).

The rationale for lotus birth is best understood through Eastern philosophy and its belief that our total being is made up of five bodies: physical, emotional, mental, etheric and spiritual. Vital energies flow through and around our bodies and are known as auras or chi. A strong auric field, extending around the physical body, is believed to preserve our integrity, while damage to the auric field is believed to weaken the immune system. Lotus birth is believed to support the continuum of life and honour the five bodies (Rachana, 2000).

METABOLIC TRANSITION

Although less dramatic than the changes occurring in the cardiopulmonary system, the metabolic adaptation at birth is equally complex and essential for survival. Colson (2002) believes that a thorough understanding of neonatal nutrition is key in the assessment of metabolic adaptive processes. Research has shown that patterns of metabolic adaptation differ depending on whether the baby is breastfed or artificially fed (Hawdon, 2016). O'Sullivan et al. (2015) state that this is largely ignored in the assessment of the newborn and that mixed feeding is common in the first week, even when the mother wants to breastfeed exclusively.

The metabolic adaptation involves intricate biochemical processes but for the majority of infants—those who are able to access, without restriction, their mother's colostrum, which is rich in medium- and long-chain fatty acids, lower in carbohydrate and perfectly designed to facilitate the transition—it will usually occur effortlessly (Colson, 2002).

A major stumbling block in the facilitation of this process is a perceived fear of hypoglycaemia on the part of health practitioners (Walker, 2015). This fear has resulted in unnecessary and untimely intervention, which can result in the supplementation of breastfeeding with artificial infant formula and even admission to neonatal intensive care units (NICU). Admission to NICU may decrease maternal confidence and consequently reduce the length of time for which she continues to breastfeed (Ericson, 2018).

The complex issue of the minimum safe level of blood glucose in the newborn—the value below which there is risk of long-term neurodevelopmental impairment—has been subject to extensive debate. As Stomnaroska-Damcevski et al. (2015) identify, 'overtreating neonatal hypoglycaemia and undertreating neonatal hypoglycaemia are poles with significant potential disadvantages'.

Yet there is no absolute universal definition of a 'normal' range for blood glucose values in the newborn. It is, however, established that blood glucose readings are influenced by birth weight, gestational age, feeding method and postnatal age (Murty and Ram, 2012).

It may be useful at this juncture to outline some of the biochemical events that facilitate this metabolic transition. Before birth, the fetus is reliant on its mother to supply its nutrients; no significant production of glucose by the fetus has been demonstrated (Ward Platt and Deshpande, 2005). The fetus prepares for the transition in the third trimester by storing glycogen, producing catecholamines and depositing brown and white fat. At birth, the blood glucose level of the baby is approximately 70% of that of the mother (American Diabetes Association, 2017).

Once the cord has ceased to provide the continuous transplacental supply of nutrients, the plasma insulin levels of the neonate fall as the hypothalamic–pituitary–adrenal axis switches on (Xiong and Zhang, 2013). As the plasma insulin levels decrease, plasma glucose levels increase. However, corresponding increases in the production of serum glucagon, growth hormone, cortisol and epinephrine create a counterregulatory effect to insulin diminution, allowing increased hepatic output by other means. This means that hepatic glycogen stores are mobilized (glycolysis) and hepatic synthesis of glucose from noncarbohydrate substrates (gluconeogenesis) ensues. These substrates, which include lactate, glycerol and amino acids, can be converted by glycolysis to pyruvate, enter the citric acid cycle and produce adenosine triphosphate (ATP), which acts as an energy source for the brain. These events augment the processes of lipolysis (mobilization of lipids stored in the adipose tissue) (Aylott, 2006). This means that for the first few days of life, blood glucose levels that would usually be considered low may be appropriate for healthy term babies of normal size and weight, particularly those who are breastfed (Hawdon, 2015).

An understanding of this physiological process confirms that transient neonatal hypoglycaemia is physiologically self-limiting in healthy term neonates, and is a

TABLE 6.3 Definitions of Hypoglycaemia in a Healthy Term Infant

Age of Neonate (Hrs After Birth)	Definition of Hypoglycaemia (mmol/l)
1–2	1.6
3–47	2.2
48–72	2.7

Adapted from Wight and Marinelli (2014).

TABLE 6.5 Categories of Infants Who May Be at Risk of Hypoglycaemia

Newborns weighing less than 2 kg or more than 4 kg
Infants born before 37 weeks' gestation
Small for gestational age, < 10th percentile for weight
Large for gestational age, > 90th percentile for weight
Babies with intrauterine growth restriction (IUGR)
Infants of mothers who are diabetic or have gestational diabetes
Newborns with suspected infections
Maternal drug treatment (e.g., beta-blockers and hypoglycaemic agents)
Intrapartum glucose administration
Newborns with symptoms suggestive of hypoglycaemia
Infants who experienced perinatal hypoxia
Hypothermia
Various syndromes (e.g., Beckwith–Wiedemann)

normal part of the adaptation process once the maternal glucose supply has been discontinued (Ward Platt and Deshpande, 2005). Practitioners should recognize that the early stages of metabolic adaptation in the normal term baby are characterized by active ketogenesis, and that the blood glucose levels of a healthy term neonate can be expected to be far lower than what we may consider to be 'normal' levels (Hawdon, 2015).

As previously stated, there does not appear to be a definitive consensus concerning the cut-off point differentiating normal blood glucose levels from hypoglycaemia in the neonate. There are guidelines, such as that included as Table 6.3 (Wight and Marinelli, 2014), which illustrates the initial fall and then rise of the neonatal blood glucose level during the early postnatal period. The signs of hypoglycaemia are nonspecific and are also associated with other common neonatal disorders (Table 6.4).

Healthy full-term infants born after a normal pregnancy and birth who do not display any of the symptoms

listed in Table 6.4 do not require screening or monitoring for hypoglycaemia. Blood glucose should not be measured too soon after birth, when levels are likely to be low in all babies. If the condition recurs or persists beyond 48 hours but is resolved by additional feeds, then a metabolic or endocrine disorder may be suspected; further steps should be taken to explore this possibility (Cornblath et al., 2000). Glucose reagent strips are not reliable and should not be used as the basis of a diagnosis. At least one laboratory value that is significantly low should be obtained when considering a diagnosis, but awaiting laboratory confirmation should not delay treatment in an infant with clinical signs (Table 6.5) (Sreenivasa et al., 2015).

HYPOTHERMIA

Thermoregulation is the ability to balance heat production and heat loss in order to maintain body temperature within a 'normal range'. This ability is very limited within the newborn. In utero, the fetus has no need to thermoregulate; it receives its heat from its mother, with its core and peripheral temperatures remaining fairly constant at 0.5°C higher than the maternal temperature (Asakura, 2004). At birth, however, the immaturity of its thermoregulatory system makes the infant vulnerable to changes of environmental temperature. Once born, wet and exposed, and often into a relatively cold

TABLE 6.4 Signs of Hypoglycaemia

High-pitched cry	Exaggerated Moro reflex	Tachypnoea/apnoea
Hypothermia	Irritability	Tachypnoea/apnoea
Poor temperature control	Lethargy	Abnormal eye movements
Sweating	Hypotonia	Tachycardia
Poor suck or refusal to feed	Seizures	Congestive heart failure
Tremors	Cyanosis	Respiratory distress

Adapted from British Association of Perinatal Medicine, 2017.

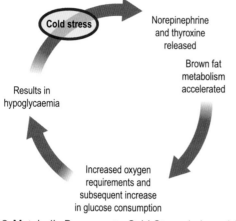

Fig. 6.2 Metabolic Response to Cold Stress (adapted from Aylott, 2006).

TABLE 6.6	Symptoms of Cold Stress	
Central cyanosis	Body cool to touch	CNS depression
Acrocyanosis	Abdominal distension	Bradycardia
Poor feeding	Increased gastric residuals	Tachypnoea
Irregular respirations	Decreased activity	Restlessness
Apnoea	Lethargy	Decreased reflexes
Mottling	Irritability	Hypotonia
Weak suck		Feeble cry
Hypoglycaemia		

environment, the baby rapidly loses heat if key actions are not undertaken immediately.

The physiological response to cold stress comprises a series of reactions including: non-shivering thermogenesis; the oxidation of brown adipose tissue (which is deposited after 28 weeks' gestation and is principally situated around the scapulae, kidneys, adrenals, neck and axillae); increased voluntary muscular activity; and vasoconstriction (Fig. 6.2). Disturbances in one or more of these elements of thermoregulation will result in an abnormal body temperature (Smith, J,. Alcock, G., Usher, K. 2013. Temperature measurement).

The healthy term baby will maintain this increased heat production for anything from a few minutes to a few hours, depending on the environmental conditions.

After this time, the energy stores of the baby will become depleted and reduced oxygen levels will soon result (Asakura, 2004).

The effects of cold stress demonstrate the interwoven relationships of the metabolic, cardiopulmonary and thermoregulatory mechanisms. This potentially detrimental state may result in an increased metabolic rate, leading to: increased oxygen consumption; increased energy expenditure and decreased glycogen stores; development of acidosis due to pulmonary vasoconstriction. The symptoms of cold stress are listed in Table 6.6. It may ultimately result in thermal shock which, if left untreated, can lead to death. Baumgart (2008) maintains that hypothermia is usually iatrogenic and there are many steps we can take to avoid it occurring. These are listed in Table 6.7.

TABLE 6.7	Steps to Avoid Hypothermia	
Forms of Heat Loss	**How to Avoid**
Evaporation: Loss of heat when water evaporates from the skin and respiratory tract	Dry the baby thoroughly after birth Remove wet towels
Convection: Heat loss to cooler surrounding air or fluid, dependent on air temperature and air movement	Place a hat on the baby's head Place skin to skin with mother, covering with a warmed blanket
Conduction: Heat loss to colder solid objects in direct contact with the body	Cover scales with warm cloth Warm hands and stethoscope prior to use Prewarm clothes, towels and linen
Radiation: Heat loss to surrounding colder solid objects not in direct contact with the body	Position cot away from wall, windows and draughts Ideally, do not bathe the baby for at least 24 hours

THE MICROBIOME

One significant development that has informed our understanding of newborn health, particularly during the transition from intrauterine to extrauterine life, is our greater understanding of the microbiome. In the 21st century, our knowledge of this complex entity has increased exponentially in a way that mirrors our emerging understanding of epigenetics. The composition of our microbiome has an extensive impact on our health and well-being throughout life by, for example, facilitating nutritional processes such as synthesizing vitamin K and detoxifying toxic elements within the enteral tract. The microbiome also assists in ensuring healthy metabolic functions and plays a key role in development of the immune system (Adams and Guttiérez, 2018). Impairment of the microbiome has been linked with the development of obesity, non-communicable disease and mental health conditions (Amon and Sanderson, 2017). Additionally, in the early-life gut maturation period of the neonate, the microbiome plays an important role in immune system development, which can also affect neurodevelopment (Dinan and Cryan, 2017).

What is the Microbiome?

Each of our bodies hosts a unique ecological community, or *microbiota*, composed of bacteria, bacteriophages, fungi, protozoa and viruses (Turnbaugh et al., 2007). The microbiota and its human host exist within a symbiotic relationship, sharing their exclusive biophysical environment. The collective genomes of the microbes are referred to as the microbiome. Each microbiome presents a collection of traits resulting from a series of complex interactions between the host and processes triggered by the microbiota, and creates what Dunn et al. (2017) have described as a composite 'human super-organism'. This is a system that has evolved over millennia and the symbiosis enables both host and microbes to reciprocate and thrive. Our microbiota is responsive to many factors including our genes, our culture, the food we eat, the medications we use, our age and our body mass index (BMI) (Wen and Duffy, 2017). All of these factors, and others, have the propensity to alter our microbiome—and with it, the potential to impact on our health and susceptibility to disease (Fig. 6.3).

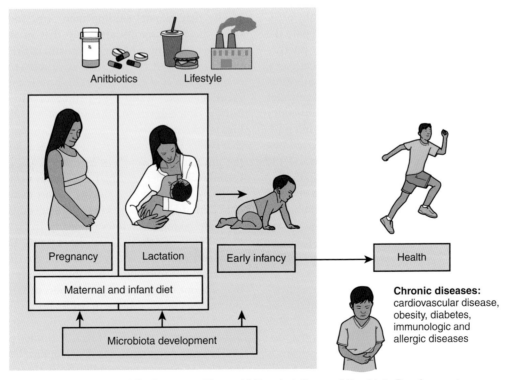

Fig. 6.3 Maternal Environment, Diet and Lifestyle Influence Microbiota Development.

The Development of the Microbiome

The development of our microbiome commences in fetal life (Collado et al., 2016) and the way in which we are born has the potential to shape both our early microbial exposure and our immune environment (Wen and Duffy, 2017). Unsurprisingly, perhaps, the initial 'microbial inoculate' received by a baby from its mother is different in every mother–baby pairing. However, it seems the inoculate is directly affected by the modality of birth. When babies are born by caesarean delivery, they are not exposed to their mother's vaginal and faecal microbes, as they would be if born vaginally. The gut environment of these babies is initially colonized by bacteria from the skin which may have an effect on the colonizing ability of other bacteria (Gritz and Bhandari, 2015). The diversity of microbial flora in babies born by caesarean has been reported as being less in the days following birth than that of those delivered vaginally (Rutayisire et al., 2016).

The inoculating or 'seeding' of the microbiome and the initiation of the early immune environment are naturally concurrent processes; the way a baby is born will not only shape the development of its microbiome but will also influence the integrity of its immune and sensitization systems (Renz et al., 2017). A healthy pregnancy and physiological birth both help to prepare the environment for further seeding in the early puerperium. When labour takes place as a physiological event, a number of antiinflammatory mechanisms are initiated. It would seem that the process of labour activates changes in the levels of endocrine and inflammatory factors, and this may impact on the maternal microbiome or the establishment of the neonatal microbiome (Renz et al., 2017). If labour does not occur and the woman has a planned caesarean delivery, the intrauterine responses do not ensue and this can affect the immune environment of the baby. By understanding the development of the early-life gut microbiota, we are able to access this short-lived window of opportunity to improve health outcomes for the baby, regardless of modality of birth.

In the complex landscape of maternity care, physiological birth is not always possible for a myriad of reasons too numerous to discuss here. However, it may be useful to view physiological childbirth as the 'default position' (Davies, 2017); this means that care is negotiated to ensure the pregnancy and birthing experience retain aspects that support physiology wherever possible, while staying within the accepted boundaries of the risk that necessitated the intervention. Such actions might include encouraging the woman to labour where possible even when caesarean delivery is essential, deferred cord clamping, and skin-to-skin contact in theatre.

Manual Seeding

A more controversial approach lies in the practice of manual seeding of the baby. This involves the transfer of some of the mother's vaginal and perianal microbiota to the baby, which theoretically serves to initiate colonization and promotes the establishment of a 'normal' infant microbiome (Dominguez-Bello et al., 2010). A sterile gauze is placed inside the woman's vagina about an hour before the planned caesarean delivery. This gauze is removed just prior to surgery, then used to swab the baby's mouth, face, hands, body and anus within a few minutes of birth. There has recently been a backlash to this practice (which was rapidly adopted by both health professionals and parents after being widely reported in the popular media). It has been argued that further robust evidence relating to efficacy and safety is needed before the practice can be sanctioned (Stinson et al., 2018). The controversy has been sparked by the possibility that manual seeding may carry some serious risks, the most significant being that of transferring pathogens that may be asymptomatic in the woman—such as Group B *Streptococcus* or *E coli*—to her baby (Cunnington et al., 2017). There is a clear counterargument that such transfer of pathogens can take place during vaginal birth and that we routinely monitor babies for the potential of infection. It can also be argued that babies who are born in the caul are not exposed to the microbial environment of the mother; should we, therefore, consider seeding these babies manually? It is probably fair to say that further robust evidence is required in order to ensure safety; to that end, at least two trials are taking place internationally. In New Zealand, Prof. Wayne Cutfield from the Liggins Institute in Auckland is leading a study 'Maternal bacteria to correct abnormal gut microbiota in babies born by C-section' that sets out to assess the effectiveness of seeding in restoring the gut microbiota in babies born this way. The babies and their stool samples are to be assessed at 1 day, 1 month, and 3 months of age. A similar prospective trial is being undertaken at Johns Hopkins University in the United States. The results from these two trials, however, will not be available for several years.

Antibiotics and Probiotics

Another factor that may assist in supporting healthy gut development in the baby is a judicious approach to the administration of antibiotics. It is well known that antibiotics disrupt the developing microbiome in the neonate and that the type, dose timing, and duration of the drug administration are influential in the degree of disruption (Berardi et al., 2018). The administration of intravenous antibiotics during caesarean delivery is a universal prophylactic measure; it is sometimes withheld until the umbilical cord has been clamped in order to minimize the exposure of the baby, but this is not an established practice in many instances (Renz et al., 2017). Consequently, the antibiotics are given the opportunity to cross the placenta and impact detrimentally on the development of the baby's microbiota. Requesting later rather than earlier administration may help to minimize this occurrence. Recognition of the importance of the neonate's microbiota has also spawned an interest in probiotic formulations of vaginal bacteria as a means of supporting a normal physiological process when intervention is required. To date, however, the only promising results available are from studies looking to mitigate the risks of necrotizing enterocolitis (NEC) in preterm babies (Olsen et al., 2016); there is little evidence that probiotics colonize the neonatal gut of healthy term infants, or influence infant health (Quin et al., 2018).

Breast Milk

Probiotics have been described as naturally fermented microbe-containing foods that can have a positive effect on health (McGuire and McGuire, 2015). It has been proposed that breast milk—particularly colostrum—meets this definition, and it certainly has many nutritional qualities that have been demonstrated to affect the microbiome of the neonate (Azad et al., 2016; Martin et al., 2012). Modification of host gene expression and the development of the immune system occur as a result of exposure to the live bacteria in breast milk (Kau et al., 2011). The supportive bacteria are derived not only from breast milk but also from the skin around the areola of the mother's nipple. The human milk oligosaccharides (HMOs) present in breast milk, whose action was unknown for many years, have been found to be metabolized by elements of the gut microbiota. The ingestion of breast milk is therefore likely to be a way of modifying some of the effects of caesarean birth on the microbiome of the newborn (Jost et al., 2015). Paradoxically, though, caesarean delivery carries a series of risks related to the establishment of breastfeeding, including delay in lactogenesis, shorter breastfeeding behaviour, and the availability of less milk in the initial days of life (Hobbs et al., 2016). This may be more likely to lead to the introduction of breast milk substitutes than would be the case following vaginal birth. In an ideal world, this substitution would come from breast milk obtained from a donor; however, donor milk is not always a readily available option and so infant formula may be introduced. Formula milk creates a more complex microbiota including *Clostridium* and *Streptococcus* species, *Escherichia coli*, and *Enterococcus faecalis*. These microorganisms would not be present naturally until the introduction of solid foods and up until the age of 3, and they have the potential to put the baby at risk of gastrointestinal tract infections. This contrasts with the beneficial *Bifido* bacteria–rich environment of the breast milk–fed baby (Adams and Gutiérrez, 2018).

Furthermore, the Canadian Longitudinal study (Azad et al., 2016) reported that when women exclusively breastfeed for the first 3 months following birth, their babies develop a microbiome profile that not only gives greater protection in terms of immunity but may protect the baby from becoming obese. The study determined that those who were fully formula fed were twice as likely to become overweight, and those who were partially formula fed still had a 63% increased risk. This suggests that even a brief introduction to formula has the potential to alter the baby's microbiota, with the potential for long-term consequences (Chapter 15).

Maternal Obesity

Women with a raised BMI are statistically more likely to be subjected to caesarean delivery (Tun et al., 2018). Obesity has been correlated with an altered microbiome during pregnancy. Both of these factors increase the odds of less than optimal microbiome development (Santacruz et al., 2010). Obesity also impacts on the microbiome of breast milk, and the microbiota of obese women contain a number of bacteria that may predispose their babies to obesity (Galley et al., 2014). These bacteria do present antenatally in those women who go on to birth vaginally, but there would appear to be an increased risk in the offspring of obese women because of all the other factors that influence the gut following caesarean birth (Tun et al., 2018). The transmission of obesogenic microbiota could be responsible for at least some of the differences in the microbiota of babies born by caesarean (Ley et al., 2006).

Supporting the Microbiome

We cannot change everything in a world where childbirth and the baby's introduction to life are subject to so many variables, but there are things we can do to help women optimize the development of the microbiome in their babies. Table 6.8 outlines some of the ways that parents can be advised or assisted in order to optimize the microbiome development of their baby, regardless of modality of birth.

TABLE 6.8 **Supporting the Microbiome**
In Pregnancy
Carry out a nutritional assessment and discuss gut health and its significance in pregnancy.
Consider colostrum harvesting prior to planned caesarean, if gestational diabetes is present, or there is any other condition that may delay milk transfer for the baby.
Educate women and their partners about the benefits of breastfeeding in relation to the microbiome.
Discuss the importance of a physiological labour and birth for optimizing the physiological preparation of the gut environment for the baby.
During Labour and Birth
Encourage a 'default' approach where normal physiological birth is not possible: discuss with obstetric colleagues the possibility of labouring to some degree in order to trigger, for example, the antiinflammatory responses of early labour.
During a caesarean, request that antibiotics are not introduced until the baby has been born and the cord clamped.
In the Early Postnatal Period
Practice skin-to-skin contact as early as is practical, wherever birth has occurred.
Use harvested colostrum where necessary but continue to put the baby to the breast as well.
Aim to assist the woman to establish breastfeeding as early as possible, and ensure that as much support as she requires is available.
Support exclusive breastfeeding wherever possible.
Avoid bathing the baby for at least the first 24 hours and longer if possible.

SKIN-TO-SKIN CARE/CONTACT

It is our role as practitioners to consider practices which may assist in bringing all the transitory processes together. Skin-to-skin contact (SSC) between the woman and her newborn could be viewed as an effective way of achieving this.

The World Health Organization's Baby Friendly Initiative (BFI) has identified SSC (sometimes referred to as Kangaroo Care) as a key factor in the establishment of breastfeeding. Indeed, a Cochrane Collaboration Review (Moore et al., 2016) found statistically significant and positive effects of early SSC on breastfeeding at 1 to 4 months post birth. We have already discussed the fact that if babies are allowed free access to colostrum, the metabolic process will usually occur spontaneously and without any need for intervention (Colson, 2002). SSC seems to influence state organization and motor system modulation of the newborn infant shortly after birth (Ferber and Makhoul, 2004), making it easier for the baby to locate the nipple and latch on to suckle.

SSC has further benefits which are reflected in the other adaptation processes and which, it is argued, may contribute to the physiological stabilization and continued well-being of the infant. The warmth of the mother's body may ensure that the baby does not have to waste precious energy on maintaining body temperature. Current data suggest that there appears to be a degree of 'thermal synchrony' between mother and baby when SSC is introduced (Phillips, 2013). This would help the infant to conserve energy, which may help to stabilize its heart and respiratory rates.

Much of the earlier research carried out on the physiological benefits of skin-to-skin contact was focused on preterm babies. However, a flurry of activity in recent years has offered evidence of the benefits of SSC for full-term healthy neonates. Babies exposed to early SSC appear to demonstrate enhanced breastfeeding behaviours and longer duration of breastfeeding (Mahmood et al., 2011; Srivastava et al., 2014). When studies on SSC following caesarean delivery have been undertaken, the findings have been equally positive. Erlandsson et al. (2007) examined term babies born by caesarean who were given immediate SSC by their fathers, and compared them with babies who were placed immediately in a cot. The skin-to-skin babies cried less, were calmer, and achieved a normal drowsy state more rapidly than the control group. Full term babies receiving SSC also show reduced pain response when exposed to painful stimuli during procedures such as blood sampling and intramuscular injections (Kostandy and Luddington-Hoe, 2016; Liu et al., 2015).

Skin-to-skin care also helps to facilitate complex neurohormonal feedback mechanisms. Moore et al. (2016) are emphatic that the mother and baby should maintain physical contact wherever possible. There is evidence demonstrating that once born, all mammals—including humans—will follow a very specific 'set sequence of behaviours' (Bergman, 2005). In the human infant, this set of behaviours presents as the active seeking of skin-to-skin contact with its mother's body; it is thought that this tactile stimulation activates the flow of affective information from the baby (Moore et al., 2016). This action therefore serves to facilitate the development of brain pathways and thus may hold the 'keys to unlocking the mysteries of parenting' (Porter, 2003).

Bergman (2005) suggests that the presence of the mother is of paramount importance, and that newborn mammals who are given breast milk from their mother but are deprived of her physical presence fail to thrive. In simple terms, he stresses that babies need their mothers and they need to enjoy SSC with them.

We cannot interview babies about their experience of early SSC; instead, we rely on scientific monitoring to indicate that the experience is positive and beneficial. However, mothers can be directly approached and questioned about the experience. Finigan and Long (2012) discovered that women in three diverse ethnic groups felt it was instinctive to experience SSC; they spoke of it as a pleasurable experience, and spoke particularly about the capacity for eye contact. This 'feel good factor' would almost certainly assist in facilitating the neurohormonal feedback mechanism by making the process a reciprocal experience.

CONCLUSION

The potential effects of actions and procedures undertaken during the hours after birth on the consequent health and well-being of the child during infanthood and beyond are complex and manifold. The iatrogenic results of perceived beneficial forms of intervention, such as early cord clamping and cutting or early mother and baby separation, may have negative and far-reaching effects, some of which we do not even recognize. These effects may manifest physically, but may equally present as emotional, psychological or even spiritual issues later in life.

This means the role of the midwife is of paramount importance during this transitional period. The midwife's responsibility should be to protect the mother and her baby by ensuring that the environment is favourable and that, as far as is possible, the pair remain undisturbed. Intervention should be kept to a minimum; the principal function of the midwife in this situation is to watchfully wait. Many of the ritualistic practices which tend to occur during the hours following birth are based on little more than custom and tradition, with little consideration of the hugely important aspects of physiology. In order to effect a paradigm shift, we need to acquire a greater understanding of the physiological processes that occur, without, of course, losing sight of the potential for pathophysiology and the need for timely referral. We also need to consider this point in time as the 'fourth' trimester, recognizing the massive significance of the mother–baby dyad and how best we may protect the integrity of this, the most profound of relationships.

In 1975, Frederick Leboyer published a book called *Birth Without Violence*. Over 40 years ago, Leboyer was aware that 'less was more'—yet we still seem to have a long way to go to achieve the optimal immediate post-birthing conditions that may prove to be a window to future health and well-being. We would do well to pay heed to the following words taken from the book:

> *We were wondering about how best to prepare the child . . . Now we can see it's not the child who needs to be prepared. It is ourselves. It is our eyes that need to open, our blindness that has to stop. If we used just a little intelligence, how simple things could be.*
>
> *Leboyer, 1975*

PARENTS' STORY

Natashia and Eve's Story

When I became pregnant, it felt like an unbelievable miracle for us. It took us quite a long time to actually believe that it had happened after trying for longer than we would have liked.

Almost immediately, my brain started putting the picture of our baby's birth together. A beautiful calm birth at home, a home we had just recently bought, surrounded by loving midwives. I could already imagine the ecstasy of birthing our gorgeous wee babe and meeting her!

As our pregnancy progressed, I found myself anxious about everything. I overanalyzed every little detail and self-diagnosed things, followed by worries that I would lose control of the perfect picture I had painted in my mind.

I developed some complications; my blood pressure played up and I got a positive gestational diabetes result—I cursed the fact that I'd had the test. My hopes and dreams for a home birth were rapidly evaporating before my eyes and I felt a lot of grief, anger and sadness about it.

I hired a private obstetrician to look after the complications I'd developed, and so from that point forward my pregnancy and birth became a medical event. I felt that control was slipping from my hands, and I really struggled to maintain some form of normality. I didn't want our birth to be just another regular event in a busy obstetrician's diary.

Our little girl decided that she really liked being head-up, so in spite of lots of upside-down time, moxibustion, an attempt by the doctor to turn her manually, she remained breech. This, combined with a diagnosis of gestational diabetes and hypertension, led to only one logical conclusion (in our minds): she was going to be born by elective caesarean, a few days before her expected date of birth.

In spite of this unplanned turn of events, my husband and I were very keen to do whatever we could to give our baby the best start we could. There were several things we ended up doing that are not routinely carried out with caesareans, but that we felt would enhance our birthing experience and gave us some degree of control over our experience.

We learned about seeding the baby's microbiome with the mother's vaginal micro-flora, as babies born by caesarean obviously bypass the vaginal canal. We learned about it by watching a film called Microbirth (https://www.fmtv.com/watch/microbirth). We had the swab ready and seeded by the time Eve was born and my husband proceeded to smear it over her body and face.

We also didn't want our baby exposed to antibiotics, either before birth or afterwards. Antibiotics are routinely used during caesarean sections and given intravenously to the mother. I was able to negotiate with the surgeon and anaesthetist, who delayed the administration of the drugs until after Eve was born. I made sure that I took plenty of probiotics in the lead-up to the birth and also had infant probiotics ready to give to Eve to help support her microbiome.

Delayed clamping of the umbilical cord was something else that was very important to me, and I made this clear to the surgeon. Because I had been diagnosed with gestational diabetes, I knew I had to make sure I had a good store of colostrum. I had 'harvested' this towards the end of pregnancy ready for when Eve was born, as I wasn't going to let her have any formula. I ended up with 20 ml of frozen colostrum for her, and her blood sugars were perfect with every check! I still have a stash in my freezer and keep it for when she might get ill—for instance, if she gets a tummy bug—so that we can help her with some liquid gold!

After lots of research about the role of vitamin K, we also decided to give her the oral dose only, as opposed to an IM injection. We enjoyed uninterrupted skin-to-skin time with Eve from just after she was born, for as long as we wanted, and we did so for at least 2 hours after she was born (Fig. 6.4).

I'm really glad we were able to do all these things to make the birth our own and give our little girl the best start, in spite of the circumstances. It was a tremendously special day, filled with joy, tears, thankfulness, laughs and cuddles.

We are so thankful to have our gorgeous Eve in our lives. Her birth was a special event that we made our own, in collaboration with the wonderful staff of our local hospital who were accommodating enough to support what could have been considered by some to be outlandish requests.

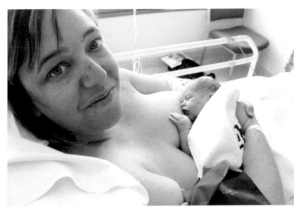

Fig. 6.4 Skin-to-Skin Time with Eve.

KEY POINTS

Practices that Support the Newborn's Physiological Adaptation

- Quiet, warm, dimly lit birthing room
- Drug- and intervention-free labour and birth
- Spontaneous physiological birth
- Physiological management of the third stage of labour
- Resuscitation with an intact umbilical cord
- Immediate skin-to-skin contact with the mother
- Baby is given colostrum as first feed
- No unnecessary separation from the mother
- Continuity of carer for mother and baby
- Calm mother due to trust in her supporters and environment

Practices that Challenge the Newborn's Physiological Adaptation

- Bright, busy, cold birthing room
- Obstetric interventions
- Practices that cause the mother to be anxious
- Active management of the third stage
- Unfamiliar caregivers of mother and baby
- Immediate cord clamping for arterial and venous pH and blood gases
- Umbilical cord blood harvesting for stem cells
- Cord cutting for resuscitation
- Separation from the mother

REFERENCES

Adams, C.A., Gutiérrez, B., 2018. Mother's Milk and Infant Formula Have Different Effects on the Microbiome in Babies. Innovations in food technology. Available from: http://jennewein-biotech.de/cms/assets/uploads/2018/11/InnovationsinFoodTechnologyNov2018.pdf. Accessed February 2019.

American Diabetes Association, 2017. 13. Management of diabetes in pregnancy. Diabetes Care. 40 (Suppl. 1), S114–S119. doi:10.2337/dc17-S016.

Amon, P., Sanderson, I., 2017. What is the microbiome? Arch. Dis. Child. Educ. Prac. Ed. 102, 257–260.

Armitage, S., Sheldon, J., Pushpanathan, P., Ellis, J., Contreras, M., 2006. Cord blood donation, testing and banking: a guide for midwives. Brit. J. Midwifery 14 (1), 6–9.

Asakura, H., 2004. Fetal and neonatal thermoregulation. J. Nippon Med. Sch. 71, 360–370.

Aylott, M., 2006. The neonatal energy triangle. Part 1: metabolic adaptation. Paediatr. Nurs. 18 (6), 38–42.

Azad, M.B., Konya, T., Persaud, R.R., Guttman, D.S., Chari, R.S., Field, C.J., et al., 2016. Impact of maternal intrapartum antibiotics, method of birth and breastfeeding on gut microbiota during the first year of life: a prospective cohort study. Br. J. Obstet. Gynaecol. 123 (6), 983–993. doi:10.1111/1471-0528.13601.

Baumgart, S., 2008. Iatrogenic hyperthermia and hypothermia in the neonate. Clin. Perinatol. 35 (1), 183–197.

Berardi, A., Pietrangiolillo, Z., Bacchi Reggiani, M.L., Bianco, V., Gallesi, D., Rossi, K., et al., 2018. Are postnatal ampicillin levels actually related to the duration of intrapartum antibiotic prophylaxis prior to delivery? A pharmacokinetic study in 120 neonates. Arch. Dis. Child. Fetal. Neonatal. Ed. 103 (2), F152–F156.

Bergman, N., 2005. More than a cuddle: skin-to-skin contact is key. Pract. Midwife 8 (9), 44.

Blackburn, S., 2007. Maternal, Fetal & Neonatal Physiology, third ed. Washington, Saunders Elsevier.

Boere, I., Roest, A., Wallace, E.M., Ten Harkel, A.D.J., Haak, M.C., Morley, C.J., et al., 2015. Umbilical blood flow patterns directly after birth before delayed cord clamping. Arch. Dis. Child. Fetal Neonatal Ed. 100, F121–F125. doi:10.1136/archdischild-2014-307144.

Bonnar, J., McNicol, G.P., Douglas, A.S., 1971. The blood coagulation and fibrinolytic systems in the newborn and the mother at birth. J. Obstet. Gynaecol. Br. Commonw. 78 (4), 355–360.

British Association of Perinatal Medicine, 2017. Identification and Management of Neonatal Hypoglycaemia in the Full Term Infant: A Framework for Practice. Available from: https://www.bapm.org/sites/default/files/files/Identification%20and%20Management%20of%20

Neonatal%20Hypoglycaemia%20in%20the%20%20
full%20term%20infant%20-%20A%20Framework%20
for%20Practice%20revised%20Oct%202017.pdf. Accessed
March 2019.

Buckley, S., 2005. Gentle Birth, Gentle Mothering. One Moon
Press, Brisbane.

Buckley, S., 2015. Hormonal Physiology of Childbearing:
Evidence and Implications for Women, Babies, and
Maternity Care. Washington DC, Childbirth Connection
Programs, National Partnership for Women and Families.
93 (12), 1560–1562.

Ciubotariu, R., Scaradavou, A., Ciubotariu, I., Tarnawski, M.,
Lloyd, S., Albano, M., et al., 2018. Impact of delayed
umbilical cord clamping on public cord blood donations:
can we help future patients and benefit infant donors?
Transfusion 58 (6), 1427–1433. doi:10.1111/trf.14574.

Collado, M., Rautava, S., Aakko, J., Isolauri, E., Salminen, S.,
2016. Human gut colonisation may be initiated in utero
by distinct microbial communities in the placenta and
amniotic fluid Nature Sci. Rep. 6, 23129.

Colson, S., 2002. Womb to world: a metabolic perspective.
Midwifery Today Int. Midwife (61), 12–17.

Cornblath, M., Hawdon, J.M., Williams, A.F., Aynsley-
Green, A., Ward-Platt, M.P., Schwartz, R., et al., 2000.
Controversies regarding definition of neonatal
hypoglycemia: suggested operational thresholds.
Pediatrics 105 (5), 1141–1145.

Cunnington, A.J., Sim, K., Deier, A., 2016. Vaginal seeding of
infants born by caesarean section: how should health
professionals engage with this increasingly popular but
unproved practice? BMJ 352, i227 doi:10.1136/bmj.i227.

Davies, L., 2017. Midwifery: A Sustainable Healthcare Profession? Unpublished Thesis. University of Canterbury,
Christchurch. Available from: https://ir.canterbury.ac.nz/
bitstream/handle/10092/14670/Davies%2C%20Lorna%20
final%20PhD%20thesis.pdf?sequence=1&isAllowed=y.
Accessed March 2019.

Dawson, J.A., Kamlin, C.O., Vento, M., Wong, C., Cole, T.J.,
Donath, S.M., et al., 2010. Defining the reference range
for oxygen saturation for infants after birth. Pediatrics
125, e1340–e1347. doi:10.1542/peds.2009-1510.

Dinan, T.G., Cryan, J.F., 2017. Gut instincts: microbiota as a key
regulator of brain development, ageing and neurodegenera-
tion. J. Physiol. 595 (2), 489–503. doi:10.1113/JP273106.

Dominguez-Bello, M.G., Costello, E.K., Contreras, M.,
Magris, M., Hidalgo, G., Fierer, N., et al., 2010. Delivery
mode shapes the acquisition and structure of the initial
microbiota across multiple body habitats in newborns.
Proc. Natl. Acad. Sci. U.S.A. 107 (26), 11971–11975.
doi:10.1073/pnas.1002601107.

Dunn, A.B., Jordan, S., Baker, B.J., Carlson, N.S., 2017. The
maternal infant microbiome: considerations for labor and
birth. MCN Am. J. Matern. Child. Nurs. 42 (6), 318–325.
doi:10.1097/NMC.0000000000000373.

Ericson, J., 2018. Breastfeeding in Mothers of Preterm Infants.
Digital Comprehensive Summaries of Uppsala Dissertations
from the Faculty of Medicine. 1398. Available from: https://
uu.diva-portal.org/smash/get/diva2:1159556/FULLTEXT01
.pdf. Accessed March 2019.

Erlandsson, K., Dsilna, A., Fagerberg, I., Christensson, K.,
2007. Skin-to-skin care with the father after cesarean
birth and its effect on newborn crying and prefeeding
behavior. Birth 34 (2), 105–114.

Farrar, D., Airey, R., Law, G.R., Tuffnell, D., Cattle, B.,
Duley, L., 2010. Measuring placental transfusion for
term births: weighing babies with cord intact. Br. J.
Obstet. Gynaecol. 118 (1), 70–75. doi:10.1111/j.1471-0528.
2010.02781.x.

Ferber, S.G., Makhoul, I.R., 2004. The effect of skin-to-skin
contact (kangaroo care) shortly after birth on the
neurobehavioral responses of the term newborn: a
randomized controlled trial. Pediatrics 113 (4), 858–865.

Phillips, R., 2013. The sacred hour: uninterrupted skin-to-
skin contact immediately after birth. Newborn and Infant
Nursing Reviews. 13 (1), 67–72.

Finigan, V., Long, T., 2012. The experience of women from
three diverse population groups of immediate skin-to-
skin contact with their newborn baby: selected outcomes
relating to establishing breastfeeding. Evid. Based
Midwifery 10 (4), 125–130.

Fogarty, M., Osborn, D.A., Askie, L., Seidler, A.L., Hunter, K.,
Lui, K., et al., 2018. Delayed vs early umbilical cord
clamping for preterm infants: a systematic review and
meta-analysis. Am. J. Obstet. Gynaecol. 218 (1), 1–18.
doi:10.1016/j.ajog.2017.10.231.

Galley, J.D., Bailey, M., Kamp Dush, C., Schoppe-Sullivan, S.,
Christian, L.M., 2014. Maternal obesity is associated with
alterations in the gut microbiome in toddlers. PLoS ONE
9 (11), e113026. doi:10.1371/journal.pone.0113026.

Gritz, E.C., Bhandari, V., 2015. The human neonatal gut
microbiome: a brief review. Front. Pediatr. 3, 17.
doi:10.3389/fped.2015.00017.

Hawdon, J.M., 2016. Postnatal metabolic adaptation and
neonatal hypoglycaemia. Paediatrics and Child Health.
26 (4), 135–139.

Hillman, N.H., Kallapur, S.G., Jobe, A.H., 2013. Physiology
of transition from intrauterine to extrauterine life.
Clin. Perinatol. 39 (4), 769–783. doi:10.1016/j.clp.2012.
09.009.

Hobbs, A.J., Mannion, C.A., McDonald, S.W., Brockway, M.,
Tough, S.C., 2016. The impact of caesarean section on
breastfeeding initiation, duration and difficulties in
the first four months postpartum. BMC Pregnancy
Childbirth 16, 90. doi:10.1186/s12884-016-0876-1.

Hooper, S.B., Morley, C.J., te Pas, A.B., Lewis, R.A., 2010. Establishing functional residual capacity at birth. Neo Reviews 11 (9), e1–e9.

Hunt, F., 2008. The importance of kangaroo care on infant oxygen saturation levels and bonding. J. Neonatal Nurs. 14 (2), 47–51.

Hutchon, D., 2014. Evolution of neonatal resuscitation with intact placental circulation. Infant 10 (2), 58–61.

Jost, T., Lacroix, C., Braegger, C., Chassard, C., 2015. Impact of human milk bacteria and oligosaccharides on neonatal gut microbiota establishment and gut health. Nutr. Rev. 73 (7), 426–437. doi:10.1093/nutrit/nuu016.

Karp, H., 2003. The Happiest Baby on the Block. Random House, New York.

Katheria, A.C., Lakshminrusimha, S., Rabe, H., McAdams, R., Mercer J.S., 2017. Placental transfusion: a review. J. Perinatol. 37, 105–111.

Kau, A.L., Ahern, P.P., Griffin, N.W., Goodman, A.L., Gordon, J.I., 2011. Human nutrition, the gut microbiome and the immune system. Nature 474, 327–336.

Kaur, N., Kaur, S., Saha, P.K., 2014. Skill development of nurses in managing the fourth stage of labour. Nurs. Midwifery Res. J. 10 (1), 16–29.

Kiserud, T., Acharya, G., 2004. The fetal circulation. Prenat. Diagn. 24, 1049–1059.

Kluckow, M., Hooper, S.B., 2015. Using physiology to guide time to cord clamping. Semin. Fetal. Neonatal. Med. 20, 225–231. doi:10.1016/j.siny.2015.03.002.

Kostandy, R.R., Luddington-Hoe, S., 2016. Kangaroo care (skin-to-skin) for clustered pain procedures: case study. World J. Neurosci. 6 (1), 43–51.

Lawton, C., Acosta, S., Watson, N., Gonzales-Portillo, C., Diamandis, T., Tajiri, N., et al., 2015. Enhancing endogenous stem cells in the newborn via delayed umbilical cord clamping. Neural Regen. Res. 10 (9), 1359–1362.

Leboyer, F., 1975. Birth Without Violence. Knopf, New York.

Lerner, E.B., Moscati, R.M., 2001. The golden hour: scientific fact or medical "urban legend"? J Soc Acad Emerg Med. 8 (7), 75860.

Ley, R.E., Turnbaugh, P.J., Klein, S., Gordon, J.I., 2006. Microbial ecology: human gut microbes associated with obesity. Nature 444 (7122), 1022–1023.

Linderkamp, O., 1982. Placental Transfusion. Can. Med. J. 93 (2), 1091–1100.

Liu, M., Zhao, L., Li, X.F., 2015. Effect of skin contact between mother and child in pain relief of full-term newborns during heel blood collection. Clin. Exp. Obstet. Gynecol. 42 (3), 304–308. doi:10.12891/ceog1831.

London, M., Ladewig, P., Ball, J. et al. (eds), 2003. Maternal-newborn and child nursing: family centred care. Prentice Hall, London.

Ludington-Hoe, S.M., Lewis, T., Cong, X., Anderson, L., Reese, S., 2006. Breast and infant temperatures with twins during shared kangaroo care. J. Obstet. Gynecol. Neonatal Nurs. 35, 223–231.

Mahmood, I., Jamal, M., Khan, N., 2011. Effect of mother-infant early skin-to-skin contact on breastfeeding status: a randomized controlled trial. J. Coll. Physicians Surg. Pak. 21 (10), 601–605. doi:10.2011/JCPSP.601605.

Martín, V., Maldonado-Barragán, A., Moles, L., Rodriguez-Baños, M., Campo, R.D., Fernández, L., et al., 2012. Sharing of bacterial strains between breast milk and infant feces. J. Hum. Lact. 28 (1), 36–44. doi:10.1177/0890334411424729.

McDonald, S.J., Middleton, P., Dowswell, T., Morris, P.S., 2013. Effect of timing of umbilical cord clamping of term infants on maternal and neonatal outcomes. Cochrane Database Syst. Rev. (7), CD004074. doi:10.1002/14651858.CD004074.pub3.

McEwan, T., 2017. Adaptation to extrauterine life 1. In: Rankin, J. (Ed.), Physiology in Childbearing with Anatomy and Related Biosciences, fourth ed. London, Elsevier, pp. 501–512.

McGuire, M.K., McGuire, M.A., 2015. Human milk: mother nature's prototypical probiotic food? Adv. Nutr. 6 (1), 112–123. doi:10.3945/an.114.007435.

Mercer, J., Skovgaard, R., 2002. Neonatal transitional physiology: a new paradigm. J Perinat. Neonatal Nurs. 15 (4), 56–57.

Mercer, J.S., Erickson-Owens, D.A., 2012. Rethinking placental transfusion and cord clamping issues. J. Perinat. Neonatal Nurs. 26 (3), 202–217.

Mercer, J.S., Erickson-Owens, D.A., Deoni, S.C.L., Dean, D.C., III., Collins, J., Parker, A.B., et al., 2018. Effects of delayed cord clamping on 4-month ferritin levels, brain myelin content, and neurodevelopment; a randomised controlled trial. J. Pediatr. 203, 266–272.e2. doi:10.1016/j.jpeds.2018.06.006.

Moore E.R., Bergman, N., Anderson, G.C., Medley, N., 2016. Early skin-to-skin contact for mothers and their healthy newborn infants. Cochrane Database Syst. Rev. 11, CD003519. doi:10.1002/14651858.CD003519.pub4.

Murty, V.Y., Ram, K.D., 2012. Study of pattern of blood sugar levels in low birth weight babies who are exclusively on breast milk. Journal of Dr. NTR University of Health Sciences. 1 (2), 90–93.

Niermeyer, S., Velaphi, S., 2013. Promoting physiologic transition at birth: re-examining resuscitation and the timing of cord clamping. Semin. Fetal Neonatal Med. 18, 385–392. doi:10.1016/j.siny.2013.08.008.

Olsen, R., Greisen, G., Schrøder, M., Brok, J., 2016. Prophylactic probiotics for preterm infants: a systematic review and meta-analysis of observational studies. Neonatology 109 (2), 105–112. doi:10.1159/000441274.

O'Sullivan, A., Farver, M., Smilowitz, J.T., 2016. The influence of early infant-feeding practices on the intestinal microbiome and body composition in infants [published correction appears in Nutr. Metab. Insights 8 (Suppl. 1), 87.]. Nutr.

Metab. Insights. 2015 8 (Suppl. 1), 1–9. doi:10.4137/NMI.S29530.

Porter, L., 2003. The science of attachment: the biological roots of love. Family Living Mothering Magazine. 119 July/August.

Quin, C., Estaki, M., Vollman, D.M., 2018. Probiotic supplementation and associated infant gut microbiome and health: a cautionary retrospective clinical comparison. Sci. Rep. 8 (1), 8283

Rabe, H., Duley, L., Diaz-Rossello, J.L., Dowswell T., 2012. Effect of timing of umbilical cord clamping and other strategies to influence placental transfusion at preterm birth on maternal and infant outcomes. Cochrane Database Syst. Rev. 8, CD003248. doi:10.1002/14651858.CD003248.pub3.

Rachana, S., (Ed.), 2000. Womb ecology becomes world ecology. In: Lotus Birth. Greenwood Press, Victoria, Australia, pp. 54–68.

Renz, H., Holt, P.G., Inouye, M., Logan, A.C., Prescott, S.L., Sly. P.D., 2017. An exposome perspective: early-life events and immune development in a changing world. J. Allergy. Clin. Immunol. 140 (1), 24–40. doi:10.1016/j.jaci.2017.05.015. Available at: https://www.ncbi.nlm.nih.gov/pmc/articles/PMC5945806/#B45.

Rutayisire, E., Huang, K., Liu, Y., Tao, F., 2016. The mode of delivery affects the diversity and colonization pattern of the gut microbiota during the first year of infants' life: a systematic review. BMC Gastroenterol. 16 (1), 86.

Saigal, S., Usher, R.H., 1977. Symptomatic neonatal plethora. Biol. Neonate 32 (1-2), 62–72.

Santacruz, A., Collado, M.C., García-Valdés, L., Segura, M.T., Martín-Lagos, J.A., Anjos, T., et al., 2010. Gut microbiota composition is associated with body weight, weight gain and biochemical parameters in pregnant women. Br. J. Nutr. 104 (1), 83–92. doi:10.1017/S0007114510000176.

Singh, Y., Tissot, C., 2018. Echocardiographic evaluation of transitional circulation for the neonatologists. Front. Pediatr. 6, 140.

Sreenivasa, B., Kumar, G.V., Sreenivasa, B., 2015. Comparative study of blood glucose levels in neonates using glucometer and laboratory glucose oxidase method. Curr. Pediatr. Res. 9 (1), 29–32.

Srivastava, S., Gupta, A., Bhatnagar, A., Dutta, S., 2014. Effect of very early skin to skin contact on success at breastfeeding and preventing early hypothermia in neonates. Indian J. Public Health 58 (1), 22–26.

Stinson, L.F., Payne, M.S., Keelan, J.A., 2018. A critical review of the bacterial baptism hypothesis and the impact of cesarean delivery on the infant microbiome. Front. Med. (Lausanne) 5, 135. doi:10.3389/fmed.2018.00135.

Stomnaroska-Damcevski, O., Petkovska, E., Jancevska, S., Danilovski, D., 2015. Neonatal hypoglycemia: a continuing debate in definition and management. Pril. (Makedon. Akad. Nauk. Umet. Odd. Med. Nauki.). 36 (3), 91–97. doi:10.1515/prilozi-2015-0083.

Sullivan, M.J., 2008. Banking on cord blood stem cells. Nat. Rev. Cancer 8, 555–563.

Tolosa, J.N., Park, D.H., Eve, D.J., Klasko, S.K., Borlongan, C.V., Sanberg, P.R., 2010. Mankind's first natural stem cell transplant. J. Cell. Mol. Med. 14 (3), 488–495. doi:10.1111/j.1582-4934.2010.01029.x.

Tun, H.M., Bridgman, S.L., Chari, R., Field, C.J., Guttman, D.S., Becker, A.B., et al., 2018. Roles of birth mode and infant gut microbiota in intergenerational transmission of overweight and obesity from mother to offspring. JAMA Pediatr. 172 (4), 368–377.

Turnbaugh, P.J., Ley, R.E., Hamady, M., Fraser-Liggett, C.M., Knight, R., Gordon, J.I., 2007. The human microbiome project. Nature 449 (7164), 804–810. doi:10.1038/nature06244.

Vali, P., Mathew, B., Lakshminrusimha, S., 2015. Neonatal resuscitation: evolving strategies. Matern. Health Neonatol. Perinatol. 1, 4. doi:10.1186/s40748-014-0003-0.

van Rheenen, P., Brabin, B., 2004. Late umbilical cord-clamping as an intervention for reducing iron deficiency in term infants in developing and industrialised countries: a systematic review. Ann. Trop. Paediatr. 24, 3–16.

van Vonderen, J.J., Roest, A.A., Siew, M.L., Walther, F.J., Hooper, S.B., te Pas, A.B., 2014. Measuring physiological changes during the transition to life after birth. Neonatology 105, 230–242. doi:10.1159/000356704.

Walker, M., 2015. Formula supplementation of breastfed infants: helpful or hazardous? ICAN: Infant, Child, Adolesc. Nutr. 7 (4), 198–207. doi:10.1177/1941406415591208.

Waller-Wise, R., 2011. Umbilical cord blood: information for childbirth educators. J. Perinat. Educ. 20 (1), 54–60. doi:10.1891/1058-1243.20.1.54.

Ward Platt, M., Deshpande, S., 2005. Metabolic adaptation at birth. Semin. Fetal. Neonatal Med. 10, 341–350.

Wen, L., Duffy, A., 2017. Factors influencing the gut microbiota, inflammation, and type 2 diabetes, J. Nutr. 147 (7), 1468S–1475S. doi:10.3945/jn.116.240754.

Wight, N., Marinelli, K.A., Academy of Breastfeeding Medicine, 2014. ABM clinical protocol #1: guidelines for blood glucose monitoring and treatment of hypoglycemia in term and late-preterm neonates, revised 2014. Breastfeed Med. 9 (4), 173–179.

Xiong, F., Zhang, L., 2013. Role of the hypothalamic-pituitary-adrenal axis in developmental programming of health and disease. Front. Neuroendocrinol. 34 (1), 27–46. doi:10.1016/j.yfrne.2012.11.002.

Yao, A.C., Moinian, M., Lind, J., 1969. Distribution of blood between infant and placenta after birth. Lancet 2, 871–873.

Yao, A.C., Lind, J., 1969. Effect of gravity on placental transfusion. Lancet 2, 505–508.

Yao, A.C., Hirvensalo, M., Lind, J., 1968. Placental transfusion-rate and uterine contraction. Lancet 1, 380–383.

7

Resuscitation of the Newborn Baby

Penny Champion

CHAPTER CONTENTS

For a number of reasons, some newborn babies do not make the transition to independent life without support, and it is the role of the midwife, neonatal nurse or paediatrician to provide that help in the form of newborn life support. This chapter will look at those babies that are more likely to need support. The pathophysiology of hypoxia will be explained, and practical measures for newborn life support will be introduced. Apgar scoring and the presence of meconium-stained liquor will also be discussed.

There are two main groups of babies who are more likely to need help:

- Those babies who have grown in utero quite healthily but are then subjected to an incident which deprives them of oxygen or depresses their natural responses. Examples of such incidents are antepartum haemorrhage caused by abruption of the placenta or placenta praevia, cord prolapse, cord compression, shoulder dystocia, breech presentation with delay, tracheal obstruction or narcotic drugs.
- Those babies who have not had a healthy start or who have a physiological abnormality, known or unknown, that makes the transition difficult for them. Examples of babies in this category are those with infections, intrauterine growth restriction, hydrops fetalis, diaphragmatic hernia, tracheo-esophageal fistula, cyanotic heart disease, pneumothorax or prematurity.

There will always be babies who are born in unexpected need of resuscitation, and the cause of their difficulty may not be identifiable.

TABLE 7.1	**Apgar Scores**		
Apgar Score	**0**	**1**	**2**
Colour	Pale/blue	Body pink/ extremities blue	Pink
Tone	Limp	Some flexion of extremities	Well flexed
Heart rate	Nil	Less than 100 bpm	More than 100 bpm
Respiratory effort	Absent	Weak cry or hypoventilation	Good
Response to stimulation	Nil	Some movement	Crying

APGAR SCORE

The Apgar score (Table 7.1) is a universally recognized and routinely utilized tool to determine a baby's condition at 1 minute after birth. The tool ascribes a score to the baby for colour, respiratory effort and heart rate, tone, activity and reflex irritability. The findings are documented at all births. The Apgar score has been subjected to some criticism regarding its accuracy as a measure of neonatal well-being; recent work by Dalili and colleagues proposes a 'combined Apgar score system' which is more sensitive in predicting birth asphyxia (Dalili et al., 2015). However, in spite of its perceived limitations, the original Apgar score continues to provide a simple baseline for monitoring the cardiorespiratory and neurological adaptation of the newborn to birth. In the absence of any tool other than the practitioner's observational skills, its continued use is guaranteed.

PHYSIOLOGY

The preceding chapter (Chapter 6) addresses the transition from uterine to extrauterine life and explains how a healthy newborn baby changes physiologically. It is important to understand the normal physiology, because the resuscitation process tries to support the baby in achieving a normal transition rather than imposing an alternative process.

Let's take a look at the physiology of hypoxia. Understanding this will help you to appreciate the physiological status of the baby you are resuscitating and what that baby needs you to do to help it. The research investigating the process was done on smaller mammals and the findings extrapolated to human physiology (Dawes, 1968).

We will look at the physiology in three areas:
- respiratory response
- blood gas and acid/base response
- cardiac response.

Respiratory Response

If the oxygen supply to a baby is cut off, the baby's immediate response is to make faster and deeper respiratory efforts. This can occur while the baby is in the uterus or when it is outside. If oxygen is not available, the pO_2 falls very quickly and the baby will become unconscious. The oxygen supply to the breathing centres in the brain is diminished and the respiratory efforts stop. This point is known as *primary apnoea*.

Cardiac Response

Up to the point of primary apnoea, the heart rate continues and sometimes rises to a tachycardic level (> 160 bpm) in order to facilitate the movement of oxygen to the vital organs. Once the breathing efforts stop, the heart rate drops to a bradycardic level (< 100 bpm). The blood pressure remains almost the same; this is achieved by shutting down the peripheral blood supply and preserving the circulation to the vital organs.

Blood Gas and Acid/Base Balance

Clearly, the pO_2 will fall very quickly if the oxygen supply to the baby is cut off. In these circumstances, the baby will work hard to compensate for the lack of oxygen and glucose coming in and the increasing amounts of carbon dioxide that cannot escape. Its condition will deteriorate if the oxygen supply is not restored. The baby retains carbon dioxide, which will make the blood more acidic (lower the pH). This initial response is called *respiratory acidosis*, because it is primarily caused by failure of respiration. So the pO_2 will fall, the pCO_2 will rise and the pH value will show increasing acidity. Remember that the oxygen supply can be restored by delivering the baby and assisting with respiration if necessary.

If the lack of oxygen continues, then the baby begins *agonal gasping*, which can occur both inside and outside the uterus. The higher respiratory centres in the brain are not functioning, which allows spinal responses to have an effect. These produce 'almost convulsive' gasping at a rate of about 12 per minute. These agonal gasps can go on for up to 10 minutes; once they have stopped, the baby has reached a point known as *terminal apnoea*. During this time, cardiac output continues but, if these gasps fail to bring oxygen into the lungs, the cardiac function will gradually cease.

The baby will become increasingly acidotic as more carbon dioxide is retained, and will begin to use *anaerobic metabolism* to provide energy for the vital organs. This is a way of producing energy without oxygen. The baby will use stores of glycogen from the heart muscle, liver and other muscles to produce energy. The waste product of this process is lactic acid, the accumulation of which will produce a *metabolic acidosis*. The increasingly acidic environment affects the function of the heart muscle and prevents it from working effectively.

A baby born in primary apnoea or during agonal gasping will, if given airway support and air, be able to 'resuscitate' itself, although the baby that has reached the gasping stage may take longer to do so.

A baby who has reached terminal apnoea will die unless an intervention in the form of resuscitation is made.

Figure 7.1 shows the cumulative effect of lack of oxygen on a human baby, but also its inherent ability to recover once oxygen is available.

In common with many other mammals, human babies have a remarkable ability to withstand lack of oxygen—much more so than adults. They can shut down their circulation, preserving blood supply to vital organs. They have the ability to respond to spinal impulses, resulting in agonal gasping, and their heart muscle has large stores of glycogen, which maintains the circulation for a long time.

Although an understanding of the pathophysiology of hypoxia will help to identify how a baby may benefit from assistance, when presented with a baby who is not breathing, how do we know whether it is in primary or terminal apnoea? The answer is that we do not—and, therefore, we have to treat all babies using the same

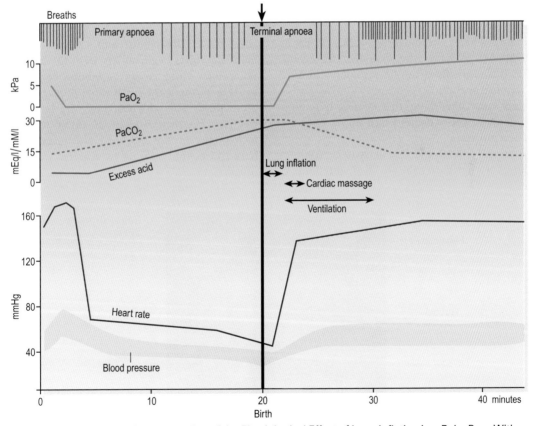

Fig. 7.1 Diagrammatic Representation of the Physiological Effect of Lung Inflation in a Baby Born With Terminal Apnoea. (Reproduced from Wyllie, 2016a with permission).

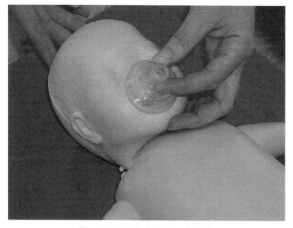

Fig. 7.2 A Well-Fitting Mask.

strategy, that is, as if they are in terminal apnoea. We will only know how far they had progressed along the graph by observing them as they recover.

A baby in primary apnoea will begin to breathe, have visibly improved colour as oxygenation increases, and recover a normal heart rate much sooner than a baby in terminal apnoea. A baby who demonstrates agonal gasping as it is resuscitated can be considered to have been in terminal apnoea.

There are some other things that we need to remind ourselves about newborn babies which may help in the resuscitation process:
- Babies are wet at birth and very likely to get cold.
- The lungs of a newborn baby are filled with fluid.

- Babies have a cartilaginous rib cage that makes chest compression easier and more effective.

The first point is crucial for *all* babies. A cold baby will have a lower oxygen tension, an increased metabolic acidosis and inhibition of surfactant production. All these factors will hamper resuscitation efforts considerably. Heat is lost by conduction, convection, evaporation and radiation, so several actions are necessary:
- Place the baby on a warm surface with an overhead heater to prevent heat loss by conduction.
- Minimize all draughts, turn off fans and shut windows to reduce heat loss by convection.
- Dry the baby thoroughly, discard the wet towel and wrap the baby in a warm dry one to minimize heat loss through evaporation.
- Put a hat on the baby and keep it covered as much as possible to prevent heat loss by radiation.

The second point is important if the baby you are resuscitating has not taken a breath. The lungs are soaked with pulmonary fluid at birth, around 30 ml/kg, which equates to about 100 ml for an average-sized baby. The labour and vaginal birth process helps the lungs begin to 'dry out'; the production of pulmonary fluid ceases as labour begins, and the squeeze through the birth canal relieves the baby of more fluid. This also explains why babies born by elective caesarean sometimes suffer with transient tachypnoea of the newborn and grunting, as they have more fluid volume to disperse with their first breaths.

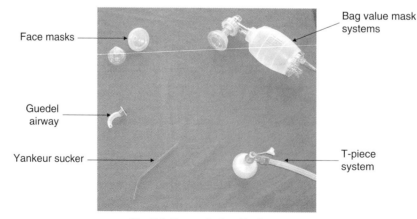

Fig. 7.3 Resuscitation Equipment.

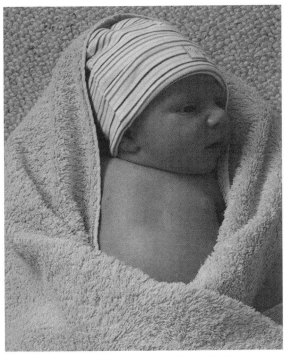

Fig. 7.4 Baby Wrapped for Resuscitation.

A healthy newborn will disperse this fluid by taking some very deep inspirations as it first breathes. If a baby does not breathe spontaneously, the resuscitator will need to give what are called *inflation breaths* to mimic those first deep inspirations. A baby's first breaths are very important because they trigger all the other physiological changes that make up the transition to extrauterine life (Chapter 6).

The final point is only relevant if cardiac compressions are required, but it should be reassuring to know that it is easier to achieve effective cardiac compressions in a newborn baby; the heart itself is larger relative to an adult and the rib cage less resistant to pressure.

Having familiarized ourselves with some babies who may need resuscitation and revised the physiological events, let's consider how we would prepare ourselves, the environment and the parents for resuscitation.

PREPARING OURSELVES

As midwives, nurses and paediatricians who may be called upon to lead or assist with newborn resuscitation, we need the necessary skills and knowledge. This may have been acquired during pre-registration education, and subsequently enhanced by hands-on experience. There are also post-registration courses for nurses, midwives and doctors, such as the NLS (Newborn Life Support) course run by the Resuscitation Council UK and similar organizations in other countries. However we acquire the knowledge, regular updating is essential. Fortunately, newborn resuscitation is not a skill we have to call upon very often, but this makes regular updates and practice even more important to maintain the skill.

As accountable practitioners, we need to bear in mind the limitations of our knowledge and skills, and know when and how to summon help in the resuscitation process.

Remember to wash your hands and put on some gloves and an apron!

PREPARING THE ENVIRONMENT

In this section, we will think about our physical environment and equipment (Fig. 7.3). Some of this depends upon where we are when the baby is born.

In both a home/community and a hospital setting, we should consider:

- Warmth: closing windows, minimizing draughts, prewarming towels, hat for the baby, heater or warming pad.
- Resuscitation surface: flat and firm (a head-down tilt is not advised, as it is more difficult to maintain an open airway).
- Bag-valve-mask: this should be a 500-ml paediatric bag in the home/community setting and may be a T-piece system on a hospital Resuscitaire. Both systems have an inbuilt safety valve which you should check before using the equipment. A functioning valve will prevent you from delivering more than 40 cm H_2O pressure into a baby's lungs. *Be careful to check because it is possible to close the valve on a bag, thus overriding the safety mechanism.*
- Mask size: it is important that the mask you use for resuscitation is the correct size to get a good seal. Use a mask with a deformable surface that fits over the baby's mouth and nose but does not overhang the chin or reach the eye sockets (Fig. 7.2).
- Stethoscope: this is the most accurate way to assess the heart rate
- Help: wherever you are, think in advance who you can call for help and how you will do it.

- Oropharyngeal airways: these may be helpful if you are having any difficulty supporting the airway, particularly if you are alone.
- Suction: this is useful but not essential in a community setting.
- Oxygen: this is helpful but not essential in a community setting and it is reasonable to start resuscitation for all babies in air.

In the hospital setting, you may also have access to the following:

- laryngoscope
- endotracheal tubes
- umbilical venous catheters
- drugs:
    1. Adrenaline (epinephrine) 1:10,000
    2. Sodium bicarbonate 4.2%
    3. Glucose 10%
    4. Saline 0.9% for volume.

PREPARING THE PARENTS

One of the key things that may make the birth experience traumatic is when parents feel that they have lost control (Green et al., 1998). In an emergency such as resuscitation, it is easy to see why practitioners feel their focus should be on the baby and its immediate needs. I acknowledge this focus fully, but there are ways to enable parents to feel a part of the process and to be active in any decision-making.

The midwife caring for them should make the parents aware in advance if she feels there may be a need for resuscitation of their baby.

The practitioner who is called to help should make every effort to introduce themselves and explain why they are there.

If possible, the midwife should ask someone to be with the parents during the resuscitation process to talk them through what is happening, using suitable language and being careful not to reassure them falsely.

If practicable, the baby should not be removed from the birth room for resuscitation.

RESUSCITATION

Table 7.2 is a flow chart based on the UK Resuscitation Council's Guideline for Newborn Life Support (Wyllie et al., 2016a). This guideline is based on current evidence and was last updated in December 2016.

Let us look at some of the actions in more detail.

Clock

Start the clock or note the time of birth. This is important for your records and for letting other helpers know how long you have been trying to resuscitate the baby.

Dry

Wrap the baby in a warm dry towel, dry it all over (including head and back), put a hat on its head and wrap it in a new warm towel, leaving only the chest exposed (Fig. 7.4). This process affords you time to assess the baby and is also a form of gentle stimulation for the baby. This is absolutely crucial for all babies, although those that are well can be put skin-to-skin with their parent and then covered.

Assess

Observe the colour, tone, heart rate and respiratory effort of the baby. These observations will help you assess what help the baby might need and what help you need. If the baby is very floppy, pale, or has a heart rate of less than 60 bpm, then it will need to be moved to the Resuscitaire.

Cord

If the baby is to be moved to a Resuscitaire, clamping and cutting the cord may become necessary; otherwise, consider leaving the cord intact if you are able to resuscitate the baby effectively. (The advantages of delayed cord clamping are discussed at length in Chapter 6.) LifeStart trolleys are now available to facilitate resuscitation without having to cut the cord (Batey et al., 2017). If the baby is being moved to a Resuscitaire, leave at least 10 cm of cord between the baby and the first clamp.

Help

You may consider calling for help after the assessment, especially if the baby looks very pale, floppy, or has a heart rate of less than 60 bpm.

Open Airway

If the baby has any loss of tone, you will need to support the airway in a neutral position (Fig. 7.5). Loss of pharyngeal tone, or an overextended or flexed neck, will close the airway and mean that the natural response to breath will not be effective (Figs 7.6 and 7.7). It is much more likely that the airway is obstructed due to poor positioning

TABLE 7.2 Newborn Life Support Algorithm

Dry the baby, remove any wet cloth, wrap and put on a hat

↓

First assessment at birth

Start the clock or note the time

Assess: COLOUR, TONE, BREATHING, HEART RATE;   DO I NEED HELP?

↓

If not breathing:

↓

Support the AIRWAY in the neutral position

↓

BREATHING

If not breathing: FIVE INFLATION BREATHS (each 2–3 seconds duration) (30–40 cm H_2O pressure)

Confirm a response: increase in HEART RATE or visible CHEST RISE

↓

If there is no response:

Check head position and apply JAW THRUST

5 more inflation breaths

Confirm a response: increase in HEART RATE or visible CHEST RISE;   DO I NEED HELP?

↓

If there is still no response:

a) Use a second person (if available) to apply two-handed jaw thrust and repeat inflation breaths

b) Inspect the oropharynx under direct vision (is suction needed?) and repeat inflation breaths

c) Insert an oropharyngeal (Guedel) airway and repeat inflation breaths

Consider intubation

Confirm a response: increase in HEART RATE or visible CHEST RISE

↓

When the chest is rising but the heart rate may still be slow or undetectable

Give ventilation breaths (30 per minute) for 30 seconds

↓

Re check the heart rate and confirm chest rise

If not detectable or less than 60 bpm, commence chest compressions   DO I NEED HELP?

↓

CHEST COMPRESSIONS

Give 3 chest compressions to 1 breath for 30 seconds

↓

Reassess heart rate

If > 60 bpm: stop chest compressions, continue ventilation if not breathing

If heart rate still slow, continue ventilation and chest compressions

Consider venous access and drugs at this stage

AT ALL STAGES, ASK: DO YOU NEED HELP ?

In the presence of meconium, remember: Screaming babies have an open airway

Floppy babies—have a look.

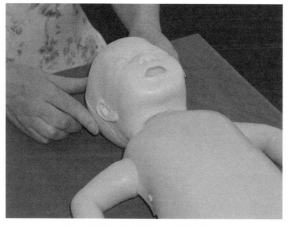

Fig. 7.5 Neutral Airway Position.

than by a physical obstruction such as blood or mucus. If a baby has poor or no tone, you may need to use *chin support* with your finger on the bony part of the chin tip, or a *jaw thrust*, where you push the lower jaw at the angle, upwards and forwards (Figs 7.8 and 7.9).

Breathing

If there is no respiratory effort, use a well-fitting mask (Fig. 7.2) and give five inflation breaths at a pressure of 30–40 cm H_2O, lasting 2–3 seconds each. Always commence resuscitation using air. If you are using a self-inflating bag, you will need to squeeze slowly with your whole hand to achieve a breath of this length and consistent pressure (Fig. 7.10).

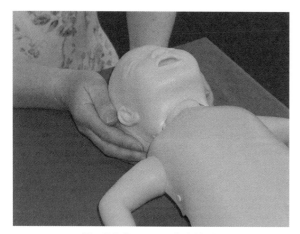

Fig. 7.6 Overextended Neck.

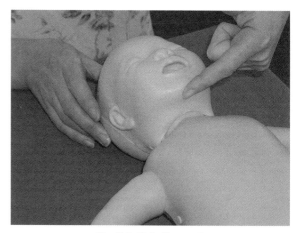

Fig. 7.8 Chin Support.

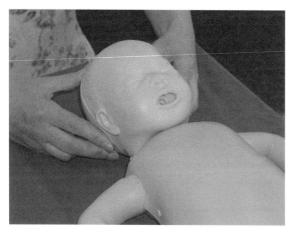

Fig. 7.7 Flexed Neck.

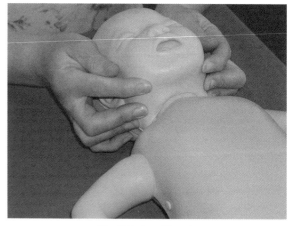

Fig. 7.9 Jaw Thrust.

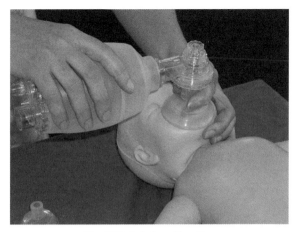

Fig. 7.10 Inflation Breaths.

TABLE 7.3 **Acceptable Right Arm Saturations After Birth**	
Time from Birth (min)	**Acceptable Saturation (%)**
2	60
3	70
4	80
5	85
10	90

These are the equivalent 'first' breaths for the baby, clearing the lung fluid and inflating the lungs. The usual response of the baby to these breaths is an increase in heart rate. Listen with a stethoscope; if you don't have one, palpate the apex. Feeling the base of the cord is not always reliable, particularly if the heart rate is slow.

Ask yourself: Has the heart rate increased? Did the chest rise?

If the heart rate is increasing, you can assume you have inflated the lungs. Continue to support the baby with ventilation breaths at a rate of 30 breaths per minute (pressure of 15–20 cm H_2O). In order to reduce the pressure if you are using a self-inflating bag, use your thumb and index finger only to squeeze the bag. Continue to ventilate until the baby starts to make its own respiratory effort.

If the heart rate is not increasing and you have not seen the chest rise, you have probably not inflated the lungs.

Help

You may wish to call for help now if you were not successful in inflating the lungs. When help arrives, consider applying a pulse oximeter so that you can see an accurate heart rate and oxygen saturation levels. The sensor should be placed on the right hand or wrist of the baby, once the skin has been thoroughly dried. See Table 7.3 for acceptable right arm saturations.

Reassess the airway position, check for overextension of the neck and *repeat the five inflation breaths*.

Ask yourself: Has the heart rate increased? Did the chest rise?

If there is still no change in the heart rate and the chest has not risen, there are three possible further actions:
- Use double jaw thrust if there are two people available to help.
- Inspect the airway under direct vision with a laryngoscope/light; if there is an obvious obstruction, remove it with suction.
- Insert an oropharyngeal airway.

After each intervention, repeat the five inflation breaths.

Suction

You will probably have noted how late suction is used in the algorithm. There are two reasons for this:
1. The airway is most likely to be obstructed by poor position and lack of tone and this should be addressed first.
2. Suction can be harmful. Blind suction into the pharynx and larynx can cause a vagal bradycardia as well as trauma.

If suction is necessary, use a paediatric Yankauer sucker or a wide-bore tube; do not let the end of the tube out of your sight during the procedure.

When the heart rate remains slow, you have to judge lung inflation by observing for chest movement. There is no point in progressing to chest compressions unless you are able to get air/oxygen into the lungs.

Circulation

If the heart rate remains slow (< 60 bpm) in spite of effective lung inflation, give the baby 30 seconds of

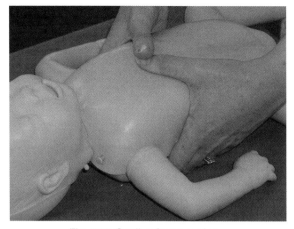

Fig. 7.11 Cardiac Compressions.

ventilation breaths before you commence chest compressions.

The aim of chest compression is to move oxygenated blood from the lungs to the heart muscle. You can achieve this in a baby by compressing the lower third of the sternum by about one-third of the depth of the chest (Fig. 7.11). The most effective way of doing this is to put your hands around the baby's chest with your fingertips along the spine, and use your two thumbs one on top of the other to compress. If you visualize a line between the nipples, your thumbs need to be just below that line, on the sternum. Be careful to press only on the sternum and not on the ribs at either side.

Compressions are given at a rate of approximately 90 per minute, and you should do three compressions to one breath. This rate is a guide; the most important thing is that you successfully ventilate the lungs and then move the oxygenated blood round to the heart. Depending upon the saturation readings, you may consider blending additional oxygen at this point.

The heart should respond within 20 to 30 seconds. Check the heart rate and chest rise every 30 seconds. Once the heart rate is increasing and above 60 bpm, you can stop compressions, but continue to ventilate the lungs and recheck the heart rate to make sure it is continuing to increase.

Drugs

These become necessary if the heart does not respond to chest compressions. It is always worth rechecking the chest movement to ensure the lungs are being inflated; this may involve intubation by the paediatrician.

If there is no circulation to carry the drugs to the heart muscle—which is where they need to be—an umbilical venous catheter (UVC) is the most effective way to get them there. The paediatrician will insert this. The drugs that may be used are listed in Table 7.4.

The current Resuscitation Council Guidelines (Wyllie et al., 2016b) suggest using adrenaline in the first instance, but with the caveat that the evidence for the appropriate dose is lacking. The same applies to the use of glucose and sodium bicarbonate.

Ongoing Care

If a baby has been asphyxiated, we can only tell how severe this has been by observing the behaviour of the baby as it recovers.

A baby who has been in terminal apnoea will have a period of agonal gasping before it establishes regular respiration; it will need continued respiratory ventilation through this time.

TABLE 7.4	**Drugs Used in Resuscitation**				
Drug	Preparation	Dose	Route	Effect	
Adrenaline (epinephrine)	1:10000 (100 μg/ml)	10μg/kg (0.1 ml/kg of 1:10000	UVC	Stimulates heart muscle	
Sodium bicarbonate	4.2% or 8.4% diluted 1:1 with 5% or 10% dextrose	1–2 mmol/kg (2–4 ml/kg of 4.2%)	UVC	Reverses intracardiac acidosis	
Glucose	10%	250 mg/kg	UVC	Provides energy to the heart muscle.	
Saline	0.9%	10 ml/kg	UVC	Replaces lost volume	

It is important that you note the time when the baby starts gasping and how long this lasts for, and also the time at which it establishes regular respiration, because these are measures of the degree of asphyxia.

The ongoing care of a baby who has needed resuscitation varies according to the speed of recovery. Each baby will need to be assessed individually and its ongoing care should be planned with the paediatric team. Most babies, however, will recover within a few minutes of birth and can remain with their parents.

Those babies who have shown signs of being in terminal apnoea are likely to have difficulty in establishing homeostasis themselves and will need ongoing care in a neonatal unit. If this happens, the midwife and paediatrician should make efforts to enable the parents to touch and talk to the baby before they are separated. It is also vital that the baby has identifying wrist/ankle bands.

COMMUNICATION

The person responsible for the resuscitation should speak to the parents as soon as they are ready, to explain what happened and what actions were required. It is important to offer the parents time to ask questions and voice their anxieties. It is not the role of the resuscitator to answer questions about the care during labour or to make any judgements about the future.

Make sure you use language that the parents understand, and check that they understand what you have said to them. It is sometimes useful to work through the written record you have made with the parents so that they can fill in any gaps in their memory. It is also useful to tell them how to contact the relevant person if they have further questions.

RECORD-KEEPING

The written record of a resuscitation procedure is likely to be scrutinized. There is an understandable connection in the minds of many laypeople between lack of oxygen and brain damage, and this concern may lead to investigation or litigation in the future.

Some key points to help you:
• Write up your notes as soon as you can after the event; include any pieces of paper on which you kept contemporaneous notes. Many hospitals have a standard proforma which is used to record actions during newborn resuscitation.

• Use factual, not descriptive, language; write down what you saw, not your interpretation of it. An example of this would be to note the fetal heart rate and any information you are told about the CTG trace, rather than calling it 'fetal distress'.
• Resuscitation Council Guidelines (2016) advise you to record the following information:
  • when you were called, by whom, and why;
  • the time you arrived, who else was there, and the condition of the baby on your arrival;
  • what you did, when you did it, and the timing and details of any response from the baby;
  • whether the baby appeared floppy and unconscious at birth;
  • the baby's heart rate at birth, and when it first exceeded 100 bpm;
  • the time at which you were first certain that the lungs had successfully been inflated;
  • whether gasping respiration preceded the onset of rhythmic breathing, when gasping started and how long it lasted;
  • when the baby started to breathe evenly, regularly and effectively 30–60 times per minute (even if still gasping intermittently);
  • if you have used a saturation monitor, it is helpful to record the initial reading of the heart rate and saturation and how these changed with your actions;
  • the date and time of writing your entry, and your role, grade, signature and registration number.

COMPLEX CASES

The algorithm we have looked at is generally appropriate for any baby who needs resuscitation. There are, however, some groups of newborns who require small adjustments in order to receive optimal care.

Preterm Babies

These babies are even more susceptible to the effects of hypothermia discussed previously; every effort should be made to prevent episodes of hypothermia occurring. Current recommendations are that any baby under 32 weeks should be placed, feet first, into a *plastic bag* without drying, then resuscitated on a thermal mattress (Wyllie et al., 2016b). Do not cover the face, but put a hat on the baby. Then place it directly under a radiant heater and do not cover with anything else.

Make sure that there is a senior neonatologist present for the birth who can intubate and give surfactant if required.

Reduce the pressures used for inflation and ventilation, and always begin resuscitation in air, with additional oxygen use being guided by saturation levels.

Meconium

In utero, babies do not inhale meconium via the normal fetal breathing movements. If we consider the physiology of hypoxia, once again we can surmise that a baby who has inhaled meconium has been gasping in utero and is therefore suffering from hypoxia.

There have been several large research studies (Wiswell et al., 2000; Vain et al., 2004) looking at the effect of suctioning on the perineum in the presence of meconium-stained liquor and this has been found to be of no benefit.

Current advice from the Resuscitation Council UK (2016) is:
- Screaming babies have an open airway
- Floppy babies—have a look.

If you can use a laryngoscope, then it is prudent to look in the airway of a baby that has other signs of hypoxia, and remove any visible meconium. If you cannot use a laryngoscope, follow the algorithm from the beginning, removing whatever meconium you can see with a swab.

UNEXPECTED RESPONSES

There are a few babies who do not respond to this approach. Always reconsider the baby's airway position in the first instance. Unexpected responses could be due to:
- A physical obstruction in the trachea—this could be a blood clot, vernix or meconium and will need removing by someone who can intubate. This is a rare event.
- The mother receiving narcotic analgesia 2–3 hours before the birth. These babies normally cry and breathe at birth, then stop a few minutes later. They need airway support and ventilation; naloxone should only be given once the airway is secure, lung ventilation is occurring and the heart rate is above 100 bpm. 200 µg IM of naloxone will reverse any opiate effects; smaller doses will not be effective for as long as the half-life of pethidine in a baby, which

is > 24 hours. Any baby who has required naloxone should be closely observed for at least 24 hours.
- A rare physical condition, such as diaphragmatic hernia, intrapartum pneumonia or pneumothorax, that may result in a baby remaining cyanosed even when there is a good heart rate. Use a pulse oximeter to check oxygen saturations, and get help from a senior colleague.
- A baby that has lost some of its circulating volume because of antepartum haemorrhage; these babies may be persistently bradycardic until you replace the volume. This is normally done with 0.9% saline, then cross-matched blood.

Finally, we have to consider when to stop resuscitation. Senior members of neonatal/paediatric staff, along with the parents, should take this decision.

This is a statement from the current NLS guideline:

if the heart rate is not detectable at birth and remains undetectable for 10 minutes (equivalent to an Apgar score of zero at 10 min despite resuscitation), it may be appropriate to **consider** *stopping resuscitation as this situation is highly predictive of death or severe morbidity for the baby…*

Wyllie et al., 2016b

I would like to end this chapter where much of the literature about resuscitation begins. Studies in Sweden (Palme-Kilander, 1992) and in the UK (Allwood et al., 2003) have shown that between two and four babies (> 2.5kg and > 37 weeks' gestation) per 1000 require intubation at birth. In the Swedish study, about eight babies per 1000 needed mask inflation. This contextual information should remind us that having the skills to manage the airway of a newborn effectively, keep it warm and inflate its lungs are crucial, and will be sufficient to help most babies recover.

KEY POINTS

- Dry the baby and keep it warm.
- Take care to position the airway correctly.
- Use inflation breaths to clear lung fluid and inflate lungs.
- Communicate with the parents before, during and after resuscitation of their baby.
- Keep careful records of your actions.
- Make sure your skills and knowledge are up to date

REFERENCES

Allwood, A.C., Madar, R.J., Baumer, J.H., Readdy, L., Wright, D., 2003. Changes in resuscitation practice at birth. Arch. Dis. Child. Fetal Neonatal Ed. 88, F375–379.

Batey, N., Yoxall, C.W., Fawke, J.A., Duley, L., Dorling, J., 2017. Fifteen-minute consultation: stabilisation of the high-risk newborn infant beside the mother. Arch. Dis. Child. Educ. Pract. 102, 235–238.

Dalili, H., Nili, F., Sheikh, M., Hardani, A.K., Shariat, M., Nayeri, F., 2015. Comparison of the four proposed Apgar scoring systems in the assessment of birth asphyxia and adverse early neurologic outcomes. PLoS ONE 10 (3), e0122116. doi:10.1371/journal.pone.0122116.

Dawes, G., 1968. Fetal and Neonatal Physiology. Year Book Publisher, Chicago, IL, pp. 141–159. (Chapter 12).

Green, J.M., Coupland, V.A., Kitzinger, J.V., 1998. Great Expectations: A Prospective Study of Women's and Experiences of Childbirth, second ed. Books for Midwives Press, Hale, UK.

Palme-Kilander, C., 1992. Methods of resuscitation in low-Apgar score in infants—a national survey. Acta Paediatr. 81, 739–744.

Resuscitation Council UK, 2016. Available from: www.resus.org.uk. Accessed August 2020.

Vain, N.E., Szyld, E.G., Prudent, L.M., Wiswell, T.E., Aguilar, A.M., Vivas, N.I., 2004. Oropharyngeal and nasopharyngeal suctioning of meconium-stained neonates before delivery of their shoulders: multicentre, randomised controlled trial. Lancet 364 (9434), 597–602.

Wyllie, J., Ainsworth, S., Tinnion, R., Hampshire, S., 2016a. Newborn Life Support, fourth ed. Resuscitation Council (UK).

Wyllie, J., Ainsworth, S., Tinnion, R., 2016b. Online Guidelines. Available from: https://www.resus.org.uk/resuscitation-guidelines/resuscitation-and-support-of-transition-of-babies-at-birth/. Accessed February 2019.

Wiswell, T.E., Gannon, C.M., Jacob, J., Goldsmith, L., Szyld, E., Weiss, K., et al., 2000. Delivery room management of the apparently vigorous meconium-stained neonate: results of the multicenter, international collaborative trial. Pediatrics 105(1), 1–7

8

Neurological, Behavioural and Growth Assessment of the Newborn

Sharon McDonald and Lindsey Rose

CHAPTER CONTENTS

A thorough neurological assessment is a critical aspect of the newborn infant physical examination (NIPE). The human baby, although extremely neurologically immature at birth, will undergo the majority of its brain growth and development for life during the first few weeks, months and early years of life. It follows that the earliest possible identification of any damage, and the earliest appropriate intervention, are key to limiting the potential for the negative outcomes of neurological injury or disease. This chapter does not set out to explore the signs of neurological conditions; rather, the scope is to observe the normal and anticipated neurological state of both the term and the preterm newborn, so that the examiner is able to recognize when deviations from the normal may have occurred.

We will begin by briefly exploring some of the neuroscientific theories relating to the newborn that have been presented since the 1970s. This may help the reader to contextualize some of the discussions that have taken place in other chapters.

The assessment of the newborn nervous system was initially based on concepts learnt from adult neurology. The baby was not seen as being able to demonstrate any significant cortical or cerebellar activity, and the study of primary reflexes was given prevalence (Smith, 2001). Throughout the last decades of the 20th century, neonatal neurologists such as Dubowitz (1970), Amiel-Tison (1986), Ballard (1991) and others worked hard to clarify this area; through their studies, practitioners became increasingly aware of the importance of neuromotor function and the behavioural state of the baby, as well as more detailed neurological signs (Heaberlin, 2019).

> While babies may not speak their first word for a year, they are born ready to communicate with a rich vocabulary of body movements, cries and visual responses: all part of the complex language of infant behavior.
>
> *(Brazelton, 2011)*

The theory relating to the early relational experiences of the newborn continues to expand and has dramatically altered the way in which we view a baby's neurological and behavioural responses. Globally, two tools—the Neonatal Behavioural Assessment Scale (NBAS) (a newborn behavioural tool) and the Newborn Behavioural Observations (NBO) (a relationship-building tool)—are utilized to understand newborn behaviour. Studies using these tools have been undertaken, exploring, for example:

- the effects of prematurity, low birthweight, undernutrition and a range of antenatal and perinatal risk factors

- the effects of obstetric medication/mode of delivery
- the effects of antenatal substance exposure
- neonatal behaviour in different cultures
- prediction studies
- primate behaviour

(Brazelton & Nugent, 2011)

In addition, there is evidence from the neurosciences that uninterrupted skin-to-skin contact has a strong link with neurological and behavioural development; the tactile stimulation offered encourages the production of signals by the autonomic nervous systems of both mother and baby, which contribute to healthy neurological development (Pearson-Glaze, 2016).

Schore (1997) says the paradigm of infant brain development accepts that it is genetically determined, it develops in linear time, brain activity increases with time, and deficits are correctable later. He argues that this is a false assumption and that we need to focus much more comprehensively on the infant's experiences within the early critical period of life, and recognize that by 3 years of age, the wiring of the brain's synapses is probably complete and the limbic system fixed. He hypothesizes, therefore, that early separation of the baby from its mother could theoretically affect the neurobehavioural responses of an individual for the remainder of their lifetime. He also suggests (Schore, 2001a; 2001b) that, at birth, the human baby has more synapses in its brain than at any other stage of life and that windows of opportunity appear in early life, when a baby's brain is 'exquisitely primed to receive sensory input in order to develop more advanced neural systems'. He suggests that interpersonal events, specifically those related to the mother, are the most significant factors that can impact both positively and negatively on the structural organization of the brain, and that intense relational stress (e.g., failure to form attachment) can alter calcium metabolism, thereby contributing to the mechanism of cell death.

GATHERING OF HISTORY AND ANTENATAL AND INTRAPARTUM EVENTS

The baby's brain and nervous system are susceptible to insult at any point during embryonic and fetal development and during the birthing process. The gathering of maternal and family history is therefore vital in order to alert the practitioner to the potential for problems relating to the neurological system—for example, if there is a family history of neural tube defect. In Chapter 3, McVicar discusses embryological development and maturation of the central nervous system and points out the sensitivity of the embryo at this stage of development. Some congenital neural tube defects are listed in Table 8.1. Davies, in Chapter 5, discusses some of the factors which may cause neurological damage during this critical period, such as environmental toxins and alcohol. During fetal development, an incident such as antepartum haemorrhage, or

TABLE 8.1	**Neural Tube Defects (NTD)**			
Failure of Neural Tube Closure				
	Incidence/ Prevalence	Presentation		Effects
Anencephaly	1:1000	Failure of neural tube to fuse in the cranial area. Occurs before 25 days post-conception. Infants have minimal development of brain tissue. Absence of skull bones.		Most infants will be stillborn. Those that survive will die during the neonatal period.
Encephalocele	1:2000	Failure of closure of a portion of the neural tube, most often in the occipital region. The sac protrudes from the back of the head or base of the neck and can vary in size. It may or may not contain neural tissue and/or parts of the cerebellum (brain) or accessory lobes.		Prognosis in these cases is poor. If cerebrospinal fluid (CSF) is leaking from the sac, surgical repair is performed to prevent infection and facilitate feeding.

Continued

TABLE 8.1   Neural Tube Defects (NTD)—cont'd

Failure of Neural Tube Closure

	Incidence/ Prevalence	Presentation	Effects
		Approximately 70% of occipital encephaloceles result in hydrocephalus. This may be present at birth or develop after repair of an encephalocele Encephalocele can occur in association with meningomylocele.	
Spina bifida		Defects in closure of the neural tube associated with malformations of the spinal cord and vertebrae. Occurs prior to or during the fourth week of development. 80% occur in the lumbar region. Certain populations have a significantly greater risk. This risk appears to be significantly high in areas of the UK.	
1. Spina bifida occulta	10% of population	A vertebral defect in the region of L5 (lumbar nerve) and/or S1 (sacral nerve) in which there is a failure of the vertebral arch to grow and fuse. Only evidence may be a dimple, tuft of hair or haemangioma. Infrequently, abnormalities of the spinal cord and/or nerve roots occur and present as a dermal sinus.	Often causes no clinical symptoms and may go unrecognized and undiagnosed. Rarely causes disability, although the degree does vary according to the site of the lesion; can be very severe in some cases, causing ambulatory problems, loss of sensation and incontinence.
2. Spina bifida cystica There are three forms:	1–4:1000	Can occur anywhere along the spinal column. Usually occurs in the lumbar or lumbosacral area. Presents as a cystic sac containing meninges and/or spinal cord.	
1. Meningocele		The sac contains meninges and CSF. The spinal cord and nerve roots are in the normal position.	Nerve damage is minimal, so there is often little disability.
2. Meningomyelocele		The most severe form of spina bifida. Sac contains meninges, CSF, spinal cord and/or nerve roots. Associated with hydrocephalus. May involve the whole of the spinal cord (also linked with anencephaly). The spinal cord is open and exposed with no cystic covering.	Typically causes some degree of paralysis, determined by where the lesion occurs in the spine. The higher the lesion, the more severe the paralysis tends to be. Children often have problems with continence; some may have attention deficit hyperactivity disorder (ADHD) or other learning difficulties, such as hand–eye coordination problems. In the case of hydrocephalus, a shunt may be surgically installed to provide a continuous drain for the cerebrospinal fluid.

TABLE 8.1 Neural Tube Defects (NTD)—cont'd

Failure of Neural Tube Closure

	Incidence/ Prevalence	Presentation	Effects
3. Myeloschisis		A tract of squamous epithelium connects to the dura mater. Found in the lumbosacral area.	
Spinal dermal sinus	1:2500	A small dimple-like opening in the midline of the spine that may connect deep into the spinal cord. The majority of dermal sinus tracts are located at the level of the sacrum or the lumbar region.	If the deficit is covered by skin, minimal neurological deficit occurs. Neurological deficit occurs below the sac. The spinal cord is damaged or not properly formed, resulting in some paralysis, bowel and bladder dysfunction. Significant neurological deficit. High risk of infection. Associated with sacral dimple.

Zaganjor et al., 2016.

any other occurrence which interupts oxygen delivery to the fetus, may lead to cerebral palsy. The intrapartum period can also offer threat: the delayed onset of breathing could potentially lead to birth asphyxia, hypoxic ischaemic encephalopathy (HIE) and a resultant neurological deficit; birth trauma may lead to intracranial haemorrhage resulting from skull fracture (Chapter 2), or conditions such as facial palsy, brachial plexus injury (of which Erb's palsy is the most common) (Fig. 8.1) or phrenic nerve palsy (Table 8.2).

It is crucial that parents are informed as early as possible of any variations in the baby's behaviours that might call for special attention and referral. If a single neurological marker is discovered, parents should be informed that although the baby may have one factor that suggests some neurological impairment, it is unlikely that one factor alone would seriously affect the baby's development; it is usually a synergistic interaction of several factors that leads to the creation of real problems in the development of the nervous system.

BEHAVIOURAL OBSERVATIONAL ASSESSMENT

Behavioural assessment of the newborn may not always be easy. Brazelton and Nugent (2011) developed the

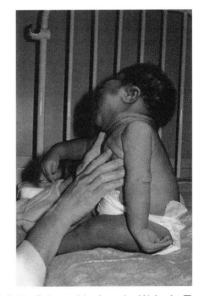

Fig. 8.1 Erb's Palsy with Arm in Waiter's Tip Position. (Reprinted from Thomas R & Harvey D, Paediatrics and Neonatology in Focus 2005, with permission from Elsevier Ltd.)

NBAS, which assesses the newborn's responses to the environment, its ability to interact with auditory and visual stimuli, and the smooth transition from one behavioural state to the next. They describe six stages of behavioural states of alertness which parents and health

TABLE 8.2	**Neurological Injuries Related to Birth Trauma**		
	Causal association	**Presentation**	**Treatment**
Facial nerve paralysis	Occurs as a result of compression of the facial nerve against the maternal sacral promontory from incorrect forceps application.	Baby presents with drooping mouth and constantly open eye on the affected side. May also have ineffective suck, swallowing problems and persistent drooling.	Traumatic facial nerve palsy will usually improve within days. However, full recovery may take weeks to months, or, if injury to the nerve is severe, several years.
Brachial plexus injury	Occurs when lateral traction is applied to the infant's neck during a difficult delivery. Particularly related to shoulder dystocia.	Erb's palsy results in paralysis of the arm and shoulder (Chapter 2); however, the hand muscles remain intact. Commonly referred to as the waiter's tip sign. In Klumpke's palsy, upper arm and shoulder movements are normal but the wrist and hand are paralysed. Injury to the entire brachial plexus is the least common type of injury; it involves paralysis of the entire upper extremity and is often associated with concurrent sensory loss.	Some injuries will resolve spontaneously; some will recover completely after physiotherapy. If this is not successful, then surgery may be attempted to improve the prognosis.
Phrenic nerve palsy	Can be injured during a difficult delivery, resulting in temporary or permanent paralysis of the diaphragm.	Cyanosis, increased work of breathing, and asymmetric chest movement.	Treatment depends on the severity. If paralysis is mild, conservative therapy, including ventilation, may be adequate. If there is recurrent pneumonia or atelectasis, or if prolonged ventilation is required, surgery may be indicated. Recovery usually occurs over 1–3 months.
Subaponeurotic (subgaleal) haemorrhage	Excessive traction (associated with vacuum-assisted birth).	This is a rare condition where the epicranial aponeurosis is pulled away from the periosteum of the skull bones, causing haemorrhage. A movable mass which crosses the suture lines and increases in size is present at birth.	Risk of excessive haemorrhage which can lead to severe shock in the baby. Associated with a high mortality rate. In smaller haemorrhages, the blood is gradually reabsorbed and swelling subsides over a number of weeks. May cause hyperbilirubinaemia.
Subdural haemorrhage	Excessive compression or traction can result in tearing of the tentorium cerebelli and rupture of the venous sinuses.	The most common lesion present in term babies. Baby may be asphyxiated and difficult to resuscitate. There may be cerebral irritation, cerebral oedema and raised intracranial pressure. Baby is likely to be nonresponsive, bradycardic, have abnormal eye movements, and may experience seizures.	Subdural haemorrhage is a serious condition which can be fatal. Diagnosis is usually confirmed with ultrasound. A subdural tap may be inserted to relieve intracranial pressure.

Tappero and Honeyfield (2019).

care professionals should be aware of in order to care and support the newborn (Table 8.3). The states of sleep and alertness consist of two sleep states, three awake states and one transitional state. The newborn's facial expressions and movements will vary with each state. There should be a smooth transition from each state to the next in a healthy newborn (Appleton, 2015; Brazelton and Nugent 2011). The interpretation of these behavioural cues may be problematic from time to time—for example, if the newborn is stressed or tired—but it is nonetheless an important part of the examination process. The behavioural assessment of the neonate helps us to evaluate aspects of its neurological status and to establish guidelines for developmental care of both the term and the preterm baby. Significantly, clear identification can help to introduce the parents to their baby's cues and is one way of adding a holistic dimension to the examination.

Observation of the newborn's behavioural state takes place before the practitioner even lays hands on the baby. The important principles of observing and listening, as outlined in Chapter 2, should alert the practitioner to any potential problems arising within the baby's neurological system.

The practitioner should always confer with the parents regarding the behavioural state of their baby. Mothers will sit gazing at the baby for prolonged periods of time, whereas assessors can only take a snapshot perspective and much can be missed. The watchword as always is 'listen to women', because they are the experts when it comes to their baby.

When observing the infant, the practitioner should consider the following:

- Are there any dysmorphic features?
- Are the facial features asymmetrical?
- Does the baby's behaviour correspond with what might be expected of the normal term neonate?
- Is the baby demonstrating the development of behavioural cues?
- Note the baby's response to arousal. Does the baby respond to stimuli?
- Is the baby asleep or awake?
- If awake, is the baby quietly alert (preterm infants have difficulty in maintaining a quiet alert state) or actively alert?
- Does the baby seem stressed or distressed?
- Is the baby demonstrating heightened sensitivity to stimuli?
- How does the baby react to sounds and movement (i.e., is the baby jittery or nonresponsive)?
- Is the baby abnormally lethargic?
- Are the baby's limb movements symmetrical? What is the quality of the movements? Are there any unusual rhythmical or jerking movements?

TABLE 8.3	**States of Sleep and Awareness**	
State 1	Deep sleep	Regular breathing; lies quietly without moving; eyes are firmly closed; no spontaneous activity; may have brief startles but will not rouse.
State 2	Active (light) sleep	Eyes are closed; moves while sleeping; startles at noises; there may be slow rotating movements of the eyes (rapid eye movement); bodily twitches with some irregular or shallow breathing; facial movements can include frowns, grimaces, smiles, twitches, mouth movements and sucking. It is believed that brain growth and differentiation may occur during active sleep.
State 3	Drowsy	Eyes may open and close, but heavy lidded appearance; variable activity with delayed responses and limited movement of limbs; breathing is regular although faster and shallower than in sleep.
State 4	Alert, awake	Baby's body and face are relatively quiet and inactive, but they will respond to sights and sounds.
State 5	Fussing	Eyes open; this is a transitional state to crying. May break down to brief fussy cries. Considerable activity with jerky, disorganized movements. Movements may produce startles.
State 6	Crying	Intense cries, perhaps screams. Motor activity is high.

- Assessment of muscle tone: is the resting posture of the baby normal (flexed arms and legs) or exaggerated (arms and legs partially or fully extended)? Are limbs floppy and hypotonic or do they appear to be hypertonic?
- Is the baby's cry abnormal?
- Does crying accompany increased motor activity?
- How is the baby feeding? Is there a poor sucking or swallowing reflex?

Influences which may alter the baby's responses include gestational age, state of alertness, degree of illness, medication and the physical environment. However, if the above questions regarding behavioural assessment highlight any unusual signs or behaviours, then the neurological health of the baby may be in question.

Other considerations when assessing the baby are:
- A variety of strong movements indicates health. Stereotyped movements indicate otherwise.
- While examining and measuring the head (Chapter 2), note:
  - any lesions resulting from birth trauma that may indicate the need for further vigilance regarding neurological health;
  - whether the fontanelles are bulging, suggesting raised intracranial pressure;
  - any excessive moulding, caput or cephalohaematomas;
  - whether there is ossification of the cranial bones or craniotabes.
- Inspect and palpate the vertebral column for evidence of neural tube defects.
- Are there any skin lesions or birth marks that may signify the presence of nerve involvement—for example, port wine stain (naevus flammeus), a flat capillary haemangioma which can occur anywhere on the body but is commonly seen on the face and in isolation causes no harm? If, however, they are cavernous, other organs may be involved (Heaberlin, 2019).

Some of the neurological neonatal alarm signals that require prompt referral and treatment are considered to be (Tucker Blackburn, 2018):
- difficulty feeding
- abnormal cry
- wide sutures and/or abnormal increase in head circumference
- persistent deviation of the head and/or eyes
- persistent irritability

- persistent asymmetry in posture and movements
- tight fisting
- opisthotonos
- apathy and immobility
- floppiness
- hyperexcitability
- convulsions
- apnoea
- jittery movements and tremors (note that this can be normal if symmetrical, generalized and stilled by flexion or sucking)

CENTRAL AND PERIPHERAL NERVOUS SYSTEMS AND CRANIAL NERVES

Although midwives are not required to diagnose specific neurological conditions, they need to have a good understanding of the anatomy of the central nervous system (the brain and spinal cord) and the physiological functions of the cranial nerves. This knowledge may alert a practitioner to a 'problem' with a particular neurological pathway. A brief introduction of the anatomy of the central nervous system (CNS) and function of the cranial nerves follows.

The CNS is the most complex system of the human body, and its role is to regulate the activities of the body. It consists of the brain and spinal cord (CNS) and the peripheral nervous system (PNS), which includes all the nerve tissues other than those of the brain and spinal cord; that is, all the nerves connecting the CNS and the other organs. The PNS carries information to the CNS through the afferent sensory nerve fibres, while some peripheral nerve fibres transmit signals in the opposite direction, away from the CNS towards distant body organs. Part of the PNS controls the activities of the viscera—for example, the heart and the gut. The visceral nervous system is referred to as the autonomic nervous system (ANS); it works outside the main nervous system. The ANS is divided into two anatomically distinct parts, the sympathetic and the parasympathetic nervous systems. The parasympathetic system maintains the body in its normal resting state, and the sympathetic system prepares it to cope with stress. Changes in the external and internal environment of the body are detected and coded into nervous impulses by sensory receptors; the CNS is therefore continuously made aware of conditions inside and outside the body. Sensory receptors convey sensations such as touch, pressure, pain, temperature, light, sound and smell.

There are 12 pairs of cranial nerves (CN): the first 2 pairs originate from the forebrain and the others from the brainstem; they all combine to coordinate and control the systems of the body (Fig. 8.2), but each has a specific function.

The physical assessment of the CNS combines observation and palpation, and considers the movement, tone and reflexes of the newborn. The absence, alteration or impairment of any of the signs listed in Table 8.4 necessitates further investigation and prompt referral. It is important to note that, in the term neonate, damage to any of the nerves will have some impact.

REFLEXES

The primary reflexes of the neonate are those inborn behavioural patterns that develop during uterine life. More than 70 primary (sometimes referred to as primitive)

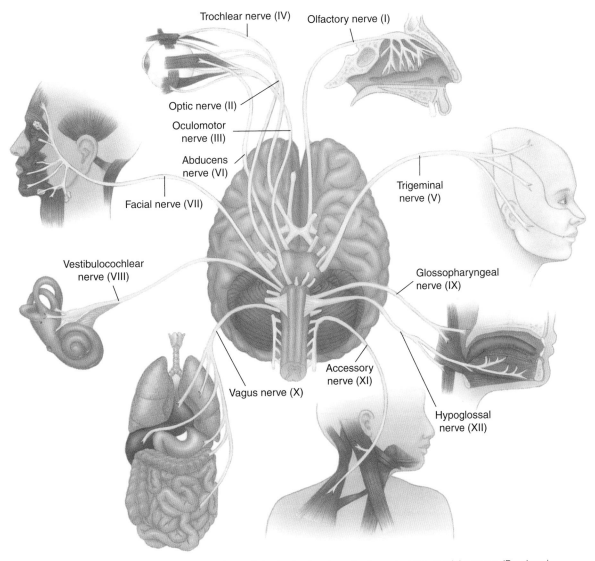

Fig. 8.2 Cranial Nerves. Ventral surface of the brain showing attachment of the cranial nerves. (Reprinted from Thibodeau GA, Patton KT, Anthony's Textbook of Anatomy & Physiology, 16th edn, 1999, with permission from Mosby.)

TABLE 8.4	**Cranial Nerves**	
Cranial Nerves (CN)	**Function**	**Examination**
CN I Olfactory nerve	Sense of smell	Not undertaken
CN II Optic nerve	Vision	Use ophthalmoscope—pupils checked for size and constriction in response to a light Blink reflex observed
CN III Oculomotor nerve	Supplies the pupil and extraocular muscles	Observe pupillary response to light for corneal light reflex which, although immature, is often present at birth; eye movement for symmetry and size; movements of eyeball and upper eyelid
CN IV Trochlear nerve		Eye movement down and outwards
CN V Trigeminal nerve	Ophthalmic nerve (sensory), maxillary nerve (sensory), mandibular nerve (mixed). Supplies jaw muscles, maxilla and mandible	General facial sensation from cornea of eyeball, upper nasal cavity, cheeks, palate, tongue, teeth. Sucking ability and later chewing
CN VI Abducent nerve	Abduction of eye	Lateral eye movement—squint. As detailed in Chapter 10, the presence of squint usually develops in the first few months. Injury to CN VI is possible but very rare
CN VII Facial nerve	Taste. Movement of facial muscles and salivation	Observe for facial asymmetry, expression, crying
CN VIII Vestibulocochlear nerve	Ear (balance and hearing)	Startle reflex Auditory—newborn hearing screening
CN IX Glossopharyngeal nerve	Mouth. Taste, tongue sensations, secretion of saliva, swallowing	Observe tongue movement and elicit gag reflex
CN X Vagus nerve	Supplies and monitors activities of all viscera—soft palate, pharynx and larynx, chest and abdominal viscera	Observe swallow reflex and ability to cry
CN XI Accessory spinal nerve	Supplies muscles of the larynx, sternocleidomastoid and trapezius	Head movement—baby should be able to move head into midline and from side to side. Sternomastoid muscles and shoulders
CN XII Hypoglossal nerve	Supplies muscles of the tongue	Observe swallow reflex and elicit suck and gag reflexes. Tongue position and movement in mouth

reflexes have been identified, and they may be classified in several ways—for example, according to function, time of appearance or the type of stimulus which releases them.

They should all be present at birth, but are gradually inhibited by the higher centres in the brain during the first 2 to 12 months of postnatal life. The presence and strength of the reflexes is an indication of the baby's neurological functioning within the first 24 hours after birth. If reflexes are absent or exaggerated, or if hypotonia is present with any of these tests, there may be significant neurological problems. However, the tests should be repeated prior to referral to ensure that compounding factors have not been the cause of a poor response—for example, in a baby who is sleepy or a baby who has a fractured clavicle resulting from a difficult birth. As with all screening tests, the findings must be recorded in the notes and appropriate referral should be made. If any of the primitive reflexes persist beyond the appropriate time frame, the baby should be referred for further neurological examination; the persistence of primary reflexes beyond their normal timespan (12 months) interferes with subsequent development and indicates neurological impairment.

In the examination of the newborn, some of the following reflexes are routinely elicited at birth (these are described in detail in Chapter 2) and some at the 6- to 8-week check. The main primary reflexes observed in the first year of life are illustrated in Table 8.5; these are the reflexes we would expect to be present in a healthy term neonate. As the nervous system develops, these

TABLE 8.5 Reflexes That Would Be Present in a Healthy Term Infant			
Primitive Reflexes	**Present from/ Established by**	**Disappears Approximately at**	**Reflexes Performed at the 6–8-Week Check**
Suck	28/34 weeks	12 months	Confirm
Swallow	Birth	Permanent. Movement seen when baby feeding	Confirm
Rooting	28/34 weeks	3–4 months. If baby's cheek, or the side of the mouth is stroked, baby will open its mouth and move head towards stimulus.	Present
Gag	Birth	Permanent	Present
Palmar grasp (hand)	28/32 weeks	2–4 months	Yes
Babinski	34/38 weeks	12–14 months	No
Plantar grasp (foot)	32 weeks	8–12 months	No
Step	35–37 weeks	3 months. Infants regain this reflex at approximately 9 months of age.	Yes
Moro and/or startle	32 weeks	3–4 months	Yes
Blinking	Birth	Permanent	Present
Ventral suspension	Birth	If the baby is held prone on the palm of your hand, the head should lift and rotate, the body should extend and the arms and legs should flex.	Yes
Tonic neck reflex	Present at birth, but continues to develop	As the baby turns to face one side, the arm and leg will extend as the opposite arm and leg flex (fencing posture). This action disappears around 2–4 months.	Yes
Incurving or Gallant	Birth	Position is the same as ventral suspension. If a finger is run gently down each side of the baby's body, the pelvis should curve to the side being stroked. Disappears 3–6 months	No
The head lag	Present in term neonates but not routinely performed. This manoeuvre should not be carried out on a preterm neonate.	Practitioners should obtain a secure hold of the baby's hands and arms with both hands. Baby should be brought forward with head in the midline. Once baby is sitting upright, head should momentarily support itself. It will then lag to one side or the other or fall backwards. This will improve with age until the baby has full head control.	Yes

initial reflexes are inhibited or transformed, and the secondary and postural reflexes emerge.

Some reflexes are simple and are mediated at the spinal cord level, whereas others are more complex and require the integration of brain centres, labyrinths and other developing nerve centres (Heaberlin, 2019).

The primary reflexes can be categorized into primitive, locomotor and postural reflexes.

The *primitive* reflexes are essential for the newborn's survival. They are involuntary, not learned, and include those associated with feeding, rooting, sucking, swallowing and urinating. Others include the grasp reflex (where the newborn grasps a finger placed in its palm) and the Moro reflex, which is activated through a sudden change of light or a loud noise. The response usually includes flexion of the legs, tensing of the back muscles and crying.

The *locomotor* reflexes are those that bear a resemblance to later voluntary movements. These include the step reflex and the closed glottis reflex that would occur if the baby were placed underwater.

Most of the *postural* reflexes are secondary and emerge after 3 months or so, but the tonic neck reflex is present from birth (Table 8.5).

6- TO 8-WEEK FOLLOW-UP ASSESSMENT

The PHE NIPE Screening Programme Standards (see the Antenatal and Newborn Screening Timeline: optimum times for testing in Chapter 4) state that all babies should be formally reviewed by 8 weeks of age at the latest (PHE, 2016). A developmental assessment at this point gives the practitioner an opportunity to ensure that the baby's neurological development is progressing as would be expected. As discussed at the beginning of the chapter, the relationship between the baby and its mother is an important consideration; the practitioner should be observing for good parent–child interaction, and for positive parenting response and parenting skills. At 6 to 8 weeks, the examiner would expect to find the features listed in Table 8.6.

GESTATIONAL AGE ASSESSMENT

In order to determine accurate gestational age, three distinct measures are usually undertaken: the mother's estimated date of conception, which is taken from the first day of the last menstrual period and the day of delivery; ultrasound scans, which are usually performed at 8 to 12 weeks for the estimated gestation for dates and

TABLE 8.6 6- to 8-Week Developmental Assessment	
Fine motor skills & vision	Palmar grip is present and equal on both sides Eyes fixate on objects—gaze follows moving persons When supine, will look at object held in midline—will follow it as it moves from side to side in the midline, up to 90 degrees
Gross motor skills	Baby lies on back with elbows flexed, knees and hips partly flexed When pulled to sitting, baby shows considerable head lag but shows some ability to raise the head, particularly at the halfway stage (45 degrees) When prone, the pelvis is fairly low on the couch and the hips partly and intermittently extended Baby can raise chin off the surface momentarily when face down When suspended in the prone position, baby can hold head in line with rest of body
6 weeks—personal and social milestones	Will smile at mother Watches faces
Signs of abnormal development	Asymmetrical neonatal reflexes Excessive head lag Failure to smile No visual fixation/following Failure to respond to sound

Table 8.7 Gestational Age	
A term baby is defined as a baby born between 37 and 42 weeks. Preterm is defined as a baby born less than 37 weeks. Post-term is defined as a baby who is born at a date beyond 42 weeks of gestation.	
Appropriate for gestation age (AGA)	Weight between 10th and 90th percentile for gestational age
Small for gestational age (SGA)	Weight less than 10th percentile for gestational age
Large for gestational age (LGA)	Weight greater than 90th percentile for gestational age
Low birth weight	Birth weight less than 2500g
Very low birth weight	Birth weight less than 1500g
Extremely low birth weight	Birth weight less than 1000g

the 18- to 20-week scan which assesses for both growth and fetal anomalies (see Table 8.7) and lastly the NIPE (Wiltgen Trotter, 2019).

During the newborn physical examination, the practitioner should be able to establish the 'developmental' age of the baby by assessing its reflexes, muscle tone, posture and vital signs in addition to its weight, length, head circumference and skin condition. If these signs do not match the anticipated gestational age, then allowances need to be made in order to meet the actual rather than the expected needs of the baby. For example, an infant born with a gestational age of 36 weeks may actually have a developmental gestational age of 38 weeks and therefore behave more like a full-term rather than a preterm infant. Conversely, a baby assessed as being 37 weeks' gestation who presents with physical and neurological signs indicative of 35 weeks' gestation may require considerably more support and possibly admission to the neonatal intensive care unit (NICU).

Gestational age assessment plays an important part in understanding the baby's behaviour. Immaturity of as little as 2 weeks may lead to behavioural differences that could possibly influence the parents' reaction to their baby if they were unclear of the reasons for them (Dubowitz et al., 1970). For example, the starved, distressed, jittery appearance of an intrauterine growth-restricted infant of 36 weeks' gestation may be at odds with the healthy-looking, chubby term baby the parents were expecting. The baby may be hypersensitive to stimuli and correspondingly appear to hyperreact to those stimuli. Alerting the parents to the reasons for this appearance and behaviour, and explaining this is likely to be a transitory stage, may help them to understand their baby's needs more effectively.

Gestational age assessment tools, which were devised in the 1950s and 1960s, have formed the basis of assessment and are still used today to estimate accurate gestational age. Dubowitz et al. (1970) developed a scoring system based on 10 neurological and 11 external criteria. The test takes on average 10 to 15 minutes to perform (Table 8.8 and Fig. 8.3). Ballard et al. revised the test in 1979 using just 6 physical and 6 neurological criteria; however, both tools were said to overestimate the actual gestational age by up to 2 weeks. Ballard et al. (1991) modified their tool (Fig. 8.4), resulting in greater accuracy. It now includes additional material for estimating the age of the extremely premature newborn (20–26 weeks) and accurately determines a newborn's gestational age to within 2 to 3 days. The test takes only 3 to 4 minutes to perform (Tappero and Honeyfield, 2019). The greater the age of the newborn, the higher the score. The consensus of opinion is that the assessment should be performed within the first 48 hours for term neonates and at less than 12 hours for extremely preterm infants because the physical criteria which are evaluated change rapidly after birth. It should be remembered, though, that labour, birth and medications may affect the assessment and it may need repeating (Thureen et al., 2004).

GROWTH CHARTS (CENTILE CHARTS)

Normal growth in individual children will, of course, vary. The height of a child, however, is generally linked

Table 8.8 External Criteria for Gestational Age Assessment

External Sign	Score*				
	0	**1**	**2**	**3**	**4**
Oedema	Obvious oedema of hands and feet; pitting over tibia	No obvious oedema of hands and feet; pitting over tibia	No oedema		
Skin texture	Very thin; gelatinous	Thin and smooth	Smooth; medium thickness; rash or superficial peeling	Slight thickening; superficial cracking and peeling, especially hands and feet	Thick and parchment-like; superficial or deep cracking
Skin colour	Dark red	Uniformly pink	Pale pink; variable over body	Pale; pink only over ears, lips, palms, soles	
Skin opacity (trunk)	Numerous veins and venules clearly seen, especially over abdomen	Veins and tributaries seen	A few large vessels clearly seen over abdomen	A few large vessels seen indistinctly over abdomen	No blood vessels seen
Lanugo (over back)	No lanugo	Abundant; long and thick over whole back	Hair thinning, especially over lower back	Small amount of lanugo and bald areas	At least half of back devoid of lanugo
Plantar creases	No skin creases	Faint red marks over anterior half of sole	Definite red marks over > anterior half; indentations over < anterior third	Indentation over > anterior third	Definite deep indentations over > anterior third
Nipple formation	Nipple barely visible; no areola	Nipple well defined; areola smooth and flat; diameter < 0.75 cm	Areola stippled; edge not raised; diameter 0.75 cm	Areola stippled; edge raised; diameter > 0.75 cm	
Breast size	No breast tissue palpable	Breast tissue on one or both sides; < 0.5 cm diameter	Breast tissue both sides; one or both 0.5–1 cm	Breast tissue both sides > 1 cm	
Ear form	Pinna flat and shapeless; little or no incurving of edge	Incurving of part of edge of pinna	Partial incurving whole of upper pinna	Well-defined incurving whole of upper pinna	
Ear firmness	Pinna soft, easily folded; no recoil	Pinna soft, easily folded; slow recoil	Cartilage to edge of pinna, but soft in places; ready recoil	Pinna firm, cartilage to edge; instant recoil	
Male genitals	Neither testis in scrotum	At least one testis high in scrotum	At least one testis down		
Female genitals with hips half abducted	Labia majora widely separated; labia minora protruding	Labia majora almost cover labia minora	Labia majora completely cover labia minora		

*If score differs on paired anatomic features (i.e., plantar creases, nipple formation, ear form), take the mean.

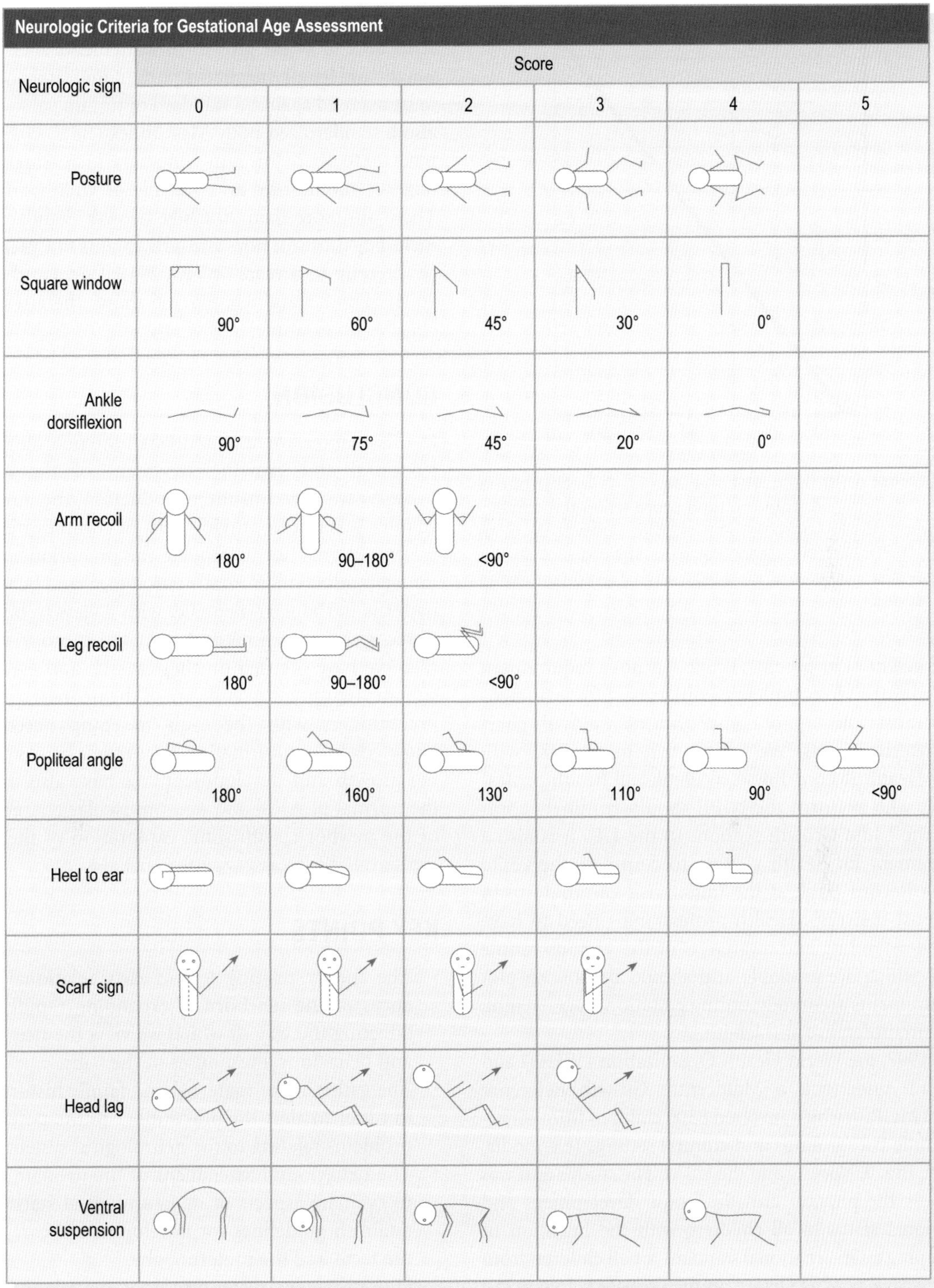

Neurologic Criteria for Gestational Age Assessment

Neurologic sign	Score					
	0	1	2	3	4	5
Posture						
Square window	90°	60°	45°	30°	0°	
Ankle dorsiflexion	90°	75°	45°	20°	0°	
Arm recoil	180°	90–180°	<90°			
Leg recoil	180°	90–180°	<90°			
Popliteal angle	180°	160°	130°	110°	90°	<90°
Heel to ear						
Scarf sign						
Head lag						
Ventral suspension						

A

Fig. 8.3 (A) Neurological criteria for gestational age assessment.

Continued

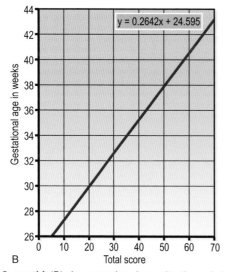

Fig. 8.3, cont'd (B) the gestational age (1–2 weeks) of the infant is determined from the total score using the conversion graph. (Redrawn from Dubovitz LMS, Dubovitz W, Goldberg C, 1970, Clinical assessment of gestational age in the newborn infant, Journal of Pediatrics 77(1): 7, with permission from Elsevier.)

to the height of its parents. While it is not a requirement in all countries to complete a centile chart for term neonates, most will require completion of a growth chart for preterm infants. We believe that in the UK, with Child Health Record Books available, all health professionals who perform the NIPE should routinely complete the Child Growth section. In the UK, it is also a requirement for health visitors to complete the Child Health Record Book at the initial visit (around 10–14 days post-delivery). Health professionals need to have an understanding and awareness of the various centile charts which are available and should be able to plot measurements accurately, noting gestational age, weight, head circumference and length.

In 1997, the World Health Organization (WHO) and UNICEF undertook a Multicentre Growth Reference Study (MGRS), which involved 8500 children from different ethnic backgrounds and cultural settings (e.g., India, Ghana, Brazil, Norway and the USA). The study's aim was to assess the physical growth, motor development and nutritional status of all children, with the intention of developing an international standard for all children from birth to 5 years of age based on the breastfed child as the norm for growth and development. The new WHO Child Growth Standards describe how babies 'should grow' with 'correct feeding practices', a healthy environment and lifestyle, and allow for growth measurements such as body weight and length/height (important indicators of health) to be assessed against a standard optimum value. There is also a standardized Body Mass Index (BMI) chart for infants up to age 5; this is proving to be increasingly important for monitoring an epidemic of childhood obesity. There are more than 30 Child Growth Standard charts, including those for boys and girls, infants to 1 year, and for children up to 5 years (WHO, 2019; Garza and de Onis, 2004) (Figs 8.5 and 8.6; Fig. 8.6 shows the girl's growth chart as an example).

CONCLUSION

In this chapter, we have addressed the neurological, behavioural and growth assessment of the newborn baby. As we stated in the introduction, the aim of this chapter was not to provide a list of complex neurological conditions, but to provide the practitioner with an understanding of 'normal' neurological and behavioural patterns in the term neonate, with a view to being able to recognize deviations and make the appropriate referrals. We have focused on the research and evidence to support best practice and care of the neonate, providing practitioners with the tools to equip parents with knowledge and information about their baby's continuing growth and development. We have also described the normal physical and neuromuscular characteristics of the newborn, with some exploration of the various tools available to assess gestational age.

KEY POINTS

- The theory relating to the early relational experiences of the newborn is expanding rapidly and is affecting the way in which we view the neurological and behavioural responses of the baby.
- The gathering of maternal and family history is vital in order to alert the practitioner to the potential for problems relating to the neurological system.
- The behavioural assessment of the neonate helps us to evaluate aspects of its neurological status and to establish guidelines for developmental care of both the term and the preterm baby.
- Observing and listening are essential and should alert the practitioner to any potential problems arising within the baby's neurological system.

The New Ballard Score

Score Sheet

Use this score sheet to assess the gestational maturity of your baby. At the end of the examination, the total score determines the gestational maturity in weeks.

NEUROMUSCULAR MATURITY

SIGN	−1	0	1	2	3	4	5	SIGN SCORE
Posture								
Square Window	>90°	90°	60°	45°	30°	0°		
Arm Recoil		180°	140°–180°	110°–140°	90°–110°	<90°		
Popliteal Angle	180°	160°	140°	120°	100°	90°	<90°	
Scarf Sign								
Heel To Ear								

TOTAL NEUROMUSCULAR SCORE

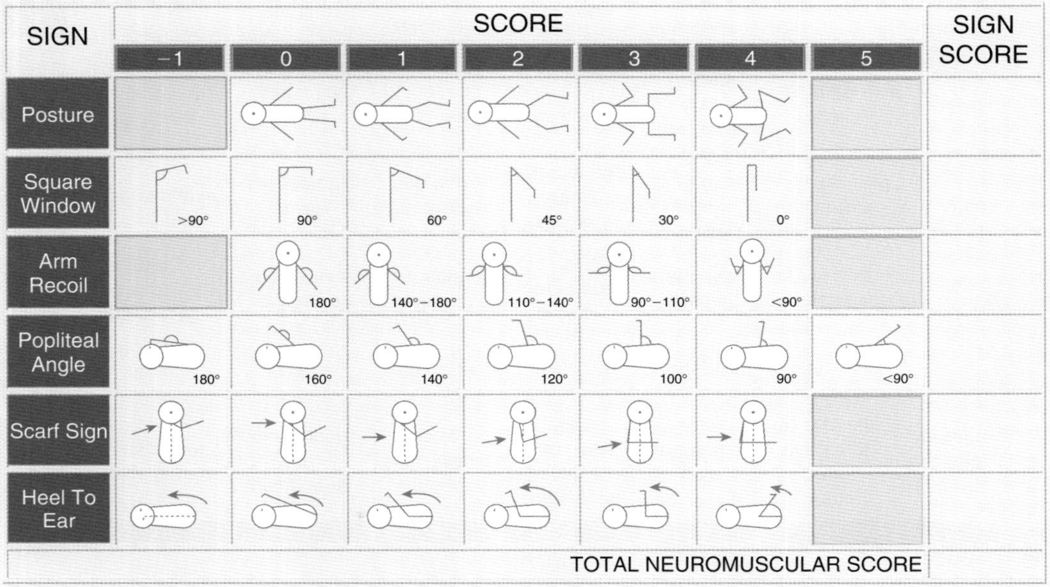

Fig. 8.4 The New Ballard Score: (A) neuromuscular maturity.

Continued

PHYSICAL MATURITY

SIGN	-1	0	1	2	3	4	5	SIGN SCORE
Skin	Sticky, friable, transparent	gelatinous, red, translucent	smooth pink, visible veins	superficial peeling &/or rash, few veins	cracking, pale areas, rare veins	parchment, deep cracking, no vessels	leathery, cracked, wrinkled	
Lanugo	none	sparse	abundant	thinning	bald areas	mostly bald		
Plantar Surface	heel-toe 40–50 mm: −1 <40 mm: −2	>50 mm no crease	faint red marks	anterior transverse crease only	creases ant. 2/3	creases over entire sole		
Breast	imperceptable	barely perceptable	flat areola no bud	stippled areola 1-2 mm bud	raised areola 3-4 mm bud	full areola 5-10 mm bud		
Eye/Ear	lids fused loosely: −1 tightly: −2	lids open pinna flat stays folded	sl. curved pinna; soft; slow recoil	well-curved pinna; soft but ready recoil	formed & firm instant recoil	thick cartilage ear stiff		
Genitals (Male)	scrotum flat, smooth	scrotum empty, faint rugae	testes in upper canal, rare rugae	testes descending, few rugae	testes down, good rugae	testes pendulous, deep rugae		
Genitals (Female)	clitoris prominent & labia flat	prominent clitoris & small labia minora	prominent clitoris & enlarging minora	majora & minora equally prominent	majora large, minora small	majora cover clitoris & minora		

TOTAL PHYSICAL MATURITY SCORE

Fig. 8.4, cont'd (B) physical maturity.

MATURITY RATING

TOTAL SCORE (NEUROMUSCULAR + PHYSICAL)	WEEKS
−10	20
−5	22
0	24
5	26
10	28
15	30
20	32
25	34
30	36
35	38
40	40
45	42
50	44

References :
Ballard JL, Khoury JC, Wedig K, et al: New Ballard Score, expanded to include extremely premature infants. J Pediatrics 1991: 119:417–423.

Fig. 8.4, cont'd (C) maturity rating. (Reprinted from Ballard JL, Khoury JC, Wedig K et al., 1991, New Ballard Score, expanded to include extremely premature infants, Journal of Pediatrics 119:417–423, with permission from Elsevier Ltd.)

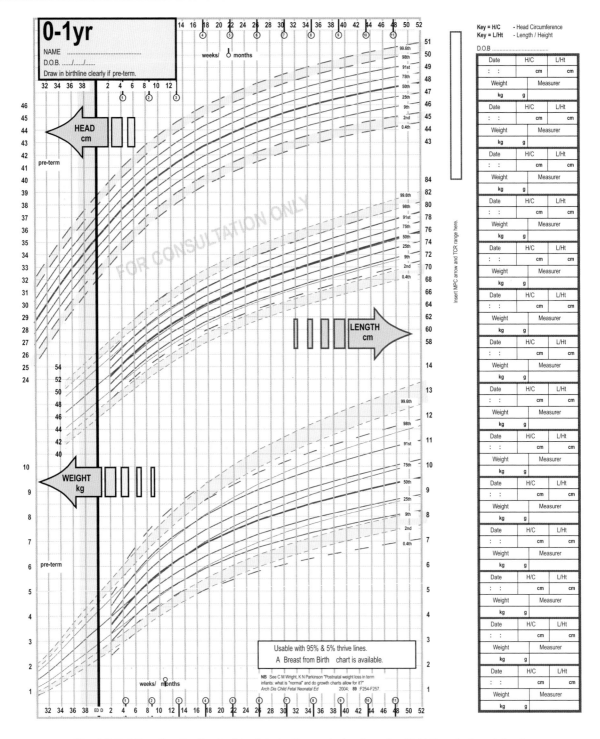

Fig. 8.5 0–1 Year Centile Charts. (Reprinted with permission from the Child Growth Foundation.)

Length/height-for-age GIRLS

Birth to 5 years (z-scores)

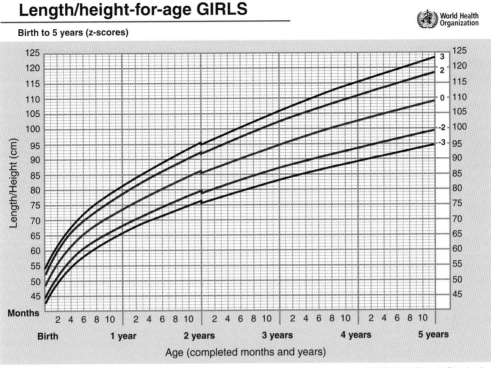

WHO Child Growth Standards

Fig. 8.6 0–1 Year Centile Charts. (Reprinted with permission from the Child Growth Foundation.)

- During the NIPE, the practitioner should be able to establish the 'developmental' age of the baby by assessing its reflexes, muscle tone, posture and vital signs.
- Health professionals who perform the NIPE should routinely complete the Child Growth Graph.

REFERENCES

Amiel-Tison, C., 1986. Neurological Assessment During the First Year of Life. Oxford University Press, Oxford, UK.

Appleton, J., 2015. Newborn behavioural aspects. In: Lomax, A. (Eds.), Examination of the Newborn: An Evidence-Based Guide. Wiley-Blackwell, London, UK, p. 192 (Chapter 8).

Ballard, J.L., Khoury, J.C., Wedig, K., Wang, L., Eilers-Walsman, B.L., Lipp, R., 1991. New Ballard Score, expanded to include extremely premature infants. J. Pediat. 119, 417–423.

Brazelton, T.B., 2011. 'Brilliant Babies' in Smidt, D., *Introducing Bruner: A Guide for Practitioners and Students in Early Years*

Education (Introducing Early Years Thinkers. Routledge, Abingdon, UK, p. 28.

Brazelton, T.B., Nugent, J.K., 2011. The Neonatal Behavioral Assessment Scale, fourth ed. McKeith/Blackwell Press, London, UK.

Dubowitz, L.M.S., Dubowitz, V., Goldberg, C., 1970. Clinical assessment of gestational age in the newborn infant. J. Pediat. 77 (1), 1–10. Available from: https://www.jpeds.com/article/S0022-3476(70)80038-5/pdf. Accessed March 2019.

Garza, C., de Onis, M., 2004. Rationale for developing a new international growth reference. Food Nutrit. Bull. 25 (Suppl. 1), S5–S14. Available from: https://www.who.int/nutrition/media_page/rationale_dev_growth.pdf?ua=1. Accessed March 2019.

Heaberlin, P.D., 2019. Neurologic assessment. In: Tappero, E.P., Honeyfield, M.E. (Eds.), Physical Assessment of the Newborn, sixth ed. Springer Publishing Company LLC, New York, pp. 167–192.

Pearson-Glaze, P., 2016. Kangaroo Care for Your Premature Baby—Breastfeeding Support [online]. Available from: https://breastfeeding.support/kangaroo-care-for-your-premature-baby. Accessed March 2019.

Public Health England (PHE), 2016. Newborn and Infant Physical Examination Screening Programme Standards. Available from: https://assets.publishing.service.gov.uk/government/uploads/system/uploads/attachment_data/file/692020/NIPE_Programme_Standards_2016_to_2017.pdf. Crown Copyright; Accessed March 2019.

Schore, A.N., 1997. Early organization of the nonlinear right brain and development of a predisposition to psychiatric disorders. Dev. Psychopathol. 9, 595–631.

Schore, A.N., 2001a. The effects of early relational trauma on right brain development, affect regulation, and infant mental health. Infant Ment. Health J. 22 (1-2), 201–269.

Schore, A.N., 2001b. Effects of a secure attachment relationship on right brain development, affect regulation, and infant mental health. Infant Ment. Health J. 22 (1-2), 7–66.

Smith, M., 2001. Review of the neurological assessment of the preterm and full-term newborn infant. Arch. Dis. Child. 84, 453.

Tappero, E.P., Honeyfield, M.E., 2019. Physical Assessment of the Newborn, sixth ed. Springer Publishing Company LLC, New York.

Thomas, R., Harvey, D., 2019. Paediatrics and Neonatology. Elsevier, Edinburgh, UK.

Thureen, P.J., Deacon, J., Hernandez, J.A., Hall, D., 2004. Assessment and Care of the Well Newborn, second ed. WB Saunders, Philadelphia, PA.

Tucker Blackburn, S., 2018. Maternal, Fetal, & Neonatal Physiology: A Clinical Perspective, fifth ed. Elsevier, UK.

Wiltgen Trotter, C., 2019. Gestational age assessment. In: Tappero, E.P., Honeyfield, M.E. (Eds.), Physical Assessment of the Newborn, sixth ed. Springer Publishing Company LLC, New York.

World Health Organization (WHO), 2019. Child growth standards. Available from: https://www.who.int/childgrowth/en/. Accessed April 2020.

Zaganjor, I., Sekkarie, A., Tsang, B.L., Williams, J., Razzaghi, H., Mulinare, J., et al., 2016. Describing the prevalence of neural tube defects worldwide: a systematic literature review. PLoS One 11 (4), e0151586. Available from: https://www.ncbi.nlm.nih.gov/pmc/articles/PMC4827875/. Accessed March 2019.

9

Congenital Cardiac Anomalies in the Newborn: Causes, Effects and Treatment

Eshita Upadhyay and Sanjay Raina

CHAPTER CONTENTS

INTRODUCTION

The assessment of a baby's cardiovascular system is an important element in the examination of the newborn. Congenital heart disease (CHD) has the potential to seriously affect the health and well-being of the newborn baby, either at the time of detection or at some point in the future. Therefore the sooner diagnosis is made and appropriate treatment commenced, the better the outcome for the baby.

This chapter aims to provide practitioners with a frame of reference for some of the clinical signs and symptoms that may be present in some forms of CHD. If identified during the Newborn Infant Physical Examination (NIPE), such identification may facilitate the initiation of prompt lifesaving medical intervention.

Congenital heart disease can be described as 'a heart condition that results in an abnormality of the actual structure of the heart or of its function, which is present at birth'. The majority of the conditions are due to malformation of the heart valves and/or vessels. There may

also be communications (holes) between the chambers of the heart (Petersen et al., 2003).

The terminology used to describe heart conditions varies widely. Although the terms differ slightly, they generally refer to the same type of problems. In different texts and articles, it is possible to encounter a variety of terms: 'congenital heart disease' (CHD), 'congenital heart defect' (CHD), 'congenital heart lesion' (CHL), 'congenital heart anomaly' (CHA). These terms are often used interchangeably. In this chapter, the author will use the term 'congenital heart disease' (CHD), and will look at some of the defects which make up the disease as a whole.

The skills required to recognize signs and symptoms of CHD in any setting include a degree of understanding of the haemodynamic effects of the disease. This chapter also provides information about the prevalence of CHD, examples of the most common types of CHD, the causes, the haemodynamic effects, the diagnosis and some of the treatment options.

PREVALENCE

Congenital heart disease occurs in approximately 8 in 1000 live births. Some of the cases are very mild and cause no problems throughout the lifespan, whereas others are very severe and cause some compromise at birth. Of those babies with defects, approximately 2–3 per 1000 will be symptomatic within the first year of life. The complexity of the disease depends on how the individual heart structure and/or function is affected (van der Linde et al., 2011). Diagnostic, palliative and corrective techniques have evolved so much over the last decade that the prognosis for a variety of heart diseases has improved considerably, resulting in more babies surviving and children with severe defects surviving into later childhood. The number of deaths in England from CHD in children under 1 year of age decreased by nearly half between 1986 and 2011, from 584 to 305 (PHE, 2018).

As ultrasound technology has become more sophisticated and technicians more skilled, our ability to diagnose CHD during the antenatal period has improved significantly. This allows time for the woman to make decisions regarding where she gives birth—which will ideally be within, or very near to a tertiary cardiac centre. Having immediate access to such a centre may significantly improve the baby's outcome. Following The Bristol Royal Infirmary Inquiry Final Report (2001), UK service provision for neonatal and paediatric cardiac surgery changed dramatically, and government-approved national standards were developed to cover all aspects of care and treatment of children with CHD.

In an attempt to improve outcomes for children undergoing cardiac surgery, the decision was made that if the cardiac centre were allowed to continue to function, then the surgeons employed there must perform a minimum number of cardiac procedures in order to maintain sufficient skill and competence.

This has resulted in fewer centres performing paediatric cardiac surgery, but with a concentration of experienced, skilled surgeons as part of a caring team, which ensures improved mortality and morbidity for the children.

CAUSES OF CONGENITAL HEART DISEASE

The specific causes of CHD are mainly thought to be idiopathic; however, certain factors would appear to predispose to its development. Babies who have associated health problems (syndromes) are more likely to have a congenital heart defect. Some of these factors are outlined in Table 9.1.

TABLE 9.1 **Factors That Increase the Risk of Congenital Heart Disease**	
Certain drugs—both therapeutic and recreational	Alcohol
Anticonvulsants: phenytoin is linked to pulmonary and aortic stenosis	Fetal alcohol syndrome to VSD, TGA, TOF and ASD
Amphetamines to ASD & VSD	
Warfarin to VSD	
Lithium to Ebstein anomaly	
Oestrogen and progesterone to TGA, VSD and TOF	
Marijuana and cocaine to VSD	
Infection	Diabetes predisposes to TGA, VSD and cardiomyopathy
Rubella to PDA and PS	
Maternal congenital heart disease increases the risk from 5% to 10% (Ewing et al., 1997; Park, 1997; Feit, 1998)	Syndromes: Trisomy 13 (Patau) 90% VSD, PDA Trisomy 18 (Edwards) 85% VSD, PDA, PS Trisomy 21 (Down) 40% AVSD Turner syndrome 35% CoAo, ASD; Klinefelter syndrome 15% PDA, ASD; Di George syndrome 10% interrupted aortic arch, truncus arteriosus; less common pulmonary atresia with VSD and TOF (Goldmutz and Emanuel, 1997; Park, 1997; Feit, 1998; Goldmutz, 1999, Grech and Gaff, 1999)

ASD, atrial septal defect; *AVSD*, atrial ventricular septal defect; *CoAo*, coarctation of the aorta; *PDA*, patent ductus arteriosus; *PS*, pulmonary stenosis; *TOF*, tetralogy of Fallot; *TGA*, transposition of the great arteries; *VSD*, ventricular septal defect.

Most congenital defects are tolerated well during fetal life, and it is only when the maternal circulation has ceased and the baby needs to sustain an independent cardiovascular system that the haemodynamic abnormality becomes apparent. The significance of various defects also changes as the child grows; for example, a large ventricular septal defect (VSD) is likely to have a lesser effect on the haemodynamics of the newborn than it would on those of the older infant/child. This is because the blood flow across the defect is reduced due to raised pulmonary resistance in the first few weeks of life.

Historically, most heart defects have been subdivided into two categories: either simple and complex, or acyanotic and cyanotic. This categorization is determined by physical examination, aided by pulse oximetry.

Babies born with simple (acyanotic) heart disease represent the majority of children affected. They remain pink in colour and their prognosis is usually good. This type of heart disease can spontaneously correct itself or can be treated nonsurgically.

Complex (cyanotic) heart disease often has a poor prognosis unless treated surgically. However, improvements in diagnosis—along with the development of heart–lung bypass machines, improved surgical techniques, safer anaesthesia, treatment via catheterization and improved postoperative care—have collectively ensured that 80% of patients will now survive into adulthood. Although they will require follow-up care by cardiac experts for the rest of their lives, as a result of these advances a new specialism has emerged, known as 'grown-up congenital heart disease' (often abbreviated to GUCH).

Practitioners can gain an alternative view of the complexities CHD creates for the child by approaching the subject from a physiological perspective. There are three main physiological effects depending on the type of heart disease. These are:

- increased pulmonary blood flow
- decreased pulmonary blood flow
- obstruction or reduction in the systemic blood flow.

Understanding these can allow practitioners a greater insight into the mechanics of the working heart.

Increased Pulmonary Blood Flow

This is the physiological effect of the most common heart defects such as:

- patent ductus arteriosus (PDA)
- atrial septal defect (ASD)
- ventricular septal defect (VSD).

The left side of the heart has a higher working pressure than the right, so connections between the two will result in blood being shunted from the left to the right (Moynihan and King, 1989).

The increase in blood being moved to the right will, in turn, increase the volume of blood being pumped to the lungs. This process will, if the volume is significant, cause congestive cardiac failure (CCF), or right-sided heart failure.

Excessive blood flow to the lungs decreases the pulmonary compliance (i.e., makes the lungs stiff and more difficult to expand and contract). The excess blood volume produces wet, boggy lungs and a reduced gas exchange. The child will naturally try to compensate for this by breathing more rapidly (tachypnoea) which will, in turn, cause tachycardia (rapid heart rate); this is the body's attempt to overcome the problem and transport blood forwards to the left side of the heart. The overloaded lungs will, on auscultation, have rales present; rales are abnormal lung sounds, audible when listening to the chest through a stethoscope. Rales can be sibilant (whistling), dry (crackling) or wet (sloshy), depending on the amount and density of fluid moving in the air passages.

The wet environment in the lungs provides a perfect medium to increase the risk of pulmonary infection. If CCF is present, accompanying symptoms will include fluid and sodium retention as the body tries to increase the blood volume to compensate for the lack of blood cells (which remain in the lungs). The child will be breathing rapidly and using more energy to do so, and the poor cell nutrition that results from decreased peripheral blood flow produces poor feeding; thus there is poor or slow weight gain, as the child uses more calories than they are taking in.

The classic picture of a child with *increased pulmonary blood flow* is of one who is thin, has episodes of diaphoresis (sweating), has feeding problems, tachypnoea, tachycardia and a degree of oedema (swelling). These children are also susceptible to frequent chest infections.

If it is not treated at an appropriate time, increased pulmonary blood flow will eventually lead to permanent changes in the pulmonary vessel (pulmonary vessel disease). Increased flow through the pulmonary vasculature causes shear forces that disrupt the vascular endothelium and activate inflammation. The changes in the pulmonary vasculature can lead to progression of pulmonary hypertension (Kliegman et al., 2016). This is an attempt by the body to decrease the flow, but it has the effect of producing muscular tissue growth around the internal diameter of the pulmonary vessels. Pulmonary hypertension can contribute to lethal complications in the postoperative period for children with CHD; it is therefore essential that surgery is undertaken prior to the development of pulmonary hypertension.

An additional effect of the increased pulmonary blood flow that creates pulmonary vasoconstriction and/or pulmonary hypertension is that it causes the right side of the heart to enlarge (right ventricular hypertrophy). This increases the pressure produced to move the blood to the lungs, which compounds the blood flow problem and worsens the existing damage. It is possible that, over time, the right ventricle will become large enough to either equalize or exceed the pressure of the left ventricle, and this will cause reverse shunting of blood from the right to the left side of the heart. The time taken for this process varies—it may occur in the first 6 months or take many years—but if it occurs, it changes the haemodynamics of the defect from acyanotic to cyanotic.

A unique feature of increased pulmonary blood flow is the risk incurred when giving oxygen. Oxygen is an effective pulmonary vasodilator and its administration causes the pulmonary vascular bed to relax, increasing the blood flow. The effect of this is to increase tachypnoea, increase fluid retention in the lungs and further decrease the oxygenation of the circulating blood. Children with defects featuring a left to right shunt and an increased pulmonary blood flow should not therefore be automatically given oxygen therapy to improve their respiratory status, as this could effectively worsen their condition (Kliegman et al., 2016).

Decreased Pulmonary Blood Flow

The symptoms exhibited by a child with decreased pulmonary blood flow are completely different from the pathophysiological symptoms of those with increased pulmonary blood flow. Hearts with a defect which results in decreased pulmonary blood flow are either those with an obstruction preventing blood flowing adequately, or those resulting from failures of embryological development which have no connection of blood flow from the right side of the heart to the lungs. Such defects include pulmonary stenosis, pulmonary atresia, Ebstein anomaly, tricuspid atresia and tetralogy of Fallot. The fact that very little (or no) blood reaches the lungs means there is a severe decrease in the number of blood cells available to carry oxygen. The failure to oxygenate the blood adequately is the telltale sign of these defects; it has the effect

of mild to severe desaturation, associated with profound cyanosis. These defects can result in the child having reduced oxygen saturation levels, ranging from 50% to 90% (Kliegman et al., 2016).

In an attempt to compensate for this lower oxygen saturation, the kidneys produce a hormone called erythropoietin which stimulates the bone marrow to produce more red blood cells. Unfortunately, this does not change the situation for the baby, because the amount of blood reaching the lungs to collect oxygen does not change. Giving additional inspired oxygen, or increasing the red cell volume, does nothing to alleviate the symptoms of desaturation and cyanosis in these cases.

An increase in red blood cell production causes polycythaemia. This is a cause for concern if the polycythaemia becomes a chronic problem, because its effects can be a diminished clotting ability in response to major insults or significant trauma, and sluggish blood flow in the small vessels. This sluggish blood flow can result in small clots forming, causing cerebral infarcts; there is also the potential for brain abscesses to form due to the presence of bacteria caught in the tiny clots. The condition puts the child at risk during any surgical intervention, because of platelet dysfunction; it also renders them an 'at-risk' patient because the viscosity of the blood causes difficulty in simple procedures such as venipuncture, due to rapid clotting in the hub of the cannula. If this condition develops into a long-term problem then, over time, the sluggish blood flow will affect the lungs, causing multiple small pulmonary clots. Ironically, the compensatory physiological changes that originally protected the lungs from overflow and pulmonary vascular disease can themselves lead to pulmonary vascular disease as a result of the formation of multiple clots (Ramaswamy, 2015).

Obstruction to Systemic Blood Flow

There is a group of congenital defects that can cause an obstruction to the systemic blood flow. These include aortic stenosis, interruption of the aortic arch, coarctation of the aorta and hypoplastic left heart syndrome (HLHS). These obstructive defects create a situation where the blood is unable to reach the body, which results in symptoms of low cardiac output such as diminished pulses, poor colour, decreased capillary filling time and decreased urinary output. There may be a poor blood supply to the gastrointestinal tract, which may cause necrotizing enterocolitis. The blood in these cases cannot move past the obstruction, and so backs up into the left atrium and then to the lungs. This results in CCF (also known as congestive heart failure, or CHF) with pulmonary oedema. As with all heart defects, the severity of the obstruction will determine the extent of the symptoms, which can range from very mild to severe. A preschool child with coarctation of the aorta, for example, may experience leg cramps, cooler feet than hands, and stronger pulses in the upper limbs than the lower, but a newborn presenting with HLHS has a severe variation with life-threatening potential. A side effect of obstructive systemic blood flow is that the left ventricle attempts to compensate for the diminished blood flow by producing a greater and greater pressure. Like any muscle, the heart becomes bigger when exercised (left ventricular hypertrophy) and grows thicker until muscle-bound; eventually the muscle will weaken to the point of left ventricular failure (LVF) with resultant poor cardiac output (Kliegman et al., 2016).

By understanding how the heart defect affects the blood flow to the lungs and body, the practitioner is able to recognize the signs and symptoms exhibited by the child. The symptoms of CHF are the most important signs to look out for in children with heart defects which cause increased pulmonary blood flow. Parents of children with these heart defects will require explanation and reassurance that a short period of cyanosis prior to surgical correction will not cause long-term damage.

Infants with obstructive blood flow heart defects are dependent on practitioners to recognize early signs in order for them to receive life-saving drugs such as prostaglandin E. Alprostadil, which is the most commonly prescribed prostaglandin E, is used to maintain patency of the ductus arteriosus in neonates with cyanotic CHD.

DIAGNOSING CONGENITAL HEART DISEASE

Common signs and symptoms of CHD that can be ascertained from clinical examination and observation are shown in Table 9.2.

A heart murmur is a sound generated from the heart over and above those which are normally present. The murmur is caused by the blood passing over an irregular surface (such as a rough-ended or defective heart valve) or flowing through a constricted opening, or by the backflow of blood through an incompetent valve. Not all murmurs are associated with a condition that requires surgery, but a murmur can be useful in monitoring any changes in a heart condition. For more

TABLE 9.2 Common Signs and Symptoms of Congenital Heart Disease That Can Be Ascertained from Clinical Examination and Observation

Heart murmur
Cyanosis: a bluish tint to the skin, lips and fingernails (due to a lower level of oxygen in the blood)
Absent or weak femoral and/or brachial pulses
Tachypnoea (fast breathing)
Shortness of breath
Poor feeding, especially in babies (tire easily while feeding)
Poor weight gain
In older children, tiring easily during exercise or play activities

detailed information regarding murmurs, refer to Chapter 2 for the examination of the heart.

The presence or absence of a heart murmur is not a reliable diagnostic tool for CHD. Infants often have transient (innocent) murmurs without heart defects; conversely, many severe forms of CHD—such as tricuspid atresia, coarctation of the aorta and transposition of the great arteries—may not produce associated murmurs. Even those murmurs that do occur with CHD cannot be relied upon to determine the severity of the defect by their intensity alone, although the nature of the murmur (harsh, musical or blowing) along with other heart sounds can be useful to differentiate severe from mild defects (van der Linde et al., 2015; Burton and Cabalka, 1994; Silove, 1994; Werner 1996).

The signs and symptoms an infant exhibits are dependent on the number and severity of the heart defects. Many types of CHD put stress on the heart, which can lead to a degree of failure; this causes the muscle of the heart to weaken and hypertrophy (enlarge). Many cases of CHD are now identified during pregnancy, but the NIPE undoubtedly still plays an extremely important role in picking up potential heart problems that might have gone undetected on, for example, ultrasound scanning. Children with less severe disease, however, may not be diagnosed until they are older, at a time when their heart is placed under greater demand. Symptoms of some disease types do not present in childhood at all, and remain undiagnosed until adulthood. Some women, for example, are diagnosed as a result of routine screening during pregnancy.

A variety of tests can be performed to help diagnose CHD; these are outlined in Table 9.3.

TABLE 9.3 **Tests That Can Be Performed to Help Diagnose Congenital Heart Disease**	
Echocardiogram	The most common diagnostic test used. The result is achieved by the machine producing sound waves that create an image of the baby's heart. The image may aid in identifying malformations of the heart as well as diagnosing whether any heart failure is present. This screening can be done during pregnancy if congenital heart disease is suspected, allowing time to plan any treatment that can be offered before the baby is born. Studies have suggested that 30%–60% of congenital heart disease can be diagnosed antenatally using high-resolution four-chamber transvaginal echocardiography; this process produces a detailed image of the fetal heart anatomy and allows the detection of major abnormalities (Allan, 1994; 1996).
ECG or EKG (electrocardiogram)	Traces the electrical activity of the heart and can measure the rate and regularity of the heartbeat.
Chest x-ray	Can be taken to show whether the heart is enlarged (hypertrophy) or if the lungs contain extra fluid.
Pulse oximeter	Can be used to assess the amount of oxygen reaching the blood from the lungs. This is a noninvasive procedure, done by placing a sensor usually on the fingertip or toe of the child.
Catheterization	An invasive test in which a thin flexible catheter (tube) is passed through an artery or vein—usually in the groin, sometimes the arm—to the heart. The procedure is observed by the doctors using x-rays. All the blood vessels of the heart can be observed clearly. The catheter is also used to measure pressure inside the heart and the vessels and can detect any mixing of blood from the two sides. During the procedure a dye that can be seen on x-ray is used to observe the flow of blood through the heart and vessels; this can identify problem areas and aid in diagnosis of the disease under investigation.

TREATMENT OF CONGENITAL HEART DISEASE

There are four main options for the treatment of CHD:
- medicines
- cardiac catheterization procedures
- heart surgery
- heart transplant.

Some infants will require just one form of therapy; others will require a combination of the treatments listed above. The choice of treatment depends on the complexity of the defect and the child's age, size and general health status.

COMMON CONGENITAL HEART DISEASE DEFECTS (CHD)

Ventricular Septal Defect (VSD)

Ventricular septal defect (VSD) (Fig. 9.1) is the most commonly occurring congenital heart defect and

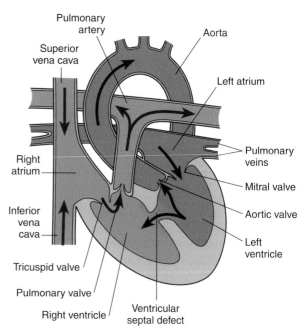

Fig. 9.1 Ventricular Septal Defect.

accounts for approximately 50% of all cases (Fulton and Saleeb, 2018; Ramaswamy, 2015).

About 5% of patients with VSD have chromosomal abnormalities, including trisomy 13 (Patau syndrome), trisomy 18 (Edwards syndrome), and trisomy 21 (Down syndrome) (Gatzoulis and Daubeney, 2011). The defect may occur along any part of the septum that separates the lower two chambers of the heart (ventricles); it allows blood to migrate from one ventricle to the other, and is thus referred to as a left-to-right shunt. The haemodynamic presentation is directly related to the size of the hole and can range from insignificant to severe (Park, 1996). Symptoms are not usually observed in neonates for the first 6 to 8 weeks because the pressures in the ventricles remain almost equal in the first 2 to 3 weeks of life. The symptoms begin to appear as the pulmonary resistance falls, allowing blood to pass through the defect from a high pressure (left side) to a lower pressure (right side) and onward to the pulmonary vascular bed.

The ventricular septum is made up of two parts: a smaller septum, which is membranous, and a muscular larger septum; 30% to 40% of defects which are membranous and muscular will close spontaneously within the first 6 months of life and are more likely to be small defects. Defects which are referred to as large can be considered to be approximately the same size as the aortic valve opening (Castaneda et al., 1994). These defects will usually require surgical or catheter intervention; this is indicated when the infant fails to grow and when medical management produces no response.

Surgery is required when the left-to-right shunt results in an increased pulmonary blood flow under high pressure, which increases the pulmonary artery pressure and causes pulmonary hypertension. In order to protect the lungs from flooding with blood, the pulmonary resistance rises initially, but if this situation is allowed to continue untreated, an irreversible change will occur in the pulmonary vasculature. If surgery has not been performed before this point, the pulmonary vascular resistance becomes so high that it exceeds the systemic vascular resistance. This results in the blood flow changing course and becoming a right-to-left shunt, causing cyanosis in the infant. This process is medically referred to as Eisenmenger complex (Kliegman et al., 2016).

Symptoms of the left-to-right shunt are determined by the amount of blood flowing to the lungs. Infants with pulmonary stenosis as well as a VSD demonstrate less severe symptoms, because this defect naturally reduces the blood flow. Any CCF that is noted usually responds to treatment with diuretics as first-line treatment. ACE inhibitors like captopril can be added to reduce the systemic vascular resistance. Commonly used diuretics are frusemide, chlorthiazide and spironolactone (Kliegman et al., 2016).

Atrial Septal Defect (ASD)

Atrial septal defect (ASD) (Fig. 9.2) is basically a hole in the septum that separates the top two chambers of the heart (atria) and allows blood to migrate from one chamber to the other. This defect is responsible for 7% of CHD.

In the heart with normal anatomy, atrial pressure is greater on the left side than the right; this difference in pressure has the effect of closing the foramen ovale which separates the two atria.

Commonly diagnosed ASDs can be referred to in three ways: an ostium secundum ASD (a defect in the middle portion of the atrial septum), an ostium primum ASD (a defect in the bottom aspect of the atrial septum), or a sinus venosus type ASD (a defect in the upper end of the atrial septum). Sinus venosus type ASDs usually have the right upper pulmonary vein draining into the right atrium through the ASD.

The majority of the secundum ASDs can be closed by cardiac catheterization; most of these children do well and are usually discharged the day after surgery. The children with large primum or sinus venosus type defects will usually require surgical intervention. Most

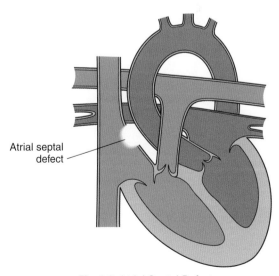

Atrial septal defect

Fig. 9.2 Atrial Septal Defect.

children with ASD will not have symptoms of CCF, and those who develop the problem usually do well with medical management using diuretics and ACE inhibitors (Kliegman et al., 2016).

Atrioventricular Septal Defect (AV Canal Defect, AVSD)

This defect (Fig. 9.3) is responsible for between 2% and 5% of CHD; it can most simply be described as a large hole in the middle of the heart. It arises when there is incomplete fusion of the endocardial cushions, and can occur below or above the atrioventricular valves (tricuspid and mitral), which can also be malformed.

Incomplete fusion of the endocardial cushions results in a lack of separation of the atria and the ventricles, and a failure of the two heart valves (the tricuspid on the right side of the heart and the mitral on the left) to separate. This results in a large connection between the atria and ventricles, and a single valve where there should be two.

There is a strong association between AV canal defects and trisomy 21 (Down syndrome); fetuses in which an AV canal defect is detected in utero have a 40% to 50% risk of Down syndrome, and approximately 40% of fetuses with trisomy 21 have an AV canal defect, usually the complete form.

The defect can present as a simple or partial AVSD, and may be referred to as complex heart disease (complete AVSD) depending on how many of the structures are involved and how they are affected (Park, 1997). The baby's symptoms are directly associated with the severity of the disease and whether treatment is prescribed accordingly (Fleishman and Tugertimur, 2018).

Patent Ductus Arteriosus (PDA)

Patent ductus arteriosus (PDA) (Fig. 9.4) is responsible for between 5% and 12% of CHD (Botto et al., 2001). The term refers to the persistence of a connection between the aorta and the pulmonary artery; this is a normal part of fetal anatomy in utero, but the transitional changes that occur at birth should ensure that this state alters once the baby is born.

The defect referred to as a PDA occurs when the normal closure does not take place after birth. The persistence of the duct may cause an excessive amount of blood to return to the lungs; depending on the size of the defect, this can cause the child problems such as CCF or pneumonia. If the PDA is small, however, the effects may be insignificant and there may be no symptoms.

This form of CHD is common in premature infants, in whom closure of the duct can occur spontaneously. If preterm infants become symptomatic and need ventilatory support, medical intervention in the form of drugs such as indomethacin or ibuprofen can be considered in the first

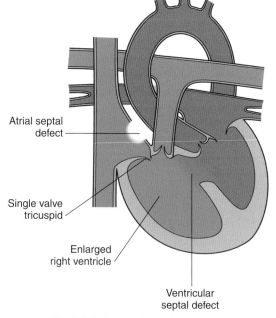

Atrial septal defect

Single valve tricuspid

Enlarged right ventricle

Ventricular septal defect

Fig. 9.3 Atrioventricular Septal Defect.

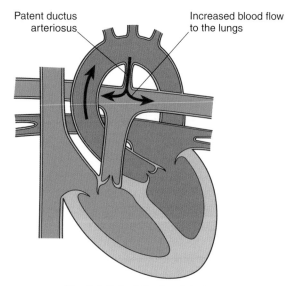

Patent ductus arteriosus

Increased blood flow to the lungs

Fig. 9.4 Patent Ductus Arteriosus.

2 weeks of life. In cases where medical treatment is not successful, surgical intervention may be considered.

In premature babies, the usual operation performed for closure of the duct takes place under direct vision and is not classed as open heart surgery. Other children will often be able to have their PDA closed under interventional cardiac catheterization, where a coil is placed in the PDA and expands to prevent all blood flow. Both forms of surgery are safe and carry a negligible risk of morbidity and mortality. Patent ductus arteriosus is considered the only CHD that is curable with no long-term complications (Lee et al., 2006).

Pulmonary Stenosis (PS)

The term *stenosis* means narrowing; pulmonary stenosis (PS) refers to a narrowing of the pulmonary artery (Fig. 9.5). There are three main locations referred to when classifying the stenosis:

- *Valvular* stenosis occurs at the level of the pulmonary valve; this is the most common type of stenosis, accounting for 90% of PS diagnosed.
- *Subvalvular* stenosis occurs below the level of the valve in the region of the infundibulum of the right ventricle; this form is commonly seen in infants and children with tetralogy of Fallot.
- *Supravalvular* stenosis is above the level of the valve and involves the actual pulmonary artery.

The right ventricle increases the pressure as it tries to pump blood up to the lungs against the constriction. If the action continues long enough, it will inevitably lead to right ventricular hypertrophy and possible tricuspid regurgitation; this could lead to an increased pressure in the right atrium, resulting in a patent foramen ovale and a right-to-left shunting of blood.

A pressure gradient develops between the right ventricle and the pulmonary artery; this is measured (in mm Hg) during echocardiography, and can be used to access the severity of the narrowing of the pulmonary valve.

The gradient increases when the cardiac output is increased; for example, when the infant or child exerts themselves or if there is pyrexia. The symptoms vary with each child, and range from mild to severe.

Severe pulmonary stenosis is most commonly seen in neonates and is sometimes referred to as critical pulmonary stenosis; it requires prompt medical intervention to relieve the narrowing. Prior to any intervention, a temporary secure systemic blood flow needs to be established and maintained. These infants depend on the patent ductus arteriosus that persists from fetal life for maintenance of their pulmonary blood flow (referred to as duct-dependent pulmonary circulation); patency of the duct can be maintained using prostaglandin E2. A percutaneous balloon valvuloplasty (which tears the valve open) is performed, but if this is not successful a more invasive surgical approach may be needed. In a few cases, this severe form can develop progressively throughout childhood.

Children with moderate pulmonary stenosis who are symptomatic will receive similar treatment at an early stage, whereas asymptomatic children with moderate and mild stenosis are likely to be monitored closely by their cardiologist and receive planned treatment; the prognosis for a full recovery is good (Jordan and Scott, 1989; Ross et al., 1992; Park, 1997).

Aortic Stenosis (AS)

Aortic stenosis (AS) (Fig. 9.6) occurs in 5% to 8% of all CHD, and is more common in males than females, with a ratio of approximately 4:1 (Kitchner et al., 1994). It is a left ventricular outflow tract obstruction and, as with pulmonary stenosis, the narrowing can be:

- *valvular* (at the level of the valve): the most common type
- *subvalvular* (below the valve): the second most common type
- *supravalvular* (above the valve): the least common type.

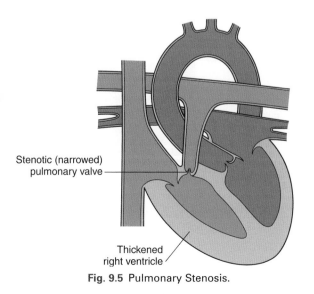

Stenotic (narrowed) pulmonary valve

Thickened right ventricle

Fig. 9.5 Pulmonary Stenosis.

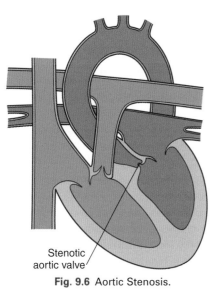

Stenotic
aortic valve

Fig. 9.6 Aortic Stenosis.

The haemodynamic effects of aortic stenosis are directly related to the degree of obstruction; this is the mean pressure gradient (measured in mm Hg) between the left ventricle and the aorta in systole. Diagnosis of a mild stenosis is made with a gradient of less than 25 mm Hg, moderate stenosis at less than 40 mm Hg, and severe stenosis with a gradient above 40 mm Hg. If left untreated, the obstruction to the blood flow out of the left ventricle will result in an increased pressure which could lead to left ventricular hypertrophy. This hypertrophy will increase symptoms; there is also an increase in the oxygen demands of the coronary arteries which cannot be sustained, leading to myocardial ischaemia and symptoms of angina (as the coronaries are supplied during diastole). Valvular aortic stenosis—seen in neonates with associated heart failure—is referred to as critical aortic stenosis and requires prompt medical intervention to relieve the narrowing. This condition is usually associated with dysmorphic aortic valves which appear thickened on echocardiography. Patients can also have a bicuspid rather than a tricuspid aortic valve; family members need to be screened in case of bicuspid aortic valve. Prior to any intervention, a temporary secure systemic blood flow needs to be established. These babies have a duct-dependent systemic circulation, and (as for babies with PS) the patency of the ductus arteriosus is maintained using a prostaglandin E2 infusion. These infants should not be administered oxygen, as that can lead to the closure of the PDA.

A percutaneous balloon valvuloplasty, which tears and separates the leaflets of the valve, can be performed on neonates and also in older children.

Surgery may be the only choice in some cases; the choice of surgery is dependent on the degree of obstruction seen at the ventricular outflow tract. The main aim of any surgery is to relieve the obstruction. Surgical treatment in infancy and childhood has significant disadvantages over such treatment in adults, because any replacement valves will not grow with the child; this may result in repeated procedures to replace the valves. The disadvantages that anticoagulant therapy for prosthetic valves may present must also be taken seriously. Only severe cases of aortic stenosis are treated with surgery, and only when no other form of treatment is available.

Tetralogy of Fallot (TOF)

This defect, first described by Fallot in 1888, is the most common heart condition seen in children beyond the infant stage (Fig. 9.7) (Kitchner et al., 1994). It has four main anomalies:
- a large VSD
- right outflow tract obstruction
- right ventricular hypertrophy
- an overriding aorta.

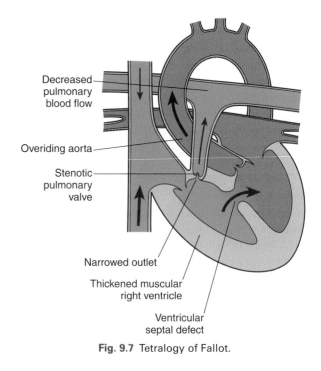

Decreased pulmonary blood flow

Overiding aorta

Stenotic pulmonary valve

Narrowed outlet

Thickened muscular right ventricle

Ventricular septal defect

Fig. 9.7 Tetralogy of Fallot.

Without surgical treatment, approximately 50% of children presenting with this condition will die.

Common symptoms of this type of defect are known as cyanotic 'spelling'. This is caused by a unique feature of TOF: a sudden, severe reduction in pulmonary blood flow. The symptom can occur at any age in infants with mild or severe cases, usually as a result of crying or feeding and most noticeably during the morning, or following other activities causing vasodilation, such as having a warm bath or being in a warm bed (Kitchner et al., 1994). Parents will usually be the first to witness the episodes which, when reported to health professionals, must be taken seriously.

The 'spell' produces an episode of hypercyanosis, accompanied by irritability and distressed crying. The infant becomes pale, breathless, sweaty, limp and eventually unconscious. Once the cycle is broken, the infundibulum relaxes and the infant will regain consciousness. This can be a life-threatening episode; once a history of spelling has been established, surgery is normally planned as a matter of urgency.

Most patients with TOF undergo intracardiac repair as their initial intervention by 1 year of age (typically before 6 months). A small minority require palliative shunts prior to surgical repair. Shunts may be necessary due to medically refractory hypercyanotic ("tet") spells or severe right ventricular outflow tract (RVOT) obstruction in infants who are not initially acceptable candidates for intracardiac repair due to prematurity, hypoplastic pulmonary arteries, or coronary artery anatomy.

Intracardiac Repair

The goals of surgical repair are:
- Relief of RVOT obstruction;
- Complete separation between the pulmonary and systemic circulations;
- Preservation of right ventricular function;
- Minimization of postprocedure pulmonary valvular incompetence.

The excellent results of primary intracardiac repair for infants with TOF have made it the treatment of choice at most centres for all patients with TOF, including asymptomatic acyanotic infants (pink variant). This is because surgical correction allows normal growth of the RVOT and pulmonary annulus.

Palliative Shunts

Although palliative shunts are no longer used routinely for surgical management of TOF, they may be required urgently for a small subset of patients, including:
- Infants who cannot undergo intracardiac repair (e.g., because they are premature);
- Infants who have severe RVOT obstruction;
- Patients with a medically refractory severe hypercyanotic ('tet') spell;
- Patients with coronary anatomy complicating initial complete repair in the neonatal period.

Palliative shunts allow deferral of elective complete repair by providing the stable pulmonary blood flow required for survival. The procedure involves creating a systemic-to-pulmonary connection. Palliative shunts include central shunts and the modified Blalock–Thomas–Taussig shunt, or Blalock–Taussig shunt (mBTS). In the mBTS, a synthetic graft is placed from the innominate or subclavian artery to the ipsilateral pulmonary artery (Doyle et al., 2019).

Surgery is usually performed electively in the first year of life, with the majority of repairs performed before the age of 6 months (Al Habib et al., 2010). The timing and choice of surgical intervention is based on individual patient characteristics and centre-specific practice.

Both time frames have advantages and disadvantages. For example, performing surgery in the newborn period prevents the infant from developing severe complications associated with the disease, but also carries a greater degree of mortality and morbidity.

Coarctation of the Aorta (CoAo)

Coarctation of the aorta (CoAo) (Fig. 9.8) is responsible for 6% to 8% of all CHD; it is more common in boys than girls, occurring at a ratio of 2:1. Approximately 50% of patients with coarctation have associated anomalies (McBride, 2005).

Coarctation (narrowing) of the aorta is primarily a congenital malformation. Increased attention is being focused on coarctation being part of a more diffuse arteriopathy; careful attention to the morphology of the aortic valve (which is often bicuspid) and ascending aorta is therefore imperative (Erbel et al., 2014).

The aetiology of congenital coarctation is incompletely understood, but two primary theories explain the narrowed segment:
- The narrowed segment is underdeveloped during fetal life due to reduced blood flow across the arch.

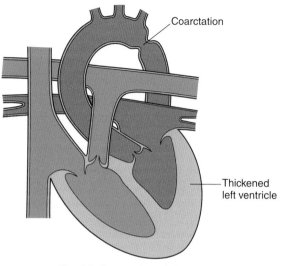

Fig. 9.8 Coarctation of the Aorta.

This is particularly thought to be the mechanism when CoAo is associated with additional left-sided lesions such as HLHS.

- Ductal tissue extends into the thoracic aorta; when the ductus arteriosus constricts and closes postnatally, the thoracic aorta is constricted (Rudolph et al., 1995).

The obstruction causes increased resistance in the blood flowing from the ascending aorta to the descending aorta, which results in a drop in systemic blood pressure. An effect of this hypotension and the hypoperfusion of the kidneys is the secretion of renin, which constricts the arteries in an attempt to increase the distal pressure; the result of this may be hypertension in the upper segment. How well the lower limbs are perfused is dependent on collateral circulation and the sufficient perfusion of vital internal organs and structures. This is of concern because a lack of perfusion can lead to further complications.

The defect is most usefully divided into two categories—preductal and postductal—as this identifies the blood flow of the defect. Preductal CoAo is found nearer to the ductus arteriosus and is commonly associated with other major abnormalities (Kumar et al., 2005). If the defect is severe, the baby will present with symptoms within the first few days of life and will become progressively worse as the ductus arteriosus closes. It should be remembered that the presentation of this condition can very easily be mistaken for septic shock, as the baby will be grey and mottled. The possibility of a CHD should always be considered and this concern voiced. Depending on the location of the narrowing, a difference in mean blood pressure may be noted, either between the right side of the body and the left or between the upper and lower limbs. There may also be differences in the right and left brachial pulses, and femoral pulses may be weak or absent.

Postductal CoAo is found further away from the ductus arteriosus; this is the most common form of CoAo. It normally presents in older children; there are not usually any symptoms evident and the problem is picked up on medical examination.

Surgery is performed to relieve the obstruction before hypertension can cause complications or before it becomes irreversible (Koehne et al., 2001).

If the baby arrives in a collapsed state due to the PDA having closed, the emergency treatment should begin with the reopening of the duct. Following successful resuscitation, a period of at least 24 hours of stabilization is needed. If the baby arrives in a stable condition with a closed duct, initial treatment will be for the hypertension. The option of treating the obstruction by nonsurgical intervention used to be kept for recoarctation after surgical intervention, but many centres now use this technique as a primary correction method outside the neonatal period. It entails a balloon coronary angioplasty catheter being placed across the coarctation via the femoral artery (Grifka, 2004). The type of surgical procedure undertaken is ultimately the choice of the surgeon and reflects their preferred choice of subclavian flap repair or end-to-end anastomosis, both of which have pros and cons.

Patients will need to be followed up for usually 6 to 12 months' monitoring for recoarctation, and antibiotic prophylaxis is required for life.

Transposition of the Great Arteries (TGA)

This is the second most common cyanotic heart defect and is responsible for 4% to 5% of all CHD (Fig. 9.9). It is commonly found in conjunction with other heart defects and is more common in boys than girls at a ratio of approximately 3:1. If the condition is not treated, 90% of patients will die during the first year of life (Kitchner et al., 1994).

In TGA, the aorta arises anteriorly from the right ventricle and the pulmonary artery posteriorly from the left ventricle. In the absence of other cardiac defects, this presentation is referred to as a simple transposition; if other cardiac defects are involved, it is a complex transposition. The aorta lies anterior to the pulmonary artery, creating two separate circulations. Deoxygenated blood

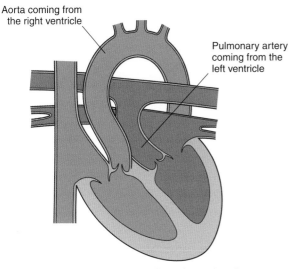

Aorta coming from the right ventricle

Pulmonary artery coming from the left ventricle

Fig. 9.9 Transposition of the Great Arteries.

enters the right atrium from the inferior and superior vena cava, and passes through the tricuspid valve into the right ventricle; from here the still deoxygenated blood is pumped into the aorta and enters the systemic circulation again. Oxygenated blood from the lungs enters the left atrium via the pulmonary veins, passes through the mitral valve and into the left ventricle; here it is pumped into the pulmonary artery and back to the lungs.

For TGA to be compatible with life, there has to be communication between the deoxygenated and oxygenated blood, allowing some mixing to occur for the passage of oxygen around the body. Complex transposition with one or more communications (e.g., ASD or VSD) would therefore seem to have an advantage over simple transposition. However, there is the potential for increased pulmonary blood flow to cause an increase in pulmonary artery pressure, with subsequent development of pulmonary vascular obstructive disease; this necessitates early surgical intervention. Infants with severe pulmonary hypertension may not necessarily have a bleak outlook because the symptoms can be reversed by surgery (Khairy et al., 2013).

Babies with simple transposition have only one viable option if there is to be any possibility of this crucial mixing taking place: maintaining a patent ductus arteriosus. If the ductus begins to close, the baby will become profoundly cyanotic, acidotic and will collapse. This is a life-threatening event; the term 'simple' belies the seriousness of the condition, and these babies are

initially the sickest of all those with CDH conditions. The babies will normally present during the first day of life. They may suffer sudden death if the ductus or foramen ovale closes completely and therefore emergency resuscitation, stabilization and transfer to a tertiary cardiac centre is vital.

Complex transposition usually does not present for several weeks if there is an ASD, VSD or PDA. If the VSD is large and there is no pulmonary stenosis, CCF develops as a result of the pulmonary vascular resistance falling, usually at 2 to 6 weeks of age. There are differing levels of cyanosis, and the other symptoms suffered are dependent on the degree of shunting. The symptoms and presentation will be very similar to those of a baby with a large VSD. The diagnosis of TGA is usually made by echocardiography, which will show the abnormal position of the great vessels.

Some cases of persistent severe hypoxia, despite a PDA, will require an urgent balloon atrial septostomy called a Rashkind procedure; this will increase the mixing of blood at the interatrial level (Wilson et al., 2007).

The arterial switch procedure (also referred to as the Jatene procedure) is a one-stop surgery, which is a great advantage. It literally takes the great vessels, places them into their anatomically correct positions, and reimplants the coronary arteries to the former pulmonary artery that is now the aorta. Any intracardiac shunts are closed.

CONCLUSION

In this chapter, we have explored a range of cardiac anomalies which may present during the initial or subsequent examinations of the newborn. We have looked at some of the causes of these conditions and their effects on the newborn baby and the slightly older infant, and considered some of the different treatments that are available.

There are many other considerations around this area, including the ethical dimensions and the need for good communication. These areas will be covered more broadly in Chapter 11, which deals with communication issues in the event of a congenital abnormality. The issues of informed choice and consent, which will usually feed into any decisions that parents have to make after diagnosis, are also given consideration in Chapter 15.

In most cases, the parents of a baby with a diagnosis of CHD will be walking into unknown territory

TABLE 9.4 Comman Critical* Congenital Heart Defects and Their Association With Cyanosis and Dependence Upon the Ductus Arteriosus

	Cyanosis	Ductal-Dependent?
Left-Sided Obstructive Lesions		
Hypoplastic left heart syndrome valvar As	Yes	Yes
• Critical As	Cyanosis or diffrential cyanosis[a]	Yes
• Moderate to severe As	No	No
COA		
• Critical COA	Differential cyanosis[a]	Yes
• Moderate to severe COA	No	No
Interrupted aortic arch	Differential cyanosis[a] (pattern of cyanosis varies based upon type)	Yes
Right-Sided Obstructive Lesions		
Tetralogy of Fallot	Variable	possibly[b]
Tetralogy of Fallot with pulmonary atresia	Yes	Yes (unless multiple or large aorto-pulmonary collaterals are present)
Pulmonary atresia with intact interventricular septum	Yes	Yes
PS		
• Critical PS	Yes	Yes
• Severe PS	No	No
Tricuspid atresia	Yes	Possibly[b]
Severe neonatal Ebstein anomaly	Yea	Possibly[c]
Parallel Circulations		
Transposition of the great arteries	Yes[d]	Yes
Other		
TAPVC	Yes	No[e]
Large VSD	No	No
AV canal defect	No	No
Truncus arteriosus	Yes	No

CHD, congenital heart disease; AS, aortic stenosis; COA, coarctation of the aorta; PS, pulmonic stenosis; TAPVC, total anomalous pulmonary venous connection; VSD, ventricular septal defect; AV, atrioventricular; RV, right ventricular; PDA, patent ductus arteriosus.

*Critical CHD refers to lesions requiring surgery or catheter-based intervention in the first year of life. The most comman lesions are listed in this table; however, there are other less common congenital heart lesions that may require intervention within the first year of life.

[a]In these lesions, the upper half of the body (preductal) is pink and the lower half (postductal) is cyanotic.

[b]Infants with tetralogy of Fallot or tricuspid atresia may have ductal-dependent circulation if there is severe RV outflow tract obstruction (i.e., critical pulmonary stenosis or artresia).

[c]In cases of severe Ebstein anomaly with extreme cyanosis, a PDA may be necessary to maintain pulmonary blood flow until pulmonary vascular resistance drops.

[d]Reversed differential cyanosis (i.e., oxygen saturation higher in the lower than upper extremity) may occur if there is coexisting coarctation of the aorta or pulmonary artery hypertension.

[e]Some patients with obstructed TAPVC may require a PDA to maintain systemic cardiac output. However, a PDA may also increase the degree of cyanosis.

(https://www.uptodate.com/contents/image?topickey=101291&search=critical%20heart%20disease&source=outline_link&imagekey=peds%2f103087) (June 2019) and will require all the support they can draw together. Most often, once the diagnosis has been made, the role of the primary carer will become that of a support person for the family. The parents' story included here serves to remind us just how enormous may be the impact of such a diagnosis on a family. We are not expected to have an expert knowledge of heart conditions, but we should ensure that we have a working knowledge of the causes, consequences and available therapies. This will enable us to play a constructive role in helping the baby and their family through what may be some difficult times ahead.

PARENTS' STORY

Amy and Logan's story

I fell pregnant with Logan in 2016. I am a type 1 diabetic and have been since I was 4 years old, and I also have polycystic ovary syndrome. So I was told 8 years ago that I couldn't have children because of those two things, and I never thought that I would get pregnant. But Logan came along anyway. My diabetes was pretty badly controlled during my teenage years when it's a really difficult time to be diabetic and you fight against it. So this time created some health issues for me.

I was getting periods once in a blue moon and they were always at different times. I had this weird gut feeling, though, and I thought I should probably carry out a test—and I was pregnant. I was referred to the hospital and had a community-based midwife for a while, but I didn't see a lot of her because I was seeing the hospital team for my diabetes at the clinic. It was suggested at one point that I should terminate the pregnancy because I wouldn't be able to cope because of my diabetes and I was like no, you're not telling me that.

Then, at 14 weeks, I got hit by a car when I was driving my moped and ended up in hospital with both arms in a cast and my leg in a brace. I couldn't have surgery so that was a challenge. When I had my anatomy scan at 21 weeks, they did a special heart scan because of the increased risk of heart issues with diabetes. We found out that he was a boy and that it looked as though there was a ventricular septal defect. I had been told there was a higher chance of the baby having a heart condition because of the diabetes—the week before that scan I just had this heavy gut feeling like there was something wrong and everyone was saying 'no, no, it's going to be fine', and I'm like 'no it's not. I can feel it'. I was in a wheelchair at the time and I just wanted to run away. I didn't want to deal with it. I am very good at suppressing my feelings, but this was one I couldn't run away from. I had to deal with it.

At 37 weeks, I had to fly up to a specialist hospital in another city to give birth to him. I had to have a C-section because they were worried that too much pressure during birth might cause me to go blind, again because of the diabetes. When I was waiting for the section, I was prepped and ready to go three times, but we were bumped twice and finally got there on the third attempt. Logan was 3.2 kg at birth and his heart had a ventricle missing and he has transposition of the great arteries. So his little heart is quite different.

Logan was taken straight to NICU for a day, then he was sent to the HDU in the kids' cardiac ward for 2 days. He had surgery at 4 days and was in recovery after that. He never had any problems with his blood sugars, although I was getting hypo quite a lot. He was in the incubator and I was only allowed to hold him a couple of times (Fig. 9.10). I was so scared I might pull his umbilical

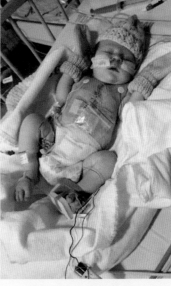

Fig. 9.10 Logan in ITU.

Continued

Amy and Logan's story—cont'd

arterial line out. He made a good recovery from that surgery but 3 weeks later his saturation levels went really low. We were all set to go home but he to have had emergency surgery. Again his healing was good and a week later the discharge was planned again. Then I noticed he was cocking his leg like a frog—I was unsure why he was doing that—and he kept crying if you tried to change his nappy or just touched him. One of the night nurses used to work in orthopaedics and she said we should push for an x-ray. That's how we found out he had osteomyelitis in the whole of his right-hand side, and he had a nice little pus gathering in his hip socket which had dislocated itself. So now he needed more surgery to do a hip washout. He ended up in a spica cast at 2 months old and we finally got to go home at 3 months. His saturation levels had to stay around the 70% to 75% mark, so we needed a special flow instrument. He needed antibiotics and so we stayed in hospital until they were finished, then went back a week later when he had the spica taken off. That was great, because he was 4 months old and he hadn't been able to find his feet or to do the little baby things that they normally do.

I never had any problems bonding with Logan. He always felt like he was mine, even when the nurses were doing so much for him. I tried breastfeeding and I managed that for 2{1/2} months, and when he got tired he had a nasogastric tube to feed him expressed milk. I would have kept going, but when I was back here at the local hospital I transmitted gastroenteritis, so that was it. But he had 3 months' worth—that was better than nothing. I was pretty privileged to be able to do that. When the spica came off, we had to work on getting his weight up to 5 kg for the next round of surgery, because they have to be 5 kg. He was 4 months and it took him up to 8 months to get there. We had to weigh him every day. There was one point where he lost 120 g over a week, so we had to get the tube in and fortifiers to get some weight on. After he had the second operation for his heart, we were out within a week. After surgery the babies get phlegmy. One night, he was lying on his back and coughing—I sat him up and he couldn't get it up and

he went blue and I lost it. I had never cried in front of the nurses before, but I'd had enough. We got through it, though, and he survived. There is one more round of surgery and he is old enough to understand now. It's kind of freaky in a way because he's quite sensitive to pain, but he's resilient and a fighter.

I'm optimistic about the future and we take each day as it comes. I'm glad I knew there was a problem before he was born, because I had time to prepare for it. I wish I'd known about the support groups on social media earlier, because you feel very lonely and isolated at times. I feel I was lucky to have some insight and understanding from working as a carer in a rest home—I've come to realize that your situation is never the same as anyone else's and that you can't really plan anything. I expected a lovely perfect birth and it didn't happen. But would I change things in terms of having Logan? No. Not at all (Fig. 9.11).

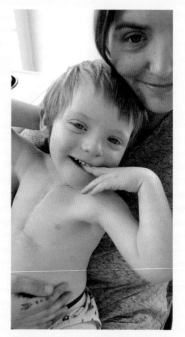

Fig. 9.11 Logan After Discharge.

KEY POINTS

- Congenital heart disease has the potential to seriously affect the health and well-being of the newborn baby either at the time of detection or at some point in the future.
- The specific causes of CHD are mainly thought to be idiopathic.
- The majority of the conditions are due to the malformation of the valves of the heart and/or vessels. There may also be anomalous communications between the chambers of the heart.
- Of those babies with defects, approximately 2–3 per 1000 will be symptomatic within the first year of life.
- The number of deaths from CHD in children under 1 year of age has decreased by about half, from 584 in 1986 to 305 in 2011.
- The parents of a baby with a diagnosis of CHD are likely to be walking into unknown territory and will require all the support they can draw upon.

REFERENCES

Al Habib, H.F., Jacobs, J.P., Mavroudis, C., Tchervenkov, C.I., O'Brien, S.M., Mohammadi, S., et al., 2010. Contemporary patterns of management of tetralogy of Fallot: data from the Society of Thoracic Surgeons Database. Ann. Thorac. Surg. 90 (3), 813.

Allan, L.D., 1994. Fetal congenital heart disease: diagnosis and management. Curr. Opin. Obstet. Gynecol. 6, 45–49.

Allan, L.D., 1996. Fetal cardiology. Curr. Opin. Obstet. Gynecol. 8, 142–147.

Botto, L.D., Correa, A., Erickson, J.D., 2001. Racial and temporal variations in the prevalence of heart defects. Pediatrics 107, E32.

Bristol Royal Inquiry Final Report. The Stationery Office Ltd, 2001. Norwich, UK.

Burton, D.A., Cabalka, A.K., 1994. Cardiac evaluation of infants. The first year of life. Pediatr. Clin. North Am. 41, 991–1015.

Castaneda, A.R., Jonas, R.A., Mayer, J.E., Hanley, F.L., 1994. Cardiac Surgery of the Neonate and Infant. WB Saunders, Philadelphia, PA.

Doyle, T., Kavanaugh-McHugh, A., Fish, F.A., 2019. Management and outcome of tetralogy of Fallot. Available from: https://www.uptodate.com/contents/management-and-outcome-of-tetralogy-of-fallot?search=Palliative%20shunts&source=search_result&selectedTitle=1~150&usage_type=default&display_rank=1#H809366402. Accessed June 2019.

Erbel, R., Aboyans, V., Boileau, C., Bossone, E., Bartolomeo, R.D., Eggebrecht, H., 2014. 2014 ESC guidelines on the diagnosis and treatment of aortic diseases: document covering acute and chronic aortic diseases of the thoracic and abdominal aorta of the adult. Task Force for the Diagnosis and Treatment of Aortic Diseases of the European Society of Cardiology (ESC). Eur. Heart J. 35 (41), 2873–2926.

Ewing, C.K., Loffredo, C.A., Beatty, T.H., 1997. Paternal risk factors for isolated membranous ventricular septal defects. Am. J. Med. Genet. 71 (1), 42–46.

Feit, L.R., 1998. Genetics in congenital heart disease: strategies. Adv. Pediatr. 45, 267–292.

Fleishman, C., Tugertimur, A., 2018. Management and outcome of atrioventricular canal defects. Available from: https://www.uptodate.com/contents/management-and-outcome-of-atrioventricular-av-canal-defects?search=management-and-outcome-of-atrioventricular-av-canal-de-fects&source=search_result&selectedTitle=1~150&usage_type=default&display_rank=1#subscribeMessage. Accessed June 2019.

Fulton, D.R., Saleeb, S., 2018. Management of isolated ventricular septal defects in infants and children. Available from: https://www.uptodate.com/contents/management-of-isolated-ventricular-septal-defects-in-infants-and-children?search=ventricular%20scanal%20defects&topicRef=5787&source=see_link. Accessed June 2019.

Gatzoulis, M.A., Daubeney, W.G., 2011. Ventral septal defect. In: Diagnosis and Management of Adult Congenital Heart Disease. Elsevier, Philadelphia, PA.

Gerraughty, A.B., 1989. Caring for patients with lesions obstructing systemic blood flow. Crit. Care Nurs. Clin. North Am. 1 (2), 231–243.

Goldmutz, E., 1999. Recent advances in understanding the genetic etiology of congenital heart disease. Curr. Opin. Pediatr. 11 (5), 437–443.

Goldmutz, E., Emanuel, B.S., 1997. Genetic disorders of cardiac morphogenesis. The Di George and velocardiofacial syndrome. Circ. Res. 80 (4), 437–443.

Grech, V., Gaff, M., 1999. Syndromes and malformations associated with congenital heart disease in a population based study. Int. J. Cardiol. 68 (2), 151–156.

Grifka, R.G., 2004. Transcatheter closure of the patent ductus arteriosus. Catheter. Cardiovasc. Interv. 61 (4), 554–570.

Hazinski, M.F., 1992. Nursing Care of the Critically Ill Child, second ed. Mosby Year Book, St Louis, MO.

Ho, S.Y., Anderson, R.H., 1979. Coarctation of the aorta. In: Godman, M.J., Marquis, R.M. (Eds.), Paediatric Cardiology. Churchill Livingstone, Edinburgh, UK, (2) pp. 173–186.

Hoffman, J.I., 1995. Incidence of congenital heart disease: postnatal incidence. Paediatr. Cardiol. 16, 103.

Jamjureeruk, V., Sangtawesin, C., Layangool, T., 1997. Balloon atrial septostomy under 2D echocardiographic control: a new look. Pediatr. Cardiol. 18 (3), 197–200.

Jordan, S.C., Scott, O., 1989. Heart disease in paediatrics, third ed. Butterworths, London. Available from: http://www.onlinejacc.org/content/58/21/2241.1989. Accessed June 2019.

Kaushall, S.K., Iyer, K.S., Sharma, R., Airan, B., Bhan, A., Das, B., et al., 1996. Surgical experience with total correction of Fallot's in infancy. Int. J. Cardiol. 56 (1), 35–40.

Khairy, P., Clair, M., Fernandes, S.M., Blume, E.D., Powell, A.J., Newburger, J.W., et al., 2013. Cardiovascular outcomes after the arterial switch operation for D-transposition of the great arteries. Circulation 127 (3), 331–339.

Kitchner, D., Jackson, M., Malaiya, N., Walsh, K., Peart, I., Arnold, R., 1994. Incidence and prognosis of left ventricular outflow tract obstruction in Liverpool (1960–1991): a study of 313 patients. Br. Heart J. 71 (6), 588–595.

Kliegman, R.M., Bonita, M.D., Stanton, J.S., St Geme, J., Schor, N.F., 2016. Nelson Textbook of Pediatrics, twentieth ed. Elsevier.

Knott-Craig, C.J., Elkins, E.C., Lane, M.M., Holz, J., McCue, C., Ward, K.E., 1998. 26 year experience with surgical management of tetralogy of Fallot: risk analysis for mortality or late reintervention. Ann. Thorac. Surg. 66 (1), 506–511.

Koehne, P.S., Bein, G., Alexi-Meskhishvili, V., Weng, Y., Bührer, C., Obladen, M., 2001. Patent ductus arteriosus in very low birthweight infants: complications of pharmacological and surgical treatment. J. Perinat. Med. 29 (4), 327–334.

Kumar, V., Fausto, N., Abbas, A., 2005. Robbins & Cotran Pathologic Basis of Disease, seventh ed. W.B. Saunders.

Lee, L.C., Tillet, A., Tulloh, R., Yates, R., Kelsall, W., 2006. Outcome following patent ductus arteriosus ligation in premature infants: a retrospective cohort analysis. BMC Pediatr. 6, 15.

McBride, K.L., Pignatelli, R., Lewin, M., Ho, T., Fernbach, S., Menesses, A., et al., 2005. Inheritance analysis of congenital left ventricular outflow tract obstruction malformations: segregation, multiplex relative risk, and heritability. Am. J. Med. Genet. A. 134A (2), 180–186.

Moynihan, P.J., King, R., 1989. Caring for patients with lesions increasing pulmonary blood flow. Crit. Care Nurs. Clin. North Am. 1 (2), 195–213.

Park, M.K., 1996. Pediatric Cardiology for Practitioners, third ed. Mosby, St Louis, MO, pp. 135–140.

Park, M.K., 1997. The Pediatric Cardiology Handbook, second ed. Mosby, St Louis, MO.

Petersen, S., Peto, V., Rayner, M., 2003. Congenital heart disease statistics. British Heart Foundation, London.

Public Health England (PHE), 2018. National Congenital Anomaly and Rare Disease Registration Service statistics NCARDRS. Available from: https://www.gov.uk/government/publications/ncardrs-congenital-anomaly-annual-data/national-congenital-anomaly-and-rare-disease-registration-service-statistics-2016-summary-report. Accessed June 2019.

Ramaswamy, P., 2015. Ventricular septal defects. Medscape. Available from: https://emedicine.medscape.com/article/892980-overview#a5. Accessed June 2019.

Reddy, V.M., Liddicoat, J.R., McElhinnery, D.B., Brook, M.M., Stanger, P., Hanley, F.L., 1995. Routine primary repair of tetralogy of Fallot in neonates and infants below three months. Ann. Thorac. Surg. 60 (6), 592–596.

Ross, D., English, C.T., McKay, R., Hyams, B., 1992. Principles of Cardiac Diagnosis and Treatment. A Surgeon's Guide, second ed. Springer-Verlag, London, UK.

Rudolph, A.M., Heyman, M.A., Spitznas, U., 1972. Haemodynamic considerations in the development of narrowing of the aorta. Am. J. Cardiol. 30, 514.

Shah, M.J., Rome, J.J., Rychik, T., et al., 1997. Outcome of primary repair of tetralogy of Fallot in the newborn period. Unpublished. The Children's Hospital of Philadelphia.

Shinebourne, E.A., Tam, A.S.V., Elseed, A.M., Paneth, M., Lennox, S.C., Cleland, W.P., 1976. Coarctation in infancy and childhood. Br. Heart J. 38, 375.

Silove, E.D., 1994. Assessment and management of congenital heart disease in the newborn by the district paediatrician. Arch. Dis. Child. Fetal Neonatal Ed. 70, F71–74.

Spilman, L.J., Furdon, S.A., 1998. Recognition, understanding, and current management of cardiac lesions with decreased pulmonary blood flow. Neonatal Netw. 17 (4), 7–18.

van der Linde, D., Konings, E.M.K., Slager, M.A., Witsenburg, M., Helbing, W.A., Takkenberg, J.J.M., et al., 2011. Birth prevalence of congenital heart disease worldwide: a systematic review and meta-analysis. J. Am. Cardiol. 58 (21), 2241–2247. Available at: http://www.onlinejacc.org/content/58/21/2241. Accessed June 2019.

Werner, J.C., 1996. Neonatal screening for congenital heart disease. Infants Children (4), 5–7.

Wilson, W., Taubert, K.A., Gewitz, M., Lockhart, P.B., Baddour, L.M., Levison, M., et al., 2007. Prevention of infective endocarditis: guidelines from the American Heart Association. J. Am. Dent. Assoc. 138 (6), 739–45, 747–760.

10

The Newborn Eye: Visual Function and Screening for Ocular Disorders

John Siderov

CHAPTER CONTENTS

INTRODUCTION

The examination of the infant eye, and in particular that of the newborn infant eye, presents a challenge even to experienced practitioners. Nevertheless, as outlined by Hall and Elliman, health surveillance for ocular disorders in newborn babies is important for a number of reasons (Hall and Elliman, 2003). For example, an ocular abnormality such as a strabismus (squint) may indicate a serious underlying systemic condition; children with ocular abnormalities have a higher prevalence of other disorders, which may also have important genetic considerations. Other abnormalities which may be sight- or even life-threatening (e.g., retinoblastoma) can be treated if detected early enough; a delay in the detection and treatment of a significant ocular abnormality

can result in a permanent loss in visual function, or even death. Therefore ocular health screening of the neonate is an important part of the more general neonatal health surveillance. The advanced neonatal nurse practitioner (ANNP) and midwife are ideally placed to conduct such examinations. With appropriate training, these practitioners are able to conduct examinations of a high quality which produce effective results.

This chapter provides the midwife, ANNP, paediatrician or other professional who examines newborn babies and young infants with the relevant basic anatomical, physiological and functional information relating to the normal newborn eye and the baby's developing visual system; a key feature is a description of the important techniques and procedures that should be employed in newborn vision screening. The chapter concludes with a description of common and/or important ocular abnormalities that may be found in infants and young children. The material assumes that the reader is familiar with general aspects of neonatal development but has little knowledge of the eye and visual development. While some common disorders of the infant eye will be discussed, the chapter is not intended to provide a comprehensive review of childhood ocular disease, and readers are referred elsewhere for this information (Taylor and Hoyt, 1997).

THE NEWBORN EYE: ANATOMY AND PHYSIOLOGY

At birth, the human eye is remarkably well developed and at first glance appears very similar to the adult eye in many ways (Fig. 10.1). The normal anatomical features present in the adult are also seen in the newborn eye and, perhaps a little surprisingly, the dimensions of the newborn eye are nearer to the adult size than those of almost any other organ in the body. Most of us will recognize the obvious external anatomical features of the human visual process. The normal newborn infant has two eyes positioned at the front of the head, appearing approximately symmetrical about the midline of the face. Apart from the small bulge at the front of each eye (the cornea), the eyes are approximately spherical and sit within each ocular orbit in a mass of fatty tissue, muscles and connective tissue. The eyes are held securely within each orbit, attached to six small extraocular muscles which are used to move them in a coordinated fashion. The eye grows rapidly up to about the first year of life, then gradually slows down during the years that follow. The normal features of the eye that are visible on external inspection are: the eyelids and eyelashes, the cornea, the sclera and conjunctiva, the iris and anterior chamber, the pupil and—depending on

the illumination used—the red reflex. The lens, vitreous and retina are visible with appropriate instrumentation.

Cornea

The cornea is a five-layered section of transparent, avascular tissue that (together with the tear film) provides the first optical surface of the eye. It is an optically clear surface, allowing light to enter the eye and providing an effective protective barrier, and has an abundance of nerve fibres which can register touch and pain. The key features to note during the NIPE are the clarity of the cornea and the corneal diameter: in the neonate, the corneas should be transparent with a healthy sheen, and the diameter is usually between 9.5 and 10.5 mm, with the vertical diameter slightly exceeding the horizontal. In premature infants, the gestational age must be taken into account, otherwise the corneal diameter may be considered too small.

A cornea that is too large (greater than about 11 mm diameter) is known as a *macrocornea* and may be a sign of infantile glaucoma, a condition that can affect the baby's vision and requires immediate further investigation. *Microcornea*, on the other hand, is defined by a corneal diameter of less than about 9 mm. It is not a common occurrence and may be associated with other problems, such as corneal neovascularization or opacification. Microcornea may also be associated with a generally smaller eye (microphthalmos).

Sclera

The sclera is an opaque whitish tissue that in newborn infants tends to have a bluish hue, although the amount of colour can be quite variable even in the normal infant eye. The sclera covers much of the eye (apart from the cornea) and provides a tough coat, although the sclera in infants tends to be thinner and more pliable than in adults. Inspection of the sclerae is important, because infants with jaundice (Chapter 12) may show evidence of it here.

Conjunctiva

The conjunctiva forms the outermost coat of the eye, surrounding the sclera and passing under the eyelid to form a thin, semitransparent membranous coat. It has the function of allowing proper positioning of the eye in the globe and maintaining the proper relationship of the eye and the eyelids. Together with the lacrimal apparatus (the tear glands) and the eyelids, the conjunctiva

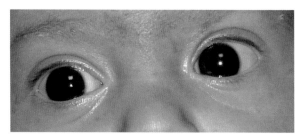

Fig. 10.1 The Normal Eye in a Young Infant.

provides a defence system to expel foreign material from the eye; it helps to maintain the normal level of microbial activity and helps to spread the tear film across the surface. While they do produce tears, newborn infants do not have the reflex tearing commonly seen in older infants and young children.

Eyelids and Eyelashes

The upper and lower eyelids form an opening known as the *palpebral aperture*; in neonates, this aperture measures about 15 mm horizontally and about half that vertically. The upper and lower lids are positioned such that they cover about four-fifths of the entire globe and leave one-fifth exposed. The lower lid margin is approximately in line with the lower limbus (the point where the cornea meets the conjunctiva); the upper lid margin tends to be slightly curved and about in line with the upper limbus in an infant, and slightly lower (1 or 2 mm below the limbus) in an adult.

Many different anomalies of the eyelid may be present in the neonate, including: a total absence of the eyelid; incomplete development of the eyelid; a *coloboma* of the eyelid, which often results in a defect in the lid margin; the absence of lashes; and congenital *ptosis*, in which the upper eyelid muscle is either absent or weakened, resulting in the lid drooping to a lower position than normal. The eyelids contain many glands that contribute to the production of tears and are important in maintaining a healthy environment on the ocular surface. The eyelashes (cilia) are formed along the leading edge of each eyelid, with about twice as many along the upper eyelid as on the lower. The eyelashes arise from small hair follicles at the base of each cilium which also contain secretory glands.

Uvea

The iris, ciliary body and choroid together form the uveal tract.

The *iris* is the most anterior structure of the uvea. It gives the eye its colour and forms the pupil, the small round aperture in the middle of the iris that allows light to enter. The iris controls the amount of light that enters the eye by changing the size of the pupil through contraction and relaxation of its two component muscles, the sphincter and the dilator.

The *ciliary body* is located posterior to the iris and the most anterior part of the retina. It is responsible for the secretion of the anterior chamber fluid which maintains the eye's intraocular pressure. The ciliary muscles are also part of the ciliary body and are used in the regulation of focusing by acting on the crystalline lens through the lens *zonules* (small specialized fibres that connect the ciliary muscle to the lens).

The *choroid* is a thin vascular layer located between the sclera and the retina which supplies the necessary nutrients to the retina's photoreceptor cells.

Lens and Vitreous

The human crystalline lens is a curved, refracting structure located just behind the iris and straddling the pupil. It is surrounded by a thin capsule and lined on its anterior surface with a single layer of cells. In the normal newborn eye, the lens is transparent.

A *cataract* is an opacity in the crystalline lens. While cataracts are usually thought of as occurring in the elderly, they can also occur in children, sometimes with profound effects on vision. Hence, one of the important aims of neonatal vision screening is the detection of infantile cataract.

The vitreous is a clear, gel-like structure that forms about two-thirds of the posterior volume of the eye. The composition of the vitreous is mostly water (99%) and it is organized so as to enhance the optics of the eye. The vitreous is strongly attached to the back of the eye near the optic nerve and anteriorly near the ciliary body.

Retina

The retina is a specialized, multilayered neural tissue at the back of the eye that is responsible for capturing light and transforming it into an electrical signal which passes along the visual pathways into the brain. The retina is more than just a conduit, however; a number of complex processes occur within the retinal cell networks that refine the information in the image before it is sent to the brain for further processing. This process begins with the capture of light by the retinal photoreceptors. These specially adapted cells are uniquely suited to capturing photons and transforming their energy into a neural signal via a chemical reaction. The neural signal is transmitted to the brain along the optic nerve. The light is focused at the retina in an area known as the *fovea*. It is this region of the retina, where the photoreceptor cells are most densely packed in adulthood, that gives the human eye its capacity for excellent, finely detailed vision.

THE NEWBORN EYE: VISUAL ACUITY AND VISUAL FUNCTION

Visual Acuity

New parents often ask, 'What can my baby see?' When this question is asked about an adult, it usually relates to the size of the smallest detail that can be clearly seen.

Light from objects passes into the eye and is focused onto the retina at the fovea. The optical system of the eye is sometimes compared to that of a camera, with a lens at the front and 'film' at the back. The eye also possesses a focusing lens, situated in the pupil just behind the iris, which can change its shape. When an infant attempts to look at (fixate onto) an object, the small ciliary muscles in the eyes contract or relax; in doing so, they alter the shape of the lens, enabling the image of the object to be focused accurately at the retina. Young infants possess the ability to alter their focusing; however, the process is not as accurate as in older children and adults. Nevertheless, an infant's visual world is not constrained so much by the optical quality of the images on the retina; rather, it is the immaturity of the neural processes in the eye and the visual areas of the brain that limit vision.

As we saw earlier, the retina contains millions of specialized photoreceptor cells which are responsible for capturing the light that enters the eye and, through a complex chemical reaction, converting the energy into an electrical signal which travels through the optic nerve, along the visual pathways and into the visual regions of the brain. The ability to see small detail depends on the proper development of all these cells and visual pathways, which takes until about the age of 5 or 6 years.

The smallest detail that is clearly resolvable by the human eye is referred to as the visual acuity and is usually measured clinically using a letter visual acuity chart, such as the Snellen chart. Visual acuity is measured in angular terms (typically minutes of arc) and expressed as a fraction (Snellen fraction), which represents the size of the smallest letter seen as a function of the distance at which it was measured. A visual acuity of 6/6 (or 20/20 in imperial measures of feet) refers to the size of the limb of the letter subtending 1 minute of arc measured at 6 metres distance (or 20 feet). A visual acuity of 6/12 (or 20/40) indicates a limb of a letter that subtends an angle of 2 minutes of arc at a 6-metre testing distance and so on. The measurement of visual acuity in an adult is therefore relatively straightforward; however, because infants are nonverbal and do not communicate in the same way as adults, they cannot be assessed by this method.

Until the 1960s, most of what was known about the visual world of infants could be summarized as follows: newborn babies start off seeing little, and their vision improves with time. As newborn infants cannot respond to subjective measurements of vision, the only way to determine a neonate's vision prior to the 1960s was to use a 'fix and follow' method. This technique employed a fixation device (e.g., a penlight or other similar object) which was used to attract the infant's attention; the clinician would monitor the infant's fixational behaviour on the penlight as it was moved about. If the infant could fix and follow the target, it was assumed that they could therefore see it. Clearly, such a method offers little quantitative information about visual acuity, but observing an infant's fixation can be a useful indicator of gross vision.

During the 1960s and later, researchers became interested in infants' vision and so this period saw the development of a number of behavioural methods for measuring visual acuity. These methods rely on infants' preference for looking at patterns rather than featureless scenes and have permitted the measurement of their visual acuity in a clinical setting. Perhaps the best known and most widely used of these is the forced-choice preferential looking (FCPL) method. The infant is presented with a series of grating patterns (stripes) that differ in size (spatial frequency or stripe width); this variation corresponds to changes in visual acuity. In practice, the infant is shown a blank plate and a plate with a grating pattern side by side. The clinician observes the infant's fixation preference without knowing the location of the grating pattern, and makes a forced-choice response based on the infant's behaviour. The size of the pattern is gradually reduced until the percentage of correct responses by the clinician falls to chance, indicating that the infant no longer exhibits a preference for the grating (i.e., it has become too small to see). The size of the grating for which performance was above chance level (taken to be halfway between the guessing rate and 100% correct) is taken as the visual acuity. Using this type of methodology, scientists determined that visual acuity in infants is about 6/180 at birth and gradually improves throughout the first few years of life to reach adult-like levels (6/6) at around 4 to 5 years of age (Fig. 10.2). During this same period, other methods to determine visual acuity in infants were also developed;

Newborn | 4 weeks

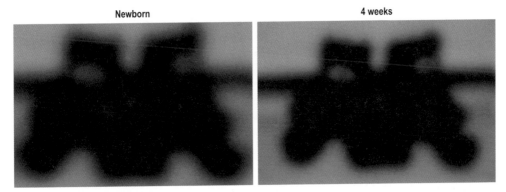

8 weeks | 3 months

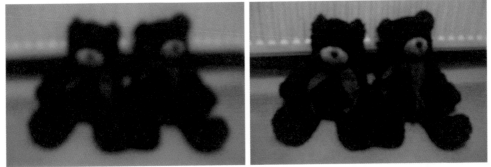

6 months | Adult

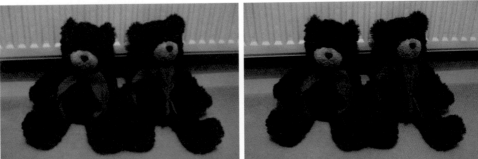

Fig. 10.2 Demonstration of the Changes in an Infant's Visual World from Newborn to 6 Months. Also shown is the original image as seen by an adult. (Infant vision simulation courtesy of TinyEyes.com.)

however, these are beyond the scope of this chapter and the reader is referred to other sources for more information (e.g., Moore, 1997).

Clinical note: newborn infants are attracted to faces.

Oculomotor Control (Eye Movements)

Infants who are born with visual impairment sometimes exhibit abnormal eye movements as a presenting sign, which is why eye movements are often used as a sign of normal visual development. Although rare in the general population, one of the most common oculomotor abnormalities in infancy is *nystagmus*, a rhythmic oscillation of the eyes around the horizontal or vertical axes. Nystagmus may occur as an idiopathic developmental disorder, but it is also associated with underlying neurological disease; any infant with nystagmus requires further detailed investigations.

In general, infants exhibit most of the same eye movements seen in adults, although they may not be as sophisticated. As discussed earlier, infants will be able to fixate an object and track (follow) its movements. They will also be attracted to objects in their peripheral visual field and be able to follow them. Infants do exhibit the fast, saccadic eye movements (the fast eye movement from one fixation target to another) seen in adults, but they usually make errors in the amplitude of the movement. They can fixate on an object with both eyes (binocularly) as long as the targets used are visually attractive and not too close to or too far from the infant. Nevertheless, the accuracy of an infant's eye movements is poor, especially within the first month or two, and it is not unusual for the eyes to appear to function independently of one another. This lack of control may result in the occasional appearance of one or both eyes 'wandering' in different directions, or 'crossed' eyes. This situation usually resolves itself within the first 2 months. Any such eye deviation noted after this time, or any deviation noted with an abnormal pupil reflex (see later), should be referred to an ophthalmologist for further investigation.

As discussed earlier, observing an infant's eye movements can give some guide as to the level of vision. An alternative to the 'fix and follow' method is a technique in which the clinician holds the infant in their arms with the infant looking up at the examiner's face. The examiner then rotates in one direction for a brief period (2–3 seconds). This has the effect of generating simple rhythmic horizontal eye movements (nystagmus) by stimulating the balance mechanisms in the ears (vestibular apparatus). The vestibular apparatus helps to keep the eyes in a stable position in the presence of any head movements. The resulting nystagmus is a normal by-product of this stabilizing mechanism. If the infant has normal vision, they will attempt to fixate onto the examiner's face and the nystagmus will stop quickly; however, in infants with impaired vision, the nystagmus will continue for many seconds after the body rotation has ceased because there is no visual input present to dampen the effect.

Clinical note: until about 2 months of age, newborn babies may occasionally appear to have eyes that wander and look crossed.

THE NEWBORN EYE: INVESTIGATIVE TECHNIQUES

History

Although the neonate cannot respond to questioning, it is important that, prior to beginning your examination,

TABLE 10.1   **Questions to Ask When Conducting a History of a Neonate**
1. Has any eye problem been noted by parents, carers or others? Do the parents have any anxieties regarding the baby's vision?
2. Does the infant suffer from any systemic abnormality?
3. Was the birth normal or was there any birth trauma?
4. Was the infant born prematurely? Babies born with a birth weight of less than 1500 g or babies that are born at 32 weeks or earlier should be screened for retinopathy of prematurity; they have an increased risk of developing significant eye and visual defects.
5. How is the infant's general health?
6. Is there any history of significant eye problems in the family (e.g., congenital cataract)?
7. Are there any other diseases or conditions that occur in the family (i.e., inherited conditions)?

a patient history be conducted; Table 10.1 lists a number of questions that should be addressed. Newborn infants who are born prematurely or suffer trauma during birth are more likely to develop problems with their vision and eyes. In addition, many systemic conditions may exhibit ocular anomalies, so it is important to try to ascertain as much relevant information in the history as possible.

General Observation

The diagnostic ability of any clinical practitioner is greatly enhanced if they are a good observer, and good observation skills are critical in screening the newborn infant.

Observation begins with a general overview of the infant's eyes and ocular areas (*adnexa*). General observation may be enhanced by using a small penlight and, if available, a magnifying loupe. A systematic approach to examination is important.

1. Begin by examining the eyelids and eyelashes, looking for symmetrical appearance and noting any irregularities, such as any redness, watery eyes, discharge or lumps.
2. The lower eyelids may be pulled down slightly to reveal the palpebral conjunctiva and lower bulbar conjunctiva. Note any roughness of the conjunctiva or lumps and bumps, as before.
3. Examine the cornea, which should appear clear with no sign of cloudiness and be free from any opacity or irregularities.

4. If possible, observe the anterior chamber, which should be free of any cells or other haze.
5. Examine the iris and the pupil. The iris should be free of any irregularities or blood vessels. The pupils should be examined, taking note of their shape and size; they should appear round and equal in size.

Remember your knowledge of the anatomy of the external eye; refer for further investigation anything you are unsure of or which looks odd or unusual.

Direct Ophthalmoscope: Principles and Uses

The ophthalmoscope was developed over 150 years ago as a device to examine the structures of the eye. The modern direct ophthalmoscope is used in routine examinations of both the external and internal eye (Fig. 10.3). It consists of an observation system and an illumination system. The observation system comprises a small aperture (to look into) and a series of optical lenses of differing powers. The lenses are used to compensate for any optical error of the patient (refractive error) and to bring into focus the various structures of the eye. For a patient and an observer with no refractive error, the lens setting on the ophthalmoscope is usually set to zero when viewing the retina. For viewing the anterior structures of the eye, the lens setting is gradually increased along the plus (positive) side. The illumination system usually comprises a light source, a high-power condensing lens, a prism reflecting system and, depending on the model used, a series of different apertures and filters.

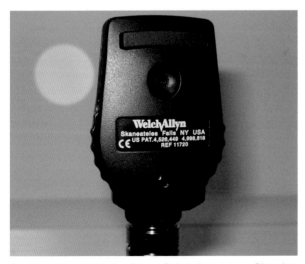

Fig. 10.3 The Back of a Direct Ophthalmoscope, Showing the Examiner's View of the Aperture and Lens Dial.

Red Reflex Test

The purpose of the red reflex test (sometimes called the Brückner test) is to detect abnormalities arising at the back of the eye (e.g., from the retina) and abnormalities of the crystalline lens (e.g., cataract) and cornea (e.g., corneal opacity).

Before attempting the red reflex test, take care to familiarize yourself with the various dials and apertures on the ophthalmoscope. For use in neonatal screening, the largest circular aperture is selected. Ensure that the infant is comfortable and awake before attempting the test; if possible, do not force open the eyelids, but allow the infant to open them voluntarily. The baby may be lying down or held in a parent's lap. The red reflex is the reflection of light from the retina that is seen in the pupil of the eye; it is often seen in photographs when a camera flash is used (the 'red eye' effect). In fact, photographs of the newborn infant which show a problem with the red reflex (e.g., where one red reflex is missing or appears different from the other) may be useful to determine the onset of a significant ocular problem. Parents expressing concern about the appearance of the red eye reflex of their child in photographs should be referred for prompt medical advice.

The red reflex in babies is easier to see when the pupils are large, so work in a darkened room to facilitate pupillary mydriasis (in some cases, it may be appropriate to have the pupil pharmacologically dilated, but such a procedure is beyond the scope of this chapter). Set the lens power to zero or about +1 to +2 (dioptres) and position yourself directly in front of the baby, at about arm's length. Hold the ophthalmoscope close to your own eye (if you normally wear glasses, keep them on; however, you may be able to perform this test without them by adjusting the lens power of the ophthalmoscope). Vary the lens power until you obtain a clear focus on the anterior eye. The red reflex should appear in the baby's pupil. The aperture should be large enough to enable you to view the red reflex in both eyes simultaneously. If not, then vary your working distance back a little until you can see both pupils (Fig. 10.4a). The two red reflexes should be equally visible and appear similar in intensity and colour (Fig. 10.4b). The colour of the reflex may differ between babies depending on their general level of pigmentation; however, for any individual infant, a symmetrical appearance is important.

To examine the red reflex further, move in towards the baby, focusing your attention on one eye and one red reflex. Be sure to adjust the power of the ophthalmoscope

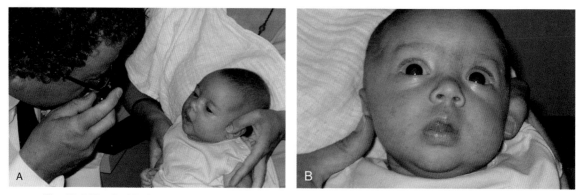

Fig. 10.4 The Red Reflex Test. (A) Performing the red reflex test on a neonate. The examiner is holding the ophthalmoscope close to his eye and is observing the red reflex in each eye of the infant. (B) The red reflex in a normal neonate. Although depicted in monochrome, a normal red reflex appears free of any spots or other colorations (e.g., whiteness) and is symmetrical between the two eyes. Also present in this image are the corneal reflexes; note that due to the angle of the camera the corneal reflexes do not appear in the middle of the pupil.

lens as you move in (typically adding a higher +1 lens). Stop moving when you are about 10 to 15 cm away (whereby the lens power will be about +7 to +10, assuming a negligible refractive error for the examiner and the patient). Examine the red reflex more closely, looking for any shadows or dark spots; such opacities may indicate a disease process such as cataract and require further investigation by an ophthalmologist. Remember that a normal red reflex appears free of any spots or other colourations (e.g., shadows or whiteness) and is symmetrical between the two eyes. Any abnormality needs prompt further attention from an ophthalmologist.

The importance of practice using an ophthalmoscope cannot be overemphasized for proficiency in observing the red reflex. Despite some concerns about the sensitivity and specificity of aspects of the red reflex test (Sun et al., 2016), it remains widely recommended (Cagini et al., 2017; Haargaard et al., 2015)

> Clinical note: the red reflex test is an effective screening test for the detection of ocular abnormalities in the newborn, and its use in screening infants' eyes should be mandatory. In infants with no ocular abnormality, the red reflex should appear clear and equal in colour and intensity in each eye and be free from any opacity.

The Corneal Reflex Test

The corneal reflex test is used to determine the relative positioning of the two eyes, and can be useful to determine the presence of a *strabismus* (a wandering eye or squint). The test relies on observing the reflection of a light source off the first corneal surface.

As for the red reflex test, the corneal reflex test is best performed in a darkened room using a small penlight or similar instrument; the ophthalmoscope can also be used. The light source is held about 50 cm away from the infant's face, in the midplane. The infant must fixate on the light for this test to succeed. Once fixation is obtained, observe the position of the corneal reflection of the light. In an infant whose eyes are both fixating properly on the light source, the corneal reflex appears just off the centre of the pupil (usually slightly towards the nose). The reflex is not exactly in the centre of the pupil because the optical axis does not coincide exactly with the visual axis. The small displacement of the corneal reflex should be identical in both eyes (e.g., both nasal by the same amount), indicating that the eyes are aligned and confirming the absence of a strabismus. If the displacement is not identical, the infant may have a strabismus and further investigation is warranted. Keep in mind that newly born babies may not have fully developed eye movements, so misalignments in the fixation positions of the two eyes may not necessarily be a problem. For infants older than about 2 months, however, any misalignment in the corneal reflex should not be dismissed and the child should be referred for further examination.

OCULAR DISORDERS: LEUKOCORIA

Leukocoria is a condition in which the pupil appears white in colour; it can be the hallmark of a significant ocular abnormality and requires urgent referral to an ophthalmologist for further investigation. Leukocoria is one of the reasons why parents bring their young babies in for eye examinations. Unfortunately, the presence of leukocoria usually indicates that the underlying pathology is advanced. For this reason, early detection through routine neonatal vision screening (using the red reflex test described earlier) is critical.

Cataract

Cataract is defined as any opacity of the crystalline lens, irrespective of size or location. Although usually associated with the elderly, cataracts also occur in infants and may be congenital (with or without a hereditary element, and sometimes associated with a chromosomal anomaly), or secondary to trauma or other intrauterine problem (e.g., rubella). Congenital cataracts can vary greatly in size and location within the lens, and may be divided into sight-threatening or non-sight-threatening categories. The red reflex test used in routine neonatal vision screening is the best way to detect congenital cataracts (Haargaard et al., 2015; Fry and Wilson, 2005; Rahi et al., 1999). Not all cataracts result in leukocoria, but all produce an abnormal red reflex, typically exhibiting a shadow or darkness. In the context of screening, all cataracts must be referred to an ophthalmologist for evaluation.

It is estimated that, globally, between 20,000 and 40,000 children are born each year with congenital cataracts. Although the incidence of congenital cataracts is relatively small at about 3 per 10,000 live births per year (Sheeladevi, 2016; Morgan, 1999), they can cause a marked loss in vision and require urgent treatment in order to prevent permanent visual impairment. The usual treatment is surgery.

Retinoblastoma

Retinoblastoma is a malignant tumour that derives from cells in the retina, and is the commonest intraocular tumour in childhood. It commonly presents as leukocoria and can occur in one or both eyes. If detection is delayed, the affected eye may also exhibit a strabismus. Immediate referral to an ophthalmologist is needed because the tumour can be life-threatening.

Persistent Hyperplastic Primary Vitreous

Persistent hyperplastic primary vitreous is a congenital condition in which the embryonic vitreous structures (the vitreous vasculature) failed to regress. It may result in the formation of a cataract and an underdeveloped eye, and can present as leukocoria.

Retinopathy of Prematurity (ROP)

Retinopathy of prematurity occurs when the retinal vascular network does not grow normally, resulting in the development of abnormal retinal blood vessels. The new blood vessel networks can lead to a detachment of the retina, which manifests as a white pupil on the red reflex test. Retinopathy of prematurity is linked to a number of factors, including the infant's gestational age and birth weight. All infants weighing less than 1500 g and of less than about 32 weeks' gestational age should be referred for ophthalmological evaluation (O'Connor et al., 2006; Taylor and Hoyt, 1997).

Coloboma

A coloboma is a malformation of the ocular structures that appears as a notch, gap or other similar anomaly, and arises due to incomplete development of the eye. It may occur as an isolated finding or may be part of a syndrome. A coloboma may be limited to only certain structures of the eye, such as the eyelid, or may involve the entire eye. Where a coloboma is large and involves the retina, choroid and optic nerve, it may be visible through the pupil and give the pupil a whitish appearance.

Uveitis

Uveitis is an inflammation of any part of the uveal tract; it may occur at the front of the eye (anterior uveitis) or at the back (posterior uveitis). It is characterized by the presence of inflammatory cells. Where the inflammatory process is substantial, sufficient material may be present in the vitreous to give rise to leukocoria.

OCULAR DISORDERS: NASAL LACRIMAL DUCT OBSTRUCTION

Obstruction of the tear duct drainage system is a relatively common problem in infants. The condition is signified by the presence of a watery eye and crustiness around the eyelashes. The child is usually comfortable and without any pain. Photophobia (aversion to light) is not present. Congenital nasal lacrimal duct obstruction may occur in one or both eyes, and usually resolves without treatment. In some cases the tear ducts may become infected, leading to the formation of a swelling around the lower lid; in such cases, prompt referral to an ophthalmologist is required.

OCULAR DISORDERS: INFANTILE GLAUCOMA

The presence of a watery eye may also be a sign of infantile glaucoma; however, unlike obstruction of the lacrimal duct, infantile glaucoma is also accompanied by photophobia and an enlarged and cloudy cornea. This condition results from a rise in the intraocular pressure, often due to a congenital blockage in the drainage of intraocular fluid, which leads to an enlargement of the globe and cornea, and changes in the optic nerve. Prompt referral to an ophthalmologist is needed.

OCULAR DISORDERS: CONJUNCTIVITIS

Conjunctivitis is an inflammation of the conjunctiva that presents with a red and sticky eye. In newborns, the most common cause is infection arising from chlamydial, gonococcal or herpes simplex infection. In these cases, the infection can cause significant and permanent corneal scarring and even systemic infection; any conjunctivitis in a neonate should be referred for prompt treatment to a general practitioner in the first instance.

SUMMARY

Examination of the newborn, although challenging, is also a rewarding experience for the practitioner. Even though the prevalence of significant visual abnormalities like congenital cataract and retinoblastoma is relatively low in UK neonates, the impact of such conditions—on not only the infant but also the family and, ultimately, the community—can be dramatic. Therefore the early detection of significant ocular abnormalities is important. The midwife or neonatal nurse is in an ideal position to conduct the appropriate visual health surveillance.

KEY POINTS

The recommendations for conducting a visual examination to detect significant and disabling ocular abnormalities in the neonatal eye examination are:
- History: be sure to ask if there is any specific history relating to ocular abnormalities.
- General observation: always employ a systematic approach.
- The red reflex test: this test should be undertaken as an essential part of every NIPE.

REFERENCES

Cagini, C., Tosi, G., Stracci, F., Rinaldi, V.E., Verrotti, A., 2017. Red reflex examination in neonates: evaluation of 3 years of screening. Int. Ophthalmol. 37, 1199–1204.

Fry, M., Wilson, G.A., 2005. Scope for improving congenital cataract blindness prevention by screening of infants (red reflex screening) in a New Zealand setting. J. Paediatr. Child Health 41, 344–346.

Haargaard, B., Nyström, A., Rosensvärd, A., Tornqvist, K., Magnusson, G., 2015. The pediatric cataract register (PECARE): analysis of age at detection of congenital cataract. Acta Ophthalmol. 93, 24–26.

Hall, D.M.B., Elliman, D. (Eds.), 2003. Screening for vision defects. In: Health for All Children. Oxford University Press, Oxford, UK, p. 408.

Moore, B.D., 1997. Eye Care for Infants and Young Children. Butterworth-Heinemann, Boston, MA.

Morgan, S., 1999. In screening for congenital cataract, many false positive referrals will occur. Br. Med. J. 319, 122–123.

O'Connor, A.R., Stewart, C.E., Singh, J., Fielder, A.R., 2006. Do infants of birth weight less than 1500 g require additional long term ophthalmic follow up? Br. J. Ophthalmol. 90 (4), 451–455. doi:10.1136/bjo.2005.083550. Available from: https://www.ncbi.nlm.nih.gov/pmc/articles/PMC1856987/#ref14. Accessed June 2019.

Rahi, J.S., Dezateux, C., 1999. National cross sectional study of detection of congenital and infantile cataract in the United Kingdom: role of childhood screening and surveillance. The British Congenital Cataract Interest Group. Br. Med. J. 318, 362–365.

Sheeladevi, S., Lawrenson, J.G., Fielder, A.R., Suttle, C., 2016. Global prevalence of childhood cataract: a systematic review. Eye (Lond) 30 (9), 1160–1169. Available from: https://www.ncbi.nlm.nih.gov/pmc/articles/PMC5023808/#bib3. Accessed June 2019.

Sun, M., Ma, A., Li, F., Cheng, K., Zhang, M., Yang, H., et al., 2016. Sensitivity and specificity of red reflex test in newborn eye screening. J. Pediatr. 179, 192–196.e4.

Taylor, D., Hoyt, C., 1997. Practical Paediatric Ophthalmology. Blackwell Science, Oxford, UK.

11

Congenital Abnormality: Screening, Diagnosis and Communication

Lorna Davies and Jacqui Anderson

CHAPTER CONTENTS

'It was as though I was on a boat crossing a lake and it was slowly sinking. I was baling out water, but it just kept sinking. I kept trying to keep it afloat, but I was fighting a losing battle. Everyone I knew was on the shore and they were shouting different things. Some were saying, "let it sink and swim back". Others were calling "keep baling, keep baling, you can get to the other side". I felt like I just wanted to go down with the boat at that time.'

Hannah, the woman whose words begin this chapter, discovered at 18 weeks that her baby had extensive congenital abnormalities. She used this analogy to express the feelings she experienced during the time between discovering her baby's condition and deciding to terminate the pregnancy.

She was given what she described as the 'most amazing support' by her midwife. She claimed it was the quietly supportive, nonjudgemental and nondirective presence of her midwife that enabled her to come through the experience and to have another child some 18 months or so later.

Hannah acknowledges that, although the midwife kept her fully informed of the nature and significance of the tests prior to the diagnosis, nothing could have prepared her for the 'sledgehammer' of discovering her baby had so many problems that he may not even survive the pregnancy. If she had continued with the pregnancy and the baby had lived, he would have been subjected to numerous surgical interventions in order to increase his chances of surviving. Hannah's decision was primarily based around the potential suffering of the baby.

This scenario will probably resonate with many health care professionals. Most practitioners who work with pregnant women and their families will have found themselves having to support women in similar situations. Sometimes, concerns raised during screening will have been confirmed by follow-up diagnostic tests; these findings usually lead to decisions of magnitude having to be made, sometimes within a cruelly short time frame. As testing methods evolve, if there is a possibility of a genetic defect—perhaps as a result of a family history—parents increasingly opt for early testing and thus are often more prepared for a less than positive outcome. It is rarer these days—although, anecdotally at least, it does still happen—for the parents and practitioners to be unaware of any abnormality until the baby presents at birth. Sometimes, the parents will have made a conscious decision not to avail themselves of the screening tests available, for whatever reason. Others will have had every test on offer, but fall within the 'false negative' category for a condition; or it may be that a problem is simply not detected on ultrasound. Even the new noninvasive prenatal testing/screening (NIPT/S; Chapter 4) cannot currently guarantee definitive results.

In this chapter, we aim to explore a range of congenital anomalies and conditions that may affect the fetus and newborn baby. Additionally, we will explore the broader professional, legal, ethical and, in particular, the communication issues at stake.

THE POWER OF LANGUAGE

Health care practitioners have developed and learned a specific language referring to the human body and its anatomical and physiological functions. We use this language comfortably to discuss what is considered 'normal' or otherwise. Practitioners use the terms 'normal' and 'abnormal' to identify a given aspect of an individual's health status, reflecting a specific identification of something as being normal or otherwise. Yet, for individuals, these terms can hold a variety of meanings depending on their personal, philosophical, cultural and societal beliefs, attitudes, values and experiences. As individuals, our understanding of what is normal or abnormal is subjective, reflecting the context of our everyday lives.

When we consider the term *normal*, our interpretation may include words like usual, standard, ordinary, common, average, routine or natural. What an individual considers normal may encompass an understanding of the physiologically normal, something that is the common or usual experience, or a situation that is routine, customary, ordinary or insignificant. Normal can also describe the typical experience or expectation of an individual or group. But the things that are regarded as normal for a particular individual may be outside the experiences of others.

If a variety of words can define 'normal', what is understood about the term *abnormal*? It can be interpreted as meaning nonstandard, atypical or unusual—in other words, 'out of the ordinary'. These words can be taken to mean 'something special' and are sometimes used to

reflect a positive perception or situation. However, other definitions of the word may reflect particular attitudes and experiences, and engender negative connotations. These definitions include strange, odd, bad, peculiar, deviant, aberrant, deformed and malformed. Unlike the words used earlier to define normal, the interpretations of 'abnormal' can be challenging; they can elicit anxiety or apprehension, especially when considered in a personal context. The use of such words, therefore, is likely to affect how we view and react to situations when what we consider to be 'normal' is absent. This has the potential to alter our behaviour and responses at both a conscious and unconscious level.

Researching this chapter, we realized the language practitioners use when describing a situation outside the usual experience is powerful and invariably negatively oriented, even if it is accurate. The words 'malformation' and 'deformation' are used routinely but, to the uninitiated, they may raise the spectre of something extremely unusual and even frightening. The reality is that these words are often used to describe any physical difference, no matter how minor; there is often no allowance for degrees of difference, and, while these variations may be explained later, it can be hard for patients and their families to move on from the initial language used.

The attitudinal perceptions of normal and abnormal that we are subject to as health professionals pervade the literature. Much of the literature relating to complications of the newborn identifies strategies for 'breaking the bad news', and this approach can set the practitioner in a position from which it can be difficult to retreat. The assumption is always that the information will be, if not devastating, then close to it. The information that needs to be conveyed may not be the best news parents will want to hear; neither is it always the worst. While it is unlikely that parents would want their baby to have a complication, practitioners who talk about the baby only in relation to that complication may not adequately develop the ability to be 'with' the parents as they try to understand what this new information means for their baby and themselves.

This was a theme identified in a study exploring parents' experiences of being told their baby has a life-threatening diagnosis (Côté-Arsenault and Denney-Koelsch, 2011). In this study, all participants identified a strong desire 'to honour and legitimize the humanity of their unborn baby'. The theme 'my baby is a person' emerged as parents struggled with the way health practitioners referred to the condition the baby had, rather than identifying the baby as a precious individual. This response was also identified in a study by McKechnie et al. (2015) including of parents' experiences of health professionals' attitudes. The study found that some professionals seemed to strike the wrong chord with parents, offering unsolicited sympathy:

I found myself, even within just a few weeks [of the diagnosis], getting mad at people … A genetic counsellor wanted to give me a big hug and [said], 'I'm so sorry'. And I'm already kind of getting defensive and getting mad because I'm like, 'She's still a baby, and we're still happy to have her'.

McKechnie et al., 2015

Practitioners often develop the communication skills they need by participating in the actual information-sharing process with parents. This may be helpful for the practitioner, but is less than optimal for the new parents who may initially find the situation incomprehensible. It is easy to resort to the use of terminology we are comfortable with when we are in an emotionally challenging situation, but this may alienate parents. We will return to this important theme later in the chapter.

INCIDENCE AND CLASSIFICATION

Congenital abnormality, by definition, is a defect present at birth. About 1 in 50babies in the UK are affected by a major congenital anomaly which is a cause of fetal, neonatal and child mortality and morbidity. Data suggest that 28% of perinatal and infant deaths in the UK are attributable to congenital abnormality (POST, 2016).

The causes of congenital abnormalities can be classified into three main groups:
- Genetic: including chromosomal anomalies such as Down syndrome, and single-gene defects such as achondroplasia. The number of congenital anomalies which originate from a genetic source is estimated to be about 28% (PHE, 2017).
- Environmental: including congenital infections, drugs, alcohol, smoking and environmental pollutants. Approximately 15% of congenital anomalies are believed to be attributable to environmental factors (Chaabane, 2013).
- Complex (multifactorial) origin: by far the largest category; represents a combination of genetic and

environmental interaction in which a predisposition is triggered by environmental risk factors. It contains the large number of idiopathic congenital abnormalities with no real known origin (LaMorte, 2016).

PREGNANCY AND SCREENING

The vast majority of women opt for antenatal screening to identify unforeseen problems with their baby. Ethical consideration should always be at the forefront of any discussion around antenatal screening, particularly when the primary—if not sole—purpose of genetic screening, ultrasound scanning and biochemical marker testing, is to determine whether the unborn child has an anomaly of some kind. The UK National Screening Committee, like its counterparts in other western health care settings, has attempted to improve the quality and coordination of antenatal screening processes, as discussed in Chapter 14 (UK NSC, 2019). Health professionals are expected to inform women about tests on offer and ensure they are fully cognizant of the risks and benefits of each test they accept (NHS England, 2017). This takes time, patience and the use of excellent communication skills in order to ensure that women are able to make informed decisions. Further discussion around this area may be found in Chapter 15.

ANTENATAL DIAGNOSIS

Once a condition is diagnosed, the midwife has the unenviable task of helping parents through the maze of the decision-making process. There are clearly some advantages for the parents in knowing that their baby has some degree of abnormality. It may allow them to plan for any special health needs before the baby is born; it can allow for pre-labour counselling so they are well prepared to meet their baby with the minimum of trauma; it may offer the opportunity for surgery in utero if appropriate, or to ensure that the appropriate treatment or surgery is available after birth, and to explore the available options. Another option offered following the diagnosis of some conditions is the termination of the pregnancy.

TERMINATION OF PREGNANCY

In legal terms, the issue of abortion in this situation is relatively uncomplicated. The Abortion Act 1967 (UK) acknowledges the need for termination of pregnancy in the event of a substantial risk of the child being born with a lethal condition, or with such physical or mental abnormalities as to condemn it to serious disability.

However, from a moral perspective, the issue of whether or not to terminate the pregnancy is a value-laden decision that a woman and her family may have to face, depending on the severity of the abnormality. It is therefore essential that parents are provided with up-to-date and unbiased information to enable them to consider the benefits and risks of abortion compared with those of continuing the pregnancy. The health professional will be with the woman and her family for a relatively short time, but the parents will have to live with their decisions for the rest of their lives and therefore must be seen to be as certain as they are ever able to be.

Evidence suggests that, in many countries, termination of pregnancy is the most likely outcome when Down syndrome or neural tube defects are diagnosed. In a systematic review published in 2012, Natoli et al. reported that rates of termination specifically for Down syndrome ranged from 61% to 92% in the United States, with a weighted mean termination rate of 67%. Denmark has a termination rate of 95% (Carstensen et al., 2018). According to a 2014 report by the UK National Down Syndrome Cytogenetic Register, 90% of women with an antenatal diagnosis of Down syndrome underwent a termination of pregnancy (NDSCR, 2014). The UK government reported that in 2017 a total of 3314 abortions were performed for congenital malformations; of these, 22% (743) of the malformations were related to the nervous system and 9% to the cardiovascular system (305). Chromosome abnormalities were reported as the principal medical condition in 34% (1131), with Down syndrome accounting for 20% of these terminations (655) (DHSC, 2017).

Each new genetic test that is developed raises serious issues for health systems as well as public health, and social policy. These issues include how the test should be used, how it is implemented, what uses are made of its results, and what the ethical implications of testing may be. The introduction of noninvasive prenatal testing/ (NIPT/S) was discussed at length in Chapter 4 , but it is worth reconsidering briefly here. Concern about the ethics of antenatal screening appears to have been heightened as a result of the introduction of noninvasive screening; some commentators have suggested that NIPT/S may lead to more terminations of pregnancies

for chromosomal abnormality and have even raised the question of whether the screening is being used as a filter to legitimize a new brand of eugenics (Thomas and Katz Rothman, 2016).

This is not a new argument with regard to the ethics of reproductive choice. Gaby (2004) argued that the notion of choice (and its role in the power relationship associated with the paternalistic medical model and the provision of knowledge) means that parents choosing to continue with a pregnancy following a less than positive prognosis may experience social sanction, stigma and discrimination. If they go on to have a child with a disability, they may be labelled as irresponsible. The argument that 'reproductive choice is not simply about the right to choose abortion, but also the right to choose not to abort' would appear to be as much an issue today as it has been for the last two decades. As Lafarge et al. (2014) discuss, societies often send conflicting messages to women, extolling the acceptance of disability while encouraging antenatal screening. Lafarge found that women identified themselves as having to make a choice between two 'alternatives, both of which are unpleasant'.

The attitudes of caregivers, and societal attitudes towards abortion and disability, colour the landscape women have to negotiate in their decision-making. Women walk a tightrope: an abortion decision may be seen as selfish, but continuing with a pregnancy may be seen as imposing a cost on society as a whole. The lack of ongoing support and enablement for families if a child is born with a disability clearly indicates the place the child will hold in that particular society. These messages must have a role in influencing decision-making. It would seem that, as health professionals, we need to develop better skills in supporting women to negotiate such life-changing decisions (Pitt et al., 2016). In both the Lafarge (2014) and the Pitt et al. (2016) studies, women valued timely, clear and unbiased information on the abnormality identified, the options available and what supports were available (no matter what decision they made), and being guided to trustworthy information which they were given time to explore.

Health economics is sometimes accused of being a covert driving force behind the decisions of women to terminate their pregnancy following a diagnosis of congenital abnormality; women have reported feeling coerced into abortion against their actual preference to continue with the pregnancy (Miller, 2016). This has been termed *reproductive coercion* and is defined as 'behaviour that interferes with the autonomous decision-making of a woman, with regards to reproductive health' (Grace and Anderson, 2016).

There have been a number of studies examining the costs and outcomes of different screening strategies for Down syndrome (e.g., Ökem et al., 2017; Walker et al., 2015; Gekas et al., 2009). These studies set out to compare the cost benefits of different types of screening, such as maternal serum screening versus NIPT/S. The measurement they generally use is based on the cost per additional liveborn baby with Down syndrome prevented as a result of termination of pregnancy following the tests. This type of cost–benefit analysis for antenatal screening has been seriously challenged, chiefly because it does not evaluate its findings in human terms; what this utilitarian line of discussion fails to address is the possibility that an individual child could become a valuable, productive member of society, rather than a social burden. However, a systematic review in 2017 examined studies from a range of countries that had introduced NIPT/S, and concluded that the introduction had resulted in little change compared with termination rates prior to the introduction. The authors found that many parents were using NIPT/S for information and were continuing with pregnancies in which Down syndrome was likely (Hill, 2017).

COMMUNICATION IN THE ANTENATAL PERIOD

In a health care world where the service is frequently understaffed and resources scarce, the fast and furious opt-out system that practitioners are obliged to provide leaves little time for individual discussion with each woman. This means that, at times, decisions may have to be made about issues that have not been fully addressed in the pre-testing phase of the process. Some women are not even aware that their 'routine' ultrasound scan is anything more than a chance for them to 'meet' their baby; Roberts et al. (2015) reported, 'Routine scan appointments have become a "not to be missed" part of the pregnancy experience, landmark events' and suggest 'it is clear that the value of ultrasound for women and families exceeds its clinical utility'. However, the introduction of NIPT/S, chromosomal microarray (CMA) and next-generation DNA sequencing (NGS) tests may be changing this perception by making women less likely

to take a perspective of optimistic bias (Richardson and Ormond, 2018).

Midwives and others who share information with women need to further consider the health literacy of the recipients, and the additional time required to provide the potential for informed decision-making. Smith et al. (2018) suggest that this calls for the development of more decision-making tools around screening, and increased opportunities for professional development. These recommendations support the findings of a Dutch study by Martin et al. (2015), who found that clients prefer antenatal counselling for congenital anomaly tests that provides health education at an understandable level, and appreciate information and tools for supporting decision-making which are tailored to clients' individual preferences rather than what the health practitioner believes is required.

SUPPORTING AUTONOMOUS DECISION-MAKING AND THE ROLE OF NONDIRECTIVENESS

One of the principal philosophical values upheld in medical ethics is that of respect for autonomy (Clarke, 2017); nondirective counselling was developed to protect the autonomy and best interests of the individual against third-party interests or societal pressure (Rehmann-Sutter, 2009). The concept of *nondirectiveness* has been considered intrinsic to ensuring that people can make the best decisions for themselves and their families. Nondirective counselling is intended to facilitate autonomous decision-making and remove the health practitioner's views about a particular course of action (Vanstone et al., 2012). Providing neutral information but no practical advice or moral judgement should theoretically enable individuals to arrive at self-determined decisions.

The aim of nondirectiveness is to communicate risk and offer support without advising individuals on what decisions to make (Arribas-Ayllon and Sarangi, 2014). This requires practitioners to explain and discuss the issues without directing the final decision; however, such neutrality is not always easy to achieve, and recognition of this problem has influenced current debates on the role of the health professional in supporting decision-making. The stance of not influencing the patient can be viewed as taking a detached attitude—which potentially affects the quality of a relationship that requires the development of trust and respect on both sides. Rehm-ann-Sutter (2009) suggests the concept of *agency* as a way to support informed decision-making. One view of agency is that it is the capacity of individuals to act independently and to make their own free choices. Rehm-ann-Sutter proposes that by allowing agency, the best parts of nondirectiveness are retained through respect for the client's values and responsible information-sharing. The health practitioner and the client develop a mutually engaged and caring interaction as partners with different roles, different knowledge resources and different decision-making responsibilities.

Self-awareness is a key characteristic for health professionals—one that we frequently need to revisit by employing a reflective approach to practice. How do we feel as practitioners if the decisions made go against our own values and beliefs, or our clinical judgement? If we are pro-life, can we offer a woman unbiased and non-judgemental advice should she decide to terminate the pregnancy? If we believe that severe disability is a burden society should not have to carry in the 21st century, how will we respond to a woman who refuses to have any screening during pregnancy?

Carlsson et al. (2015) explored the experiences of parents and their need for information when congenital heart disease was discovered antenatally in their baby. Parents reported that receiving early and honest information, along with practitioners ascertaining their preferences, was crucial to supporting decision-making regarding the future of the pregnancy. They also identified that the use of illustrations of the condition was very helpful and increased their comprehension and acceptance of the oral information. The participants described the 'emotional chaos' or acute stress reaction experienced when trying to 'grasp the facts today while reflecting on the future' and at the same time grieving the loss of their anticipated 'perfect baby'. Parents described the first days after the diagnosis as being psychologically 'disordered' and said that trying to make any decisions was very difficult. Repeated information was considered as being of great importance. One couple in the study commented that 'Your reactions and feelings have such a big impact on the information you take in. You see, we've noticed when we get together, me and my husband, that we have understood things differently'. The study participants also reported that the perceived trustworthiness of the health practitioner giving the information was vital and affected the parents' ability to

trust the information they were being given. Continuity of care was identified as a key component in developing trustworthiness.

There is a balance to be worked towards between giving parents enough information to make decisions and not overwhelming them with the sheer amount of information available. Supporting parents to decide for themselves what they need to know, rather than deciding for them, is a key component of autonomous decision-making and compassionate care.

POSTNATAL COMMUNICATION

One of the most potentially life-changing events for parents is the discovery that their child has a birth defect. What they do with this news depends on many factors, but a key element is the knowledge, attitude, and communication style of the practitioner who gives the diagnosis (Lemacks et al., 2013). The responses and attitudes of health care professionals also carry considerable significance once the baby has been born; these responses have been shown to affect both short- and long-term parental coping and adjustment (Côté-Arsenault and Denney-Koelsch, 2011; Lemacks et al., 2013; McKechnie et al., 2015). When a baby is born with an unexpected condition or abnormality, responses and reactions are immediate, and the initial attitude of practitioners stays with the parents. Unfortunately, when disability is suspected or confirmed, it seems that many health care providers remain uncomfortable and ill-prepared to talk to parents, and tend to liken the outcome to a tragedy (Wright, 2008). In her discussion on the ethics of antenatal screening for Down syndrome, Alderson (2001) identifies that parents of babies born with this condition 'felt that the maternity staff expressed shock and distress, which they, the parents, did not particularly share'.

Before diagnosis, parents have a vision of life with their child that changes drastically when an abnormality is identified; the ideal of the perfect baby leaves and forces a new reality on them (Welch, 2018). It is normal for parents to experience the typical stages of grief as they mourn the loss of what they expected, and it is important that this process is acknowledged (Lemacks et al., 2013). Health care practitioners' words and responses have been shown to have an impact at this time when the woman is most vulnerable to others' reactions (McKechnie et al., 2015). Research has shown that parental responses to the disclosure of disability or abnormality are complex and variable, but it is clear that parents attach importance to the attitude and approach of the health practitioners who inform them of their baby's condition (Côté-Arsenault and Denney-Koelsch, 2011; Lemacks et al., 2013; McKechnie et al., 2015).

These studies also identify that many parents experience reactions similar to a grieving process but, unlike the situation where a baby has died, these babies are still here; most parents also felt love and concern for their baby. They worried that their baby would be suffering and wanted to know how they could ease it. Parents also felt guilt, anger, shame and blame, similar to bereaved parents. However, the potential for health practitioners to enter into 'loss' counselling when disclosing disability can reinforce negative stereotypes and encourage feelings of rejection towards the baby.

Despite the literature identifying good practice for sharing information on congenital abnormality, researchers continue to find that the discovery and disclosure of disability or abnormality is often handled less than optimally by health practitioners (McKechnie et al., 2015). An example of this is related by da Silva et al. (2015) in their study identifying maternal perceptions of newborn congenital malformations. The woman relates that when she was told her baby had (what she now knows was) an imperforate anus: 'I was there on the delivery table; they were stitching me and the paediatrician came and spoke to me in a gentle way, you know? He said that my baby was born with a closed anus, so he would have to do surgery; he said it's very difficult to do a surgery like this.' While this woman acknowledges the kindness of the way she was spoken to, her first comments relate to the context, which was obviously completely inappropriate for discussing such news.

The birth of a baby with an unexpected abnormality is a shock for the practitioners as well as the parents, and sometimes the initial reaction is to take the baby away from the parents. This can give the practitioner time to compose themselves, but inevitably creates distress in the parents, who guess something is wrong and commonly think the baby has died. This experience was reported by a woman in the Kerr and McIntosh (1998) study, who describes her baby being 'whipped away into the corner of the room … I thought he was dead actually. They didn't say anything, eventually I had to ask them to tell me what was wrong'. Even if a clear diagnosis cannot be made initially, an explanation of the

suspected (or obvious) condition should be given to the parents immediately; the more open the practitioner is, and the less drama that surrounds the disclosure of abnormality, then the less the parents experience feelings of panic and trauma. Another participant in the Kerr and McIntosh (1998) study articulates her experience '… and put her in my arms and said she's got a slight problem … there was no great fuss … There was no drama, they didn't try to cover anything up'.

Unfortunately, it is not uncommon for parents to be told about an abnormality but not to be shown it; neither is it unusual for parents to be given information that does not accurately describe the condition. Conversely, some parents may be given what amounts to a lecture on the condition at a time when they are not emotionally or physically able to take in a large amount of information.

Many parents, especially mothers, experience feelings of guilt when their baby has an abnormality, and these feelings can be reinforced when practitioners question the mother on whether she 'took' anything in pregnancy, or imply that the problem may have been caused by something she did. This apparent placing of blame is unfair on the mother and will ultimately result in her not feeling safe to express her true feelings; it will contribute to the potential for psychological and emotional distress.

WHAT DO PARENTS WANT FROM HEALTH PROFESSIONALS?

The literature on the needs of parents when being informed of their baby's condition identifies a number of aspects important to parents (Côté-Arsenault and Denney-Koelsch, 2011; Lemacks et al., 2013; McKechnie et al., 2015). Although not an exhaustive list, these aspects include:

- Being told of their baby's condition as early as possible, with both parents and the baby present, in an unhurried manner with privacy;
- In the case of an unexpected condition at birth, practitioners not taking the baby away or trying to cover up a visible abnormality and then waiting for someone else to explain;
- Practitioners using the correct terminology when identifying the abnormality or condition rather than euphemisms;
- Practitioners not using jargon;

- Practitioners using a variety of tools/diagrams to illustrate the abnormality or condition;
- Being told in a sympathetic and honest manner;
- Being given the opportunity to express their feelings;
- Having someone who is willing to listen without giving advice;
- Being given early and frequent opportunities for follow-up meetings, and time to assimilate information;
- Being given information (both verbal and written) and illustrations about what the condition is, what caused it and how their child may be affected (if known);
- Identifying the support (both professional and community) available at an early stage.

An empathetic attitude is acknowledged as being particularly helpful and appreciated by parents. Empathy involves being supportive and being able to be with the parents at a confusing and often distressing time; it requires time, understanding and acceptance of the gamut of emotions parents may experience, and the ability to allow them the time and space they need. Being in an obvious hurry and offering quick-fix solutions rather than listening are detrimental to parents' well-being and their ongoing relationship with health practitioners.

CONDITIONS THE PRACTITIONER MAY ENCOUNTER

This section introduces some of the more common conditions the practitioner may encounter. There are three tables that outline the conditions, their usual presentation and the care or treatment currently available, but we acknowledge that this is not by any means an exhaustive list. For further information, the reader is encouraged to access specialist paediatric texts that cover the topics in much greater depth.

The tables are separated into three categories:
- Congenital anomalies: some of the more common interruptions in normal embryonic and fetal development, such as cleft lip/palate and talipes equinus. Fig. 11.1 identifies the gestation at which some of these anomalies occur.
- Congenital infections: antenatal and intrapartum infections that may cause short- and long-term problems for the neonate.
- Chromosomal conditions: common trisomies and monosomies that contribute to the catalogue of genetic conditions.

The anomalies listed may have been identified antenatally and the paediatric team may already be alerted and prepared for the baby; conversely, the practitioner and the family may be unaware of any problem until after the baby has been born. Either way, any abnormality would clearly warrant a referral to a paediatrician; practitioners need to be fully aware of local referral procedures and the pathways which are in place after referral, in order to keep the family informed of what is likely to happen.

Congenital Anomalies

Congenital anomalies (Table 11.1) may be described as:
- Lethal: conditions which result in stillbirth or perinatal death (e.g., anencephaly);
- Severe: conditions which may cause disability or death without medical intervention (e.g., exomphalos, cardiac anomaly);
- Mild: conditions which may require some medical intervention, but have a good prognosis (e.g., developmental dysplasia of the hip) (Czeizel, 2005).

Congenital Infections

Antenatally, infection of the fetus may occur via the transplacental route or by an ascending genital tract infection (Table 11.2). Invasive procedures for the diagnosis and treatment of fetal conditions, which are increasingly used, also have the potential to introduce infective organisms through, for example, amniocentesis or intrauterine transfusion. Intrapartum infections are most commonly acquired through ascending organisms, contact with infected secretions (as in the case of herpes simplex virus) and monitoring procedures such as fetal scalp electrodes and fetal blood sampling.

Transplacental transmission of most bacteria is uncommon, although any illness suffered by the mother has the potential to affect fetal growth and development by compromising placental function. But because of their small size, certain microorganisms—in particular protozoa and viruses—are able to cross the placental barrier, infect the fetus and interfere with growth and/or development, depending on the gestational age at the time of infection (Simpson, 2004).

The teratogenic effects of viruses are well recognized, but the mechanisms involved in pathophysiological responses to infection, such as hyperthermia and inflammation, have also been implicated in neonatal

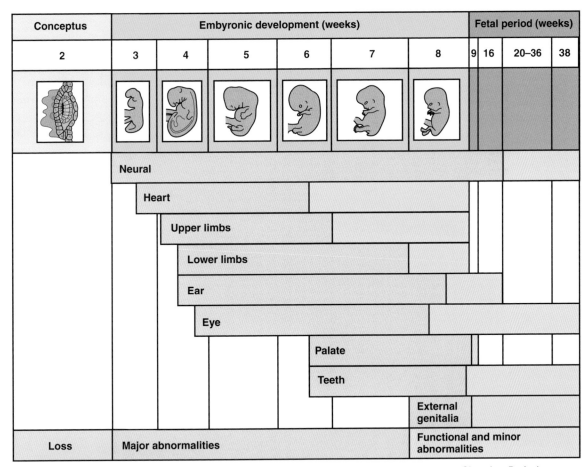

Fig. 11.1 Schematic Illustration of Critical Periods in Human Prenatal Development, Showing Periods of Sensitivity to Teratogens. (Redrawn from Stables D, Rankin J, Physiology in Childbearing, 2nd edn, 2005, with permission from Elsevier Ltd.)

neurological dysfunction (Petrova et al., 2001; Seri et al., 2012).

Infection of the embryo or fetus may result in miscarriage, stillbirth or premature birth of a live baby, with or without apparent abnormality. Low birth weight, developmental abnormalities or congenital disease may reflect in utero infection. Antenatal infections may persist after birth, causing the baby to be severely ill, or may cause abnormality that does not become apparent until later in infancy, such as vision, hearing or neurological disturbances.

Chromosomal Disorders

Table 11.3 presents some of the many chromosomal disorders that can occur, and lists the symptoms that may be exhibited during the NIPE. Chromosome disorders can be classified into two main types: numerical and structural. Numerical disorders occur when there is a change in the number of chromosomes (more or fewer than 46); most numerical disorders are trisomies, in which there is an extra copy of one chromosome. Structural chromosome disorders arise from breakages within a chromosome during gametogenesis which result in the presence of duplications or deletions (more or less than two copies of a group of genes). This difference in number of copies of genes may lead to clinical differences in affected individuals (GARD, 2017). Chromosome disorders are discussed in greater depth in Chapter 3; the selection here represents only a small number of the many disorders that can occur, and further reading around

TABLE 11.1   Common Congenital Anomalies

Condition	Incidence	Association	Clinical features/presentation	Ongoing care and management
Cleft lip and palate	1:300–600 60% include the lip. 1:20 if either parent has the condition.	Associated with other congenital malformations, most commonly with Pierre Robin sequence.	Cleft lip can range from a slight notch in the red part of the upper lip to complete separation of the lip extending into the nose. Can occur on one or both sides of the upper lip. Cleft palate may occur as part of the cleft lip deformity or as an isolated midline entity involving the secondary palate.	Paediatric and surgical referral. Feeding may be an issue, depending on severity. Surgical repair usually commenced after 3 months of age.
Choanal atresia	1:7000–8000	Approximately 50% of bilateral cases associated with CHARGE syndrome: C: coloboma (eye) H: heart defects A: atresia (choanal) R: restricted growth G: genital defects E: ears (deafness).	Anomaly of the anterior skull base characterized by closure of one or both posterior nasal cavities. Approximately 60% of reported cases are unilateral with a right-sided predominance. Respiratory distress may be evident at birth with bilateral presentation, or baby may become cyanotic at a later stage.	Bilateral condition requires early intubation and urgent referral to ENT specialist for CT scan to diagnose. Unilateral lesions may go undiagnosed until the child presents with persistent unilateral nasal drainage. Repair at around 2 to 3 years of age for unilateral atresia.
Oesophageal atresia	1:3000–4000	Associated with VACTERL syndrome which involves birth defects affecting several organs: V: vertebral defects A: anal deformities C: cardiac problems TE: tracheoesophageal fistula R: renal abnormalities L: limb deformities.	Incomplete formation of the oesophagus in early fetal development results in atresia. Newborn accumulates excessive saliva and frothy mucous secretions in the mouth and pharynx, causing obstructed breathing and possibly cyanosis.	NG tube to clear build up of fluid and for feeding. Main risk to the baby is from pneumonia if there is a fistula present. Urgent operative repair is essential.
Duodenal atresia/ stenosis	1:5000–10,000	Associated with isolated cardiac defects. 30% of fetuses with DA have Down syndrome.	Absence or complete closure of a portion of the duodenum, or partial obstruction due to stenosis. May be detected antenatally by the presence of a 'double bubble' due to a dilated fluid-filled stomach and proximal duodenum. Sustained vomiting is the most common symptom, within 24 hours of birth. Fullness in the epigastrium, caused by the dilated duodenum and stomach, may be noted.	Congenital intestinal obstruction is associated with gastric aspirates that measure greater than 30 ml. Urgent surgical referral should be instigated.

	Incidence	Associated anomalies		
Pyloric stenosis	Incidence 1:500 With parental history: 1:5–20 for a boy, 1:15–40 for a girl	Associated anomalies have been described in the central nervous system, gastrointestinal tract and heart. Also recently associated with VUR.	Major feature is vomiting, usually between 3–5 weeks but sometimes earlier. Gradually becomes projectile occurring immediately after feeding. Weight loss and small infrequent bowel motions. Visible gastric peristalsis in the left upper abdominal quadrant after feeds.	Referral for further investigation, generally ultrasound. Will require surgical treatment.
Diaphragmatic hernia	1:2200–1:5000	Associated with oesophageal atresia, tracheoesophageal fistula and truncus arteriosus.	Diaphragm fails to develop properly, abdominal organs fill the chest space. More commonly on the left side (almost 90% of cases) so displaces the heart to the right. Respiratory distress and hypoxia at birth. Presents at delivery as a difficult resuscitation or later with tachypnoea.	Intermittent positive pressure for resuscitation will compound respiratory distress. Survival is now greater than 80% although a poor prognosis is associated with polyhydramnios and presence of the fetal stomach in the chest. Long-term complications include persistent pulmonary hypertension, recurrent lung infections and gastrointestinal problems.
Imperforate anus	1–3:5000	Incidence of renal and urinary tract abnormalities increases with the severity of the imperforate anus.	Ranges from anal atresia to the absence of a normal anal opening. Continued communication between the urinary tract and rectal portions of the cloacal plate causes rectourethral or rectovaginal fistulas. Presents as inability to pass meconium within first 24 hours.	Diagnosis confirmed by examination of the perineum. Surgical treatment of infants with imperforate anus depends upon the severity of the condition. A low imperforate anus can be repaired in the newborn period but if high imperforate anus occurs, a colostomy is usually performed.
Exomphalos	1:4000–5000	Associated with chromosomal defects, usually trisomy 18 but also trisomy 13 and Beckwith–Wiedemann syndrome.	Protrusion of part of intestine through a defect in the abdominal wall at the umbilicus. The hernial sac is composed of an outer layer of amnion and an inner layer of peritoneum. There are two types of the condition: minor: sac is relatively small with attached to its summit; major: sac is larger and umbilicus is attached to its inferior aspect. It contains small and large bowel and often liver.	Cover with a saline-soaked sterile dressing or cling film to prevent fluid loss. In exomphalos minor, the hernia can be pushed back into the peritoneal cavity through the umbilical opening. It is retained by firm strapping for 14 days. In exomphalos major, immediate surgery is necessary before the hernial sac ruptures. Prognosis varies according to size of defect.

Continued

TABLE 11.1 Common Congenital Anomalies—cont'd

Condition	Incidence	Association	Clinical features/presentation	Ongoing care and management
Gastroschisis	1:5000	Correlation with Beckwith–Wiedemann syndrome. More common in preterm babies.	Congenital defect in the anterior abdominal wall lateral to the umbilical cord, usually to the right. There is no peritoneal sac so evisceration of the bowel occurs throughout intrauterine life. Amniotic fluid irritates the exposed bowel wall and may cause peritonitis.	Hypothermia, hypovolaemia and sepsis resulting from exposure of the eviscerated bowel are major problems. Lower half of baby should be placed in a sterile bag and fluids rapidly administered. An orogastric tube should be passed to aspirate intestinal contents. Antibiotics should be given. Surgery will be required.
Hirschsprung disease	1:5000–7000	More common in males and preterm infants. 20% of infants will have one more or associated abnormality.	Developmental disorder of enteric nervous system, involving neurological, cardiovascular, urological, or gastrointestinal system. Characterized by absence of ganglion cells in distal colon resulting in functional obstruction. May present with distended abdomen and/or spasm of the anus. Should be considered in newborn who fails to pass meconium within 24–48 hours after birth. Other symptoms include bilious vomiting, abdominal distension, poor feeding and failure to thrive.	Contrast enema and rectal biopsy may be used to confirm diagnosis. Intravenous hydration, nasogastric decompression and antibiotics. Colostomy may be indicated and reversed at a later stage or a 'pull-through' procedure may be performed.
Meconium ileus		Strong association with cystic fibrosis. Occasionally seen in association with pancreatic atresia or stenosis of the pancreatic duct	Failure of a full-term newborn to pass meconium in the first 24 hours may signal intestinal obstruction. Classic signs progressive include abdominal distension, refusal to feed and vomiting of bilious intestinal contents. Abdominal examination often reveals distended loops of bowel, which may be visible or palpable. Anal inspection is essential to exclude defects such anal atresia or fistula.	Treatment may be operative or non-operative. Mild cases may respond to 'gastrograffin' enemas. If not, then surgical operation is required to remove the impacted meconium. Complications may include volvulus, atresias, gangrene, perforation or peritonitis.

Inguinal hernia	1:50–100 live births. Usually left-sided. Sometimes bilateral.	Incidence is increased in premature and low birth weight infants. Can be associated with CHD, meningomyelocele, malrotation of gut.	Usually presents with intermittent groin lump. In girls, lump is in upper part of the labia majora. Hernias can be difficult to detect in a quiet child. Increases in size with straining or crying. May reach into the scrotum.	Complications include hernia incarceration and strangulation. Elective surgical repair is recommended as soon as possible after diagnosis.
Umbilical hernia	1:100	Incidence is increased with low birth weight, Down syndrome and Beckwith–Wiedemann syndrome.	Hernia is usually symptomless. Strangulation is extremely rare.	95% spontaneously close by 2 years of age. Surgical repair only needs to be considered if present beyond this age.
Undescended testes	1:200 Incidence increased in premature babies.	Can be unilateral or bilateral. In 70% of children with this condition, there is an associated hernia.	In most cases self-correcting. The testis may be felt in the groin or inguinal region, or may not be felt at all. If testis is not palpable, may be inside the abdomen, deep in the inguinal region, or rarely, may be absent.	Surgery may be required if undescended at 1–1.5 years of age to gain best results. Long-term problems include impaired fertility, torsion of the testis leading to infarction, and testicular cancer.
Hypospadias	1:500 Increased risk for siblings.	Other anomalies associated with hypospadias include cryptorchidism and inguinal hernia, which are more likely to occur with proximal hypospadias.	Hypospadias (proximally displaced urethral meatus) varies from a mild glandular form to a more severe perineal form. Chordee (ventral curvature of the penis) without hypospadias occurs less frequently and may be due to skin tethering or a short urethra.	Circumcision should not be performed as extra foreskin may be needed for surgical repair. Can be repaired with surgery. Usually, the surgical repair is done when baby is between 6 and 12 months old.
Vesicoureteric reflux (VUR)	1:200	Strong association with renal abnormalities in the absence of urinary infection.	Congenital urinary tract defect caused by the failure of the ureter to insert correctly into the bladder. Urinary reflux from the bladder to the kidney can lead to renal damage, resulting in pyelonephritis or hydronephrosis. Babies may present with pyelonephritis, cystitis or uraemic symptoms.	May present later in life as proteinuria, hypertension or renal failure. It is the commonest cause of end-stage renal failure in children. Lesser grades frequently just disappear. Ultrasonography is a simple method of diagnosing VUR of grades III–IV. Treatment of high grades IV–V is surgical correction by ureteric reimplantation.

Continued

TABLE 11.1   Common Congenital Anomalies—cont'd

Condition	Incidence	Association	Clinical features/presentation	Ongoing care and management
Hydrocele	1:100		Painless, tense, fluctuant scrotal mass that transilluminates when a light source is used. Upper border is usually movable away from inguinal canal. The testis may not be palpable.	No treatment usually needed, because hydroceles generally decrease in size and resolve over the first year of life; if not resolved by the age of 1 to 2 years, consideration of elective surgical repair for hydrocele that fluctuates in size, same treatment as for inguinal hernia.
Ambiguous genitalia	1:5000	May be linked with true or pseudohermaphroditism, mixed gonadal dysgenesis, congenital adrenal hyperplasia, chromosomal abnormalities (including Klinefelter and Turner syndromes). Maternal ingestion of androgenic steroids. Lack of testosterone cellular receptors.	In females: enlarged clitoris; urethral opening anywhere along, above, or below surface of the clitoris; labia may be fused, resembling a scrotum. Baby may be thought to be a male with undescended testicles. In males: small penis that resembles an enlarged clitoris; urethral opening may be anywhere along, above or below the penis; it can be placed as low as on the perineum, making the infant appear to be female; there may be a small scrotum with any degree of separation, resembling labia. Undescended testes commonly accompany ambiguous genitalia.	Genetic testing will confirm genetic sex. Laparoscopy, x-ray, exploratory laparotomy, or biopsy of the gonads may be needed to determine the presence or absence of internal genital structures. Hormone replacement is frequently used although surgery may be required in extreme cases.
Talipes	1:1000 3:100 if family history. More common in boys than girls.	Associated with joint laxity, developmental dysplasia of the hip, tibial torsion, ray anomalies of the foot (oligodactyly), absences of some tarsal bones and a history of other foot anomalies in the family.	May be unilateral or bilateral. Features include a fixed plantar flexion (equinus) of the ankle, characterized by the drawn-up position of the heel and inability to bring the foot to a flat standing position. This is caused by a tight Achilles tendon. Adduction (varus), or turning in of the heel or hindfoot and adduction of the forefoot and midfoot give the foot a kidney-shaped appearance.	Treatment may involve serial plaster casting and splinting, gentle manipulations and toe-to-thigh cast (Ponsetti method), physiotherapy and taping of the limb. Surgical treatment may be considered: posteromedial release aims to loosen and lengthen tightened ligaments and tendons in the medial and posterior parts of the feet.
Syndactyly and polydactyly	1:2250	May be present with malformation syndromes.	Supernumerary digits occur more often than true polydactyly (which occurs more commonly on the feet). Often lateral to the fifth digit on hands or feet. Extra digits may have a nail and are attached by a small pedicle, which differentiates the defect from true polydactyly. Syndactyly (fused digits) may involve soft tissue (simple synostosis) or fusion of bone (complex synostosis).	With supernumerary digits, if bony tissue is not palpable, the application of a ligature around the pedicle allows the digit to fall off. X-rays are necessary to determine the degree of fusion. In cases of both syndactyly and true polydactyly, affected newborns should be referred to an orthopaedic surgeon.

TABLE 11.2   Congenital Infections

Viral

Rubella	Rates of congenital rubella syndrome vary depending on the gestational age at which the infection occurred. Can incorporate a number of anomalies: cardiac defects (particularly if contracted between 5th and 8th weeks), hearing loss, cataracts, retinopathy, microphthalmia, microcephaly. Newborn rubella may be evidenced by hepatosplenomegaly, jaundice, thrombocytopenia, low birth weight, rubella osteitis. Diagnosis via viral culture from stools or CSF. Care depends on clinical features.
Cytomegalovirus (CMV)	Member of the herpes virus group. Occurs in 0.4%–2.3% of all births. Approximately 1% of primary infection occurs in pregnancy, resulting in 40% of fetuses affected at any stage of pregnancy. Can occur in primary or recurrent infections. Can cause miscarriage, stillbirth, low birth weight, jaundice, purpura, hepatosplenomegaly, respiratory distress, pneumonia. Approximately 10% of infected newborns are symptomatic at birth and the majority of these (80%–90%) will go on to have long-term neurological disorders: cerebral palsy, hearing or vision loss, or seizures. 10% of asymptomatic newborns will develop late-onset complications, most commonly hearing loss, poor coordination and intellectual developmental delays. Diagnosis is via viral cultures of urine and throat swab. Antivirals may be of some assistance for active infection. Neonatal mortality of 20–30% from disseminated intravascular coagulation, sepsis or liver disease.
Herpes simplex virus (HSV)	Primary infection in pregnancy most severe as no antibodies have been developed. Infection can affect the fetus at any stage of pregnancy but main risk of transmission is during labour and birth, which accounts for 85% of neonatal HSV infection (5% intrauterine and 10% postnatal). Signs of infection may include prematurity, low birth weight, chorioamnionitis and skin lesions. Usual age of onset of symptoms is between 5 and 21 days postnatally. May present with irritability, fever, lethargy, respiratory distress and seizures. Vesicles may or may not be present. May exhibit signs of encephalitis, vesicles on skin, eyes or mouth. Disseminated infection involves multiple organs: CNS, lungs, liver, adrenals and haemodynamic instability. Cultures are taken at 48 hours of age from eyes, throat, rectum and skin lesions (if present). LFTs and PCR of CSF. Babies treated with IV antivirals. Usually severe illness with a high mortality rate, especially in babies with decreased conscious state, DIC and prematurity.
Hepatitis B (HBV)	Transmission rates with a primary infection in the third trimester are 80%–90%, although it is rare to develop fulminant hepatitis. 25% of chronic infection will result in long-term liver disease (cirrhosis/cancer). Immunoglobulin and vaccination should be offered within 12 hours of birth with vaccination follow-up at 6 weeks and 3 months. Breastfeeding not contraindicated.

Continued

TABLE 11.2   Congenital Infections—cont'd

Viral

Hepatitis C (HCV)	Rate of maternal–fetal transmission is dependent on level of viraemia and varies from 6%–12% (up to 20% in women co-infected with HIV). Maternal–fetal transfer most commonly occurs in labour and birth. Avoid use of invasive techniques including artificial rupture of the membranes (ARM) and use of FSE or forceps. Most infants have no symptoms until later in life. May result in long-term liver disease: cirrhosis, carcinoma. HCV is not transmitted via urine or stools in the newborn.
Varicella zoster virus (chickenpox)	If contracted <20 weeks then 2%–5% of newborns will have congenital varicella syndrome. Maternal infections within 7 days before and 28 days after birth are serious, with nearly 25% of babies developing the infection. Consider offering VZV immunoglobulin to mother within 92 hours of contact (if known). Varicella syndrome: skeletal abnormalities, chorioretinitis, cataracts, skin lesions, encephalitis and neurological damage. Mortality rate approximately 30%. If born with or develop the infection in first few weeks, complications include encephalitis, renal and hepatic disorders and pneumonia. If active infection at or soon after birth or mother has infection within 7 days of birth, neonatal varicella zoster immunoglobulin is recommended. Treatment is with IV antivirals.
Erythrovirus (Erythema infectiosum B19; parvovirus B19; slapped cheek syndrome; fifth disease)	50%–60% of adult population have immunity (evidence of previous infection). Affects human erythroblasts and therefore the fetus may develop anaemia. If mother not immune, there is approx. 30% transmission rate. Low birth weight, prematurity, diffuse oedema, anaemia (nonimmune hydrops fetalis), visual impairment and CNS abnormalities. Serology from mother, antenatal ultrasound to detect oedema or effusion, e.g., pericardial ascites. Neonate may require transfusion.
Zika virus	Closely related to dengue and transmitted by mosquitos; also a risk of sexual transmission as virus is found in semen. Probable cause of microcephaly and other severe fetal brain abnormalities, as well as Guillain–Barré syndrome. Congenital Zika syndrome includes: severe microcephaly, decreased brain tissue, damage to the back of the eye with a specific pattern of scarring and increased pigment, limited range of joint motion, such as club foot and too much muscle tone restricting body movement soon after birth.

Bacterial

Treponema pallidum (syphilis)	Infection of fetus does not occur before 16 weeks. 50% of babies born where infection was recent have an active infection. Maternal treatment with benzathine penicillin G has been shown to reduce transmission rates. May lead to stillbirth, preterm birth and/or congenital syphilis and low birth weight. Commonly asymptomatic at birth, but can have skin lesions (especially palms and soles), hepatosplenomegaly, eye infection, jaundice, rhinorrhoea, osteochondritis, periostitis, anaemia and thrombocytopenia. Clinical features often appear between 2nd and 6th weeks. IM penicillin bd for 10 days.

TABLE 11.2 Congenital Infections—cont'd

Bacterial

Listeria monocytogenes (listeriosis)	Listeria has a unique predilection for pregnant women. 20% of infections result in miscarriage or stillbirth. The placenta is directly infected. Aggressive treatment in pregnancy with high-dose penicillin or trimethoprim has been useful. May cause unexplained stillbirth; premature labour may follow chorioamnionitis. May present with petechial rashes, hepatosplenomegaly, leucopenia and thrombocytopenia. Neonates develop pneumonia, general sepsis and meningitis with 50% mortality rate. 50% of those who survive have significant neurological deficit.
Streptococcus agalactiae (group B beta-haemolytic streptococcus (GBS))	Prevalence of colonization of pregnant women ranges from 15% to 40%. Approximately 1%–2% of babies born to GBS-colonized women will develop early-onset infection (early-onset GBS <7 days and usually within first 24 hours). Usually acquired through vertical transmission during labour and birth. Women often asymptomatic antenatally, therefore important to identify risk factors for perinatal infection if no routine screening: previous baby with sepsis, maternal fever and/or tachycardia, fetal tachycardia, prelabour or prolonged rupture of membranes, premature labour, chorioamnionitis, long labour and increased interventions. If risk factors present or GBS cultured in late pregnancy, prophylactic antibiotics in labour are recommended. Early-onset GBS: signs of septicaemia may develop immediately after birth or over a few hours: respiratory distress including grunting, intercostal recession and nasal flaring, irritability, tachycardia or bradycardia, high or low temperature, tachypnoea, pallor, poor tone, hypotension. Baby's condition will deteriorate rapidly. Lethargy and poor feeding may be later signs. Late-onset GBS (>7 days) usually presents with signs of meningitis. Often a prolonged hospitalization. 6% mortality rate for early-onset GBS and higher in preterm babies. May have neurological and/or sensory deficits.

Protozoa

Toxoplasma gondii (toxoplasmosis)	Usually acquired by ingesting sporocysts from unwashed fruit or vegetables from soil contaminated by cat faeces, or tissue cysts from raw or uncooked meat. Does not always cause congenital disease. Overall rate of transmission is about 50%. Highest risk of transmission is when infection occurs in third trimester, but infection anytime between 10 and 24 weeks may result in intrauterine fetal death. Generally asymptomatic infection. Up to 85% of infected neonates are asymptomatic at birth, but most will develop complications later in life. Fulminating illness may present with low birth weight, purpura, thrombocytopenia, jaundice, hepatosplenomegaly and anaemia. More common to present with seizures and other signs of cerebral irritation, development of hydrocephalus and choroidoretinitis leading to blindness. Antenatal ultrasound may identify cerebral ventricular dilation and liver and intracranial calcifications. Diagnosis confirmed by identifying organism in CSF. Pharmacological treatment including folic acid for up to 1 year to reduce risk of choroidoretinitis.

CNS, Central nervous system; CSF, Cerebrospinal fluid; DIC, Disseminated intravascular coagulation; FSE, Fetal scalp electrode; IM, intramuscular; IV, Intravenous; LFT, Liver function test; PCR, Polymerase chain reaction test; VZV, Varicella Zoster virus

TABLE 11.3   **Chromosomal Anomalies**

Condition	Incidence	Features that may be identified at Newborn Infant Physical Examination	Prognosis and related problems
Down syndrome (trisomy 21)	1:800–1000	Frequently small for gestational age and low birth weight Microcephaly and abnormally shaped head Atypical facial features, flattened nose, protruding tongue and upward slanting eyes with epicanthal folds Short, broad hands with short fingers. Single palmar crease Growth and development are usually delayed Congenital heart disease (CHD) Gastrointestinal abnormalities (e.g., oesophageal atresia and duodenal atresia)	Obstruction of the gastrointestinal tract may require major surgery shortly after birth. Varying degrees of impaired intellectual and motor function. Life expectancy averages 55 years depending on related conditions such as CHD. Acute lymphocytic leukaemia is also more common in children with DS.
Patau syndrome (trisomy 13)	1:5000	Microcephaly (small head) Scalp defects: absent skin Microphthalmia (small eyes) and coloboma (Chapter 10) Holoprosencephaly (failure of the embryo's forebrain to divide to form bilateral cerebral hemispheres, causing defects in the development of the face and in brain structure) Profound intellectual disability. Cleft lip and palate Low-set ears Haemangiomas Skeletal abnormalities including polydactyly Malformations of the function of the CNS DDH	Most embryos with trisomy 13 will abort spontaneously. More than 80% of children born with trisomy 13 die in the first month and 90% within the first year.
Edwards syndrome (trisomy 18)	1:6000	Low birth weight Microphthalmia (small eyes), micrognathia (small jaw), small mouth, low-set ears Cleft lip and palate Clenched fists with overlapping fingers DDH Failure to thrive 'Rocker bottom' feet Scoliosis	About half die in utero. Of liveborn infants, only 50% live to 2 months, and only 5%–10% will survive their first year of life. Profound developmental delays.
Turner syndrome (45,X i.e., monosomy X; structural X chromosome variants and mosaicism are common) Females missing some or all of one X chromosome.	1:2500 females	Lymphoedema Neck webbing Cystic hygroma Low hairline at the back of the neck Asymmetry of shape and position of the ears Broad chest and widely spaced nipples Increased number of naevi Cardiovascular anomalies, particularly coarctation of the aorta Renal anomalies (horseshoe kidney) Narrow, high-arched palate Short stature	Poorly formed or absent ovaries results in incomplete sexual development. Greater incidence of diabetes, high blood pressure and a higher incidence of cardiovascular, renal and thyroid disease.

TABLE 11.3	Chromosomal Anomalies—cont'd		
Condition	Incidence	Features that may be identified at Newborn Infant Physical Examination	Prognosis and related problems
Klinefelter syndrome (47,XXY or XXY syndrome) Males with an extra X sex chromosome	1:500–1000 males	Hypotonia Hypogonadism Microorchidism (small testes)	Affected males usually infertile as a result of decreased testicular hormone/endocrine function. Language learning impairment may be evident. Increased risk of breast cancer and osteoporosis
Cri-du-chat syndrome (5p deletion syndrome, 5p minus) Loss of part of one chromosome 5	1:20,000–50,000	Cry sounds like a mewing kitten Low birth weight Hypotonia Microcephaly Unusual facial features Micrognathia (small jaw) Low-set ears Single palmar creases CDH	Severe cognitive, speech, motor delays and behavioural problems. Failure to thrive as a result of poor feeding
Fragile X syndrome, (Martin-Bell syndrome; mutation of the FMR1 gene on the X chromosome)	1:3600 males 1:4000–6000 females	Macroorchidism in boys (large testes) Prognathism (pronounced jaw) Hypotonia Elongated face with large ears High-arched palate, and malocclusion (misalignment of teeth) Lordosis (spine curvature) CDH Pectus excavatum (deformity of the sternum, causing concave chest appearance) Flat feet Joint laxity	Impaired intellectual functioning including attention disorders, hyperactivity, anxiety and language-processing problems Females tend to be less seriously affected by fragile X than males. Autism.

CHD, Congenital heart defect; CNS, Central nervous system; DDH, Developmental dysplasia of the hip; DS, Downs syndrome

these is recommended. With the increasing use of whole-genome sequencing in routine diagnostic testing, it is also important to realize that, although 'traditional' chromosome disorders will make up the majority of those diagnosed, some of the conditions identified may be unique to a particular baby and conclusive evidence about prognosis may be difficult to find. The National Library of Medicine (2019) offers a comprehensive list of conditions which is accessible at https://ghr.nlm.nih.gov/search?query=chromosome+disorders.

CONCLUSION

When a baby presents with a congenital abnormality at any stage of pregnancy or at birth, it can raise a variety of challenges for even the most experienced practitioners.

It is important that we are aware of how and where to seek appropriate support for the family, who may feel engulfed by insurmountable future obstacles. There are many community support groups, agencies and charities with expertise in dealing with a huge range of conditions and who can offer condition-specific advice, information and support. The health care professional should be sure they have knowledge of and access to the appropriate contacts in their locality.

The practitioner should also consider their own emotional well-being in relation to dealing with a baby with a congenital abnormality. Journeying with a woman and her family in such a situation can be an emotional and sometimes harrowing experience; good collegial support and the opportunity to reflect on and debrief about the experience are vitally important.

PARENTS' STORY

Hazel and Harry's Story

We always wanted to have our children close together, so when Florence was barely a year old and I became pregnant, we were very excited and told everyone the good news. I had my 12-week dating scan and it was fine—then my midwife called and told me that my screening results showed I had a 1 in 5 chance that the baby was going to have Down syndrome. I was offered an amniocentesis or a CVS and we decided to go for the amnio. I thought it would be OK and I know so many people have it, but I found it really invasive—horrible. The clinic said we'd hear within a couple of days, but we never heard anything, and then a week later the doctor called to say it had been confirmed that Harry did have Down syndrome. Strangely, she said she'd rather tell me on the phone than have me crying in the clinic rooms. Anyway, I just cried and cried on the phone. She was a locum doctor and I said to her, 'Look, my husband and I have always said that if any of our children had any problems we wouldn't contemplate abortion', just so she knew when we got in there that termination wasn't an option. Caleb, my husband, always says there's no such thing as 'perfect' and he's right. You could have what we would term as a perfect child that gets some illness when they are older, passes away or causes a lot of stress because of substance abuse or similar. Caleb and I believe that Harry is perfectly imperfect, like all of us (Fig. 11.2).

We found it interesting when we went to the first appointment after Harry's diagnosis—after welcoming us, one of the first things the doctor offered us was some pamphlets on abortion and dealing with loss. We said that wasn't what we wanted, as previously stated, but it felt as though we were being pushed down that road. It felt like the decision for us to keep Harry was not encouraged, and it was surprising that the doctor didn't offer any encouragement or support in our decision. We decided to tell our friends and family about Harry's diagnosis as the conversations came up. It was difficult at times, as understandably people weren't always on the same page as us. However, the differing opinions have been hard to deal with at times—I can't forget the times people said, 'you shouldn't have had him' or 'if it was me and my husband, we would abort' or 'think of how it will affect your daughter's life'. I look back now and think, how naïve they are. Harry is great! He brings so much joy to our lives and those around us. Florence, our older daughter, adores him. You can't look at Harry and not see that he is 'life'.

There were a few medical professionals throughout the process who were really encouraging. My midwife,

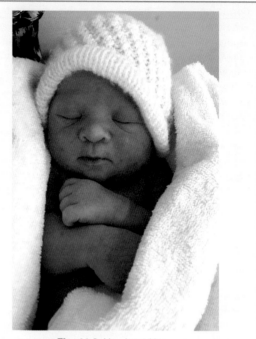

Fig. 11.2 Newborn Harry

Michelle, was amazing! As soon as we told her our decision to keep Harry, she said, 'I thought that would be the decision you'd make' and she never questioned it, ever. Michelle seemed to go the extra mile, making sure we were fully informed so we could make the right decisions for our family. We so appreciated her support. We also had an amazing sonographer who would often do the additional anatomy scans for Harry—he had a family member with Down syndrome, who he adored. He thought Harry was perfect and was genuinely pleased to know there would be a Harry in the world.

I had a normal pregnancy other than having the extra scans; it was difficult to know whether they were necessary or not. The first scan after the diagnosis at 16 weeks was doom and gloom. The baby had an AVSD, which would have meant major surgery in Starship hospital. Even though I work in health, I'm no expert on unwell babies or (at that time) what it's like to have a child with a disability. Michelle helped us a lot with this and would always question the systems, which was helpful. Two weeks later the next scan showed it only to be a tiny wee hole in the heart—nothing to worry about.

Hazel and Harry's Story

Throughout the pregnancy, Caleb was my greatest source of support. We didn't feel we needed any other external support from groups and things. Family and friends are awesome, but he was my rock to stand on.

I went into labour naturally at 37 weeks. We agreed for the baby to be born in the tertiary hospital so medical support was on hand. There's risk in anything—you can't eliminate it, but you can minimize it to some degree. I had a water birth with Florence; they suggested I might be better not to give birth in water with Harry, but that labouring in water would be fine. Florence was born in a birthing unit and I felt so uncomfortable in hospital with the lights and the sounds; it felt so invasive. At the birth, Michelle kept people out of the room. Just two other midwives came in, but I know that staff were on alert outside. The birth was straightforward and Harry only needed a little bit of support with breathing. The first thing I said was, 'Oh yes, you do look like you've got Down syndrome'—wish I could take that back actually, as I don't really care what he looks like! Anyway, I was thrilled with him, and by that time I didn't care about his diagnosis. He was just my baby. The plus side of screening meant that we knew already and were prepared—well, as prepared as you can ever be. However, the journey to get him home was going to be a long one.

Once he was born, we went to the postnatal ward and he breastfed beautifully. I've had a breast reduction, so I knew supply would be a problem and I'd planned to introduce a bottle at 2 to 3 days as he needed more. However, he couldn't take any more than 20 ml and that seemed odd. He had also been born with a rash, which was a bit unusual; it turned out to be a rare blood disorder that only Down syndrome people can get that can turn into leukaemia. Thankfully, this did not progress. Harry then began to lose weight, so was transferred to NICU and a nasogastric tube was inserted to feed him. After a couple of days, we said we wanted to take him home. We spent the night before discharge with him in hospital, which ended up being really challenging as Harry was vomiting after every NG feed. Caleb and I had a gut feeling something was not right. We asked for a meeting with his paediatrician and a big multidisciplinary meeting was organized. I said, 'I can't cope with this kid at home', and they offered a scan to rule out any issues. He was 10 days old when we found he had a duodenal web and a malrotation of his bowel. Harry underwent surgery and then he started making a recovery and was heading for home when he was diagnosed with hand, foot and mouth disease—he was terribly

unwell, and put back into an incubator. His oxygen requirements were high and it took 40 days to get out of NICU (Fig. 11.3). I was really trying to pump to produce milk, and he was going to the breast and having NG feeds. It's so hard to pump when you're stressed like that. I wanted to teach him to bottle-feed but they said it would confuse him further, which really bugged me, as I had breast- and bottle-fed my daughter. I didn't agree with the staff on this.

When he got home, Harry slept well but it was hard using the NG tube to feed, and with pumping and coping with a 2-year-old who'd become slightly more demanding than normal, it was a really difficult time. Florence went into preschool for an extra day a week—everything changed because she was so much happier and we just carried on. Harry went on to take the bottle at just 4 months so I didn't have to keep pumping all the time. I just felt we had to keep the palate working and keep his tongue moving, and getting him to take the bottle was a game changer.

He ended up on CPAP overnight because sleep studies showed his saturation levels were dropping anything up

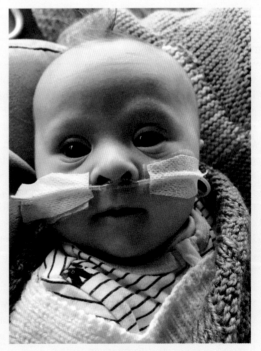

Fig. 11.3 Harry following surgery

Continued

PARENTS' STORY—cont'd

Hazel and Harry's Story

to six times an hour, and down to 80%. He'd also begun to have strange breathing episodes which I began to video to show the doctors. I went to see a paediatrician who suggested it was a cold—but I knew as his mother that this was not a cold. I requested a second opinion and saw an ENT specialist who suggested they look at what was going on under general anaesthetic. They found he has tracheomalacia, which means that he has a very floppy trachea and lungs. It was suggested that he might need a tracheostomy, but CPAP was stopping the desaturations and so we're using that at night and it seems to be working.

He's eating solids now, which is great, although he's still very small and still looks very much like a young baby. He got sick again recently with a virus and had his third ambulance ride in 8 months. It has been a tough time but he's brought more to our lives than we could ever imagine. He brings so much joy! Florence loves him to pieces and wants him to grow up so he can play with her (Fig. 11.4). Harry started attending a specialist centre once a week recently and they are so supportive. They will text me and check how he is if we're not in that week. I so appreciate their help. Harry may end up having to have a tracheostomy and we have to face that possibility. I'm an expert on things I would never have known I would be. I think one of the most important things I would like to leave with people in health care is how important it is for the family to see past the condition and really see the baby. I want him to be treated as a regular kid who happens to have Down syndrome.

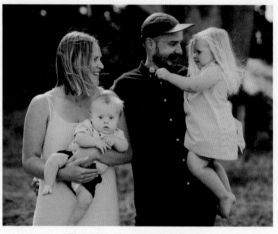

Fig. 11.4 Harry and his family.

KEY POINTS

- It is estimated that 2%–3% of newborn babies in the UK are affected by a major congenital anomaly; these anomalies are a cause of fetal, neonatal and child mortality and morbidity.
- Congenital anomalies may be the result of one or more genetic, infectious, nutritional or environmental factors and it is often difficult to identify the exact causes.
- Health professionals must inform women about the antenatal tests on offer and ensure they are fully cognizant of the risks and benefits of each test.
- Research has shown that parental responses to the disclosure of disability or abnormality are complex and variable.
- Parents require clear, nonmedical, jargon-free information about their baby's condition, in a variety of formats. They want to be told of any unexpected problems with their baby in a sympathetic and unhurried manner, and to be given time to take in the information and revisit that information frequently.

REFERENCES

Abortion Act 1967, UK. Available from: http://www.legislation.gov.uk/ukpga/1967/87/contents.

Alderson, P., 2001. Prenatal screening, ethics and Down's syndrome: a literature review. Nurs. Ethics 8 (4), 360–374.

Arribas-Ayllon, M., Sarangi S., 2014. Counselling uncertainty: genetics professionals' accounts of (non)directiveness and trust/distrust. Health Risk Soc. Soc. 16 (2), 171–184. doi:10.1080/13698575.2014.884545.

Carlsson, T., Bergman, G., Melander Marttala, U., Wadensten, B., Mattsson, E., 2015. Information following a diagnosis of congenital heart defect: experiences among parents to prenatally diagnosed children. PLoS ONE 10 (2), e0117995. doi:10.1371/journal.pone.0117995.

Carstensen, K., Lou, S., Petersen, O.B., Nielsen, C.P., Hvidman, L., Lanther, M.R., et al., 2018. Termination of pregnancy following a prenatal diagnosis of Down syndrome: a qualitative study of the decision-making process of pregnant couples. Acta Obstet. Gynecol. Scand. 97 (10), 1228–1236. doi:10.1111/aogs.13386.

Chaabane, S., Bérard, A., 2013. Epidemiology of major congenital malformations with specific focus on teratogens. Curr. Drug Saf. 8 (2), 128–140.

Clarke, A., 2017. The Evolving Concept of Non-directiveness in Genetic Counselling. In: Petermann H., Harper P., Doetz, S. (Eds.), History of Human Genetics. Springer, Cham.

Côté-Arsenault, D., Denney-Koelsch, E., 2011. 'My baby is a person': parents' experiences with life-threatening fetal diagnosis. J. Palliat. Med. 14 (12), 1302–1308.

Czeizel, A.E., 2005. Birth defects are preventable. Int. J. Med. Sci. 2 (3), 91–92. doi:10.7150/ijms.2.91.

da Silva,, P., Ayres Soares, A., Tadeu, N.F., 2015. Maternal perception in terms of newborns with congenital malformations: a descriptive study. Online Braz. J. Nurs. 14 (2). Available from: http://www.objnursing.uff.br/index.php/nursing/article/view/5199/html_688.

Department of Health and Social Care, 2017. Abortion Statistics England and Wales. Available from: https://assets.publishing.service.gov.uk/government/uploads/system/uploads/attachment_data/file/763174/2017-abortion-statistics-for-england-and-wales-revised.pdf.

Gaby, S., 2003. The ethical pregnancy: reproductive choice in the context of prenatal testing. Unpublished PhD thesis, Maquarie University.

Genetic and Rare Diseases Information Center (GARD), 2017. Chromosome Disorders. National Institutes of Health. Available from: https://rarediseases.info.nih.gov/guides/pages/73/faqs-about-chromosome-disorders.

Gekas, J., Gagné, G., Bujold, E., Douillard, D., Forest, J.C., Reinharz, D., et al., 2009. Comparison of different strategies in prenatal screening for Down's syndrome: cost effectiveness analysis of computer simulation. BMJ 338, b138 doi:10.1136/bmj.b138.

Grace, K.T., Anderson, J.C., 2016. Reproductive coercion: a systematic review. Trauma Violence Abuse 19 (4), 371–390.

Hill, M., Barrett, A., Choolani, M., Lewis, C., Fisher, J., Chitty, L.S., 2017. Has noninvasive prenatal testing impacted termination of pregnancy and live birth rates of infants with Down syndrome? Prenat. Diagn. 37 (13), 1281–1290.

Kerr, S.M., McIntosh, J.B., 1998. Disclosure of disability: exploring the perspective of parents. Midwifery 14, 225–232.

Lafarge, C., Mitchell, K., Fox, P., 2014. Termination of pregnancy for fetal abnormality: a meta-ethnography of women's experiences. Reprod. Health Matters 22 (44), 191–201.

LaMorte, W.W., 2016. Residual confounding, confounding by indication, & reverse causality. Boston University School of Public Health. Available from: http://sphweb.bumc.bu.edu/otlt/MPH-Modules/BS/BS704-EP713_Confounding-EM/BS704-EP713_Confounding-EM4.html.

Lemacks, J., Fowles, K., Mateus, A., Thomas, K., 2013. Insights from parents about caring for a child with birth defects.

Int. J. Environ. Res. Public Health 10 (8), 3465–3482. doi:10.3390/ijerph10083465.

Martin, L., Hutton, E.K., Gitsels-van der Wal, J.T., Spelten, E.R., Kuiper, F., Pereboom, M.T., et al., 2015. Antenatal counselling for congenital anomaly tests: an exploratory video-observational study about client-midwife communication. Midwifery 31 (1), 37–46.

McKechnie, A.C., Pridham, K., Tluczek, A., 2015. Preparing heart and mind for becoming a parent following a diagnosis of fetal anomaly. Qual. Health Res. 25 (9), 1182–1198.

Miller, B., 2016. Down syndrome: parents say they feel pressured to terminate pregnancy after diagnosis. ABC News. Available from: https://www.abc.net.au/news/2016-11-22/down-syndrome-parents-pressured-to-terminate-pregnancy/8033216.

National Down Syndrome Cytogenetic Register (NDSCR), 2014. Annual Report. London. Online. Available from: http://www.binocar.org/content/annrep2013_FINAL_nologo.pdf.

Natoli, J.L., Ackerman, D.L., McDermott. S., Edwards, J.G., 2012. Prenatal diagnosis of Down syndrome: a systematic review of termination rates (1995–2011). Prenat. Diagn. 32 (2), 142–153. doi:10.1002/pd.2910.

NHS England, 2017. Better Births: improving outcomes of maternity services in England. from: https://england.nhs.uk/wp-content/uploads/2016/02/national-maternity-review-report.pdf.5, 2020.

Ökem, Z.G., Örgül, G., Kasnakoglu, B.T., Çakar, M., Beksaç, M.S., 2017. Economic analysis of prenatal screening strategies for Down syndrome in singleton pregnancies in Turkey. Eur. J. Obstet. Gynecol. 219, 40–44.

Parliamentary Office of Science and Technology (POST), 2016. Infant Mortality and Stillbirth in the UK (POSTnote 527). Available from: http://researchbriefings.files.parliament.uk/documents/POST-PB-0021/postpn527_UK_Infant_Mortality_and_Stillbirth_online.pdf.

Petrova, A., Demissie, K., Rhoads, G.G., Smulian, J.C., Marcella, S., Ananth, C.V., 2001. Association of maternal fever during labor with neonatal and infant morbidity and mortality. Obstet. Gynecol. 98, 20–27.

Pitt, P., McClaren, B.J., Hodgson, J., 2016. Embodied experiences of prenatal diagnosis of fetal abnormality and pregnancy termination. Reprod. Health Matters 24 (47), 168–177.

Public Health England (PHE), 2017. National Congenital Anomaly and Rare Disease Registration Service. PHE Publications. Available from: https://assets.publishing.service.gov.uk/government/uploads/system/uploads/attachment_data/file/716574/Congenital_anomaly_statistics_2015_v2.pdf.

Rehmann-Sutter, C., 2009. Why non-directiveness is insufficient: ethics of genetic decision making and a model of agency. Med. Stud. 1 (2), 113–129. doi:10.1007/s12376-009-0023-7.

Richardson, A., Ormond, K.E., 2018.Ethical considerations in prenatal testing: Genomic testing and medical uncertainty. Semin. Fetal Neonatal Med. 23, 1–6.

Roberts, J., Griffiths, F.E., Verran, A., Ayre, C., 2015. Why do women seek ultrasound scans from commercial providers during pregnancy? Sociol. Health Illn., 37, 594–609. doi:10.1111/1467-9566.12218.

Seri, L., Rossiter, J.P., MacNair, L., Flavin, M.P., 2012. Impact of hyperthermia on inflammation-related perinatal brain injury. Dev. Neurosci. 34, 525–553.

Simpson, C., 2004.. Infection. In: Henderson, C., MacDonald, S. (Eds.), Mayes Midwifery: A Textbook for Midwives, thirteenth ed. Bailliere Tindall, Edinburgh, UK (Chapter 39).

Smith, S.K., Cai, A., Wong, M., Sousa, M.S., Peate, M., Welsh, A., et al., 2018. Improving women's knowledge about prenatal screening in the era of non-invasive prenatal testing for Down syndrome—development and acceptability of a low literacy decision aid. BMC Pregnancy Childbirth 18 (1), 499. doi:10.1186/s12884-018-2135-0.

Thomas, G.M., Katz Rothman, B., 2016. Keeping the backdoor to eugenics ajar? Disability and the future of prenatal screening. AMA J. Ethics 18 (4), 406–415. doi:10.1001/journalofethics.2016.18.4.stas1-1604.

United Kingdom National Screening Committee (UK NSC), 2019. Online. Available from: https://www.gov.uk/government/groups/uk-national-screening-committee-uk-nsc.

US National Library of Medicine, 2020. Genetics Home Reference. Your Guide to understanding Genetic Conditions. http://www.ghr.nlm.gov.conditions.

Vanstone, M., Kinsella, E.A., Nisker, J., 2012. Information-sharing to promote informed choice in prenatal screening in the spirit of the SOGC clinical practice guideline: a proposal for an alternative model. J. Obstet. Gynaecol. Can. 34 (3), 269–275.

Walker, B.S., Nelson, R.E., Jackson, B.R., Grenache, D.G., Ashwood, E.R., Schmidt, R.L., 2015. A cost-effectiveness analysis of first trimester non-invasive prenatal screening for fetal trisomies in the United States. PLoS ONE 10 (7), e0131402. doi:10.1371/journal.pone.0131402.

Welch, S.B., 2018. Navigating infant death from life-limiting congenital anomaly: a classic grounded theory study. Grounded Theory Review: An Int. J. 17 (1) Online. Available from: http://groundedtheoryreview.com/2018/12/27/navigating-infant-death-from-life-limiting-congenital-anomaly-a-classic-grounded-theory-study/.

Wright, J.A., 2008. Prenatal and postnatal diagnosis of infant disability: breaking the news to mothers. J. Perinat. Educ. 17 (3), 27–32. doi:10.1624/105812408X324543.

12

Neonatal Jaundice: Implications for Newborn Health

Angela Deken and Maggie Meeks

Nature does nothing uselessly.
        Aristotle (384–322 BCE)

INTRODUCTION

Jaundice can be normal in up to 60% of term and 80% of preterm newborns for the first 3 to 5 days as they transition from using fetal haemoglobin to adult haemoglobin (Lancet, 2010; Juretschke, 2005). There is a growing understanding that jaundice may confer several benefits that protect and promote health in both the short and long term (Gazzin et al., 2016). The challenge for the midwife is to recognize when the physiological is at risk of becoming pathological, because the consequences of unrecognized pathological jaundice can be significant (Juretschke, 2005); they include brain damage and hearing loss (from severe early unconjugated jaundice) and pituitary dysfunction or liver failure (as causes of late-onset conjugated jaundice) (Boskabadi et al., 2018; Weiss and Vora, 2018).

The aim of this chapter is to provide an overview of the issues relating to jaundice and hyperbilirubinaemia in the newborn. This will be approached in a holistic manner that acknowledges the potential benefits of mild jaundice, as supported by a growing body of evidence. We will begin by discussing the production and excretion of bilirubin (the jaundice pigment) and the importance of establishing breastfeeding in the transition from in utero to ex utero life. We will also explore the purpose of physiological jaundice and discuss the pathological causes and management of jaundice, with some new areas of interest.

THE PHYSIOLOGY AND BIOLOGY OF BILIRUBIN IN HUMANS

Introducing Haemoglobin and Bilirubin

Haemoglobin is an important molecule, responsible for the oxygen-carrying capacity of red blood cells; it comes in a variety of forms, including the adult and fetal subtypes. As discussed in Chapter 6, newborn babies go through many physiological transitions in their adjustment to extrauterine life, including changes in their haemoglobin. In utero, they have a higher concentration of haemoglobin and this is made up of fetal and adult haemoglobin: 50% to 85% is fetal haemoglobin and 15% to 40% is adult haemoglobin. The presence of fetal haemoglobin facilitates the diffusion of oxygen across the placenta because it has a higher oxygen binding capacity than the adult haemoglobin of the maternal circulation. This enables unborn babies to obtain sufficient oxygen for normal metabolism, growth and development.

Any increase in the breakdown of red blood cells and haemoglobin contributes to the accumulation of bilirubin (jaundice), which in the presence of a normally functioning liver and gut will be predominantly *unconjugated* (as discussed later in the chapter). This increased breakdown can occur as a direct consequence of the normal physiological processes, or because there is an immune-facilitated breakdown (e.g., Rhesus or ABO) or an inherited problem with the red blood cells (e.g., spherocytosis or G6PD deficiency).

The spleen begins the process of red blood cell breakdown into haemoglobin and protein. The haemoglobin is broken down by macrophages into its component parts of *haem* and *globin*. The iron molecule is then removed from the haem to be recycled along with the protein and globin components, and the haem molecule is oxidized to carbon monoxide and biliverdin. Biliverdin is then reduced by the enzyme biliverdin reductase to form *unconjugated bilirubin* (Dennery et al., 2001; Vitek, 2005). This unconjugated bilirubin (indirect) is not water soluble but is highly lipid soluble; this has two main consequences:

- Unconjugated bilirubin easily crosses lipid membranes, such as those within the brain, which is why bilirubin-induced neurological dysfunction (BIND), potentially leading to kernicterus (discussed later), occurs with high levels of unconjugated jaundice.
- Its insolubility in water means that bilirubin must be transported in the bloodstream linked to albumin; in this protein-bound state, it is not available to be filtered by the glomeruli into the urine.

Bilirubin Excretion and the Enterohepatic Circulation

Unconjugated bilirubin is transported to the liver and converted into *bilirubin diglucuronide* (otherwise known as *conjugated* or *direct* bilirubin) by the enzyme *UDP glucuronosyltransferase*. Conjugated bilirubin is water soluble and actively excreted by the liver into the intrahepatic bile ducts with bile salts, cholesterol and phospholipids, forming *bile*. The bile then flows down the extrahepatic ducts into the small intestine, where it has a role in activating lipases to break down fat, providing more easily available nutrition for the baby. Within the colon, some of the conjugated bilirubin is converted back to unconjugated bilirubin by the enzyme *beta-gluconidase* and absorbed back into the circulation. It has been estimated that a single molecule of bilirubin completes this whole circuit up to six times a day before being excreted (Beath, 2003); this is known as the enterohepatic circulation (Fig. 12.1).

The remaining conjugated bilirubin is metabolized by gastrointestinal bacteria into *stercobilinogen* and *urobilinogen*. Stercobilinogen is a brown pigment that is excreted within the faeces and contributes to their colour. Urobilinogen is mostly reabsorbed in the enterohepatic circulation and converted back to unconjugated bilirubin, but a small amount of urobilinogen is carried in the bloodstream and excreted by the kidneys.

The Gastrointestinal Microbiome

As discussed in Chapters 5 and 15, the microbiome of a women's vagina and breastmilk alters as pregnancy progresses, in preparation for birth (Moreno and Franasiak,

Enterohepatic and Systemic Circulation

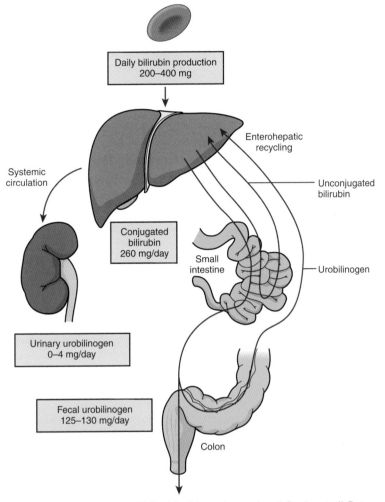

Fig. 12.1 Diagram Showing the Flow of Bilirubin (Unconjugated and Conjugated) Between the Liver, Small and Large Intestine and the Kidneys. This makes up the enterohepatic circulation.

2017). It was previously thought that the newborn's gut was sterile but recent work suggests the fetus may begin to establish its microbiome in utero (Gensollen et al., 2016). Optimal bacterial colonization of the newborn intestines can take several months (stabilizing by 3 years of age) and can be affected by multiple factors, including the method of birth, type of feeding, and antenatal or postnatal exposure to antibiotics (Pannaraj et al., 2017; Ho et al., 2018; Moossavi et al., 2019; Hermansson et al., 2019; Azad et al., 2016). Colonization with these health promoting bacteria that feed on oligosaccharides enhances the baby's ability to conjugate bilirubin into urobilinogen and can reduce serum levels of unconjugated bilirubin (Dong et al.,

2018). A greater understanding of the microbiome's importance and its significant lifelong impacts is important for all health professionals. In the absence of medical contraindications, professionals involved in newborn care should promote a spontaneous labour and vaginal birth (Gensollen et al., 2016; Ding and Schloss, 2014; Peters et al., 2018) with unrestricted skin-to-skin and support for breastfeeding following birth (Widström et al., 2019).

Breastfeeding

Breastfeeding reduces bilirubin levels in several ways:
- Breast milk has many components that assist in the postnatal development and adaptation of the baby's gut.

- Breast milk contains factors which protect against infection, such as enzymes, lactobacillus, oligosaccharides, immunoglobulins, leukocytes, lactoferrin and glycoconjugates which have anti-infective properties (Hanson, 2007; Ruiz et al., 2017).
- Exclusively breastfed babies have a more stable and less varied gut microbiome compared with those who received formula milk (Ho et al., 2018).
- Regular early breastfeeding (up to 12 times per day is normal) will increase gut motility and ensure the early and frequent passage of stools; colostrum also has a laxative effect (Lawrence and Lawrence, 2011).
- There is a direct correlation between the number of breastfeeds in the early postpartum period and the levels of jaundice. The more a baby breastfeeds, the less likely it is to experience significant hyperbilirubinaemia.

It is acknowledged that some women are unable to breastfeed due to a wide range of anatomical, functional and psychological considerations. In these situations, feeding can be with donated human milk where available (e.g., from milk banks) or with modified cow's milk (infant formula).

JAUNDICE IN THE NEWBORN

Once serum bilirubin levels reach concentrations of 34.2–51.3 μmol/l (2–3mg/dl), a yellow discoloration of the baby's skin and eyes becomes evident (Askin and Diehl-Jones, 2003). This is known as *jaundice* or *icterus* and is visible in 60% to 80% of healthy babies, usually fading by 2 weeks after birth. *Physiological jaundice* refers to the appearance of jaundice at 3 to 5 days which occurs because:

- The newborn baby begins life with 6 to 7 million red cells per cubic millimetre (compared with the adult level of 5 million). The increased cellular oxygenation that occurs after birth leads to reduced red cell production (erythropoiesis) and the destruction of inactive, immature red blood cells in the liver, spleen and bone marrow.
- There is a reduction in fetal haemoglobin and an increase in the percentage of adult haemoglobin over the first 6 to 12 months of life. Fetal red blood cells also have a shorter life span compared with those of adults (80 vs. 120 days).
- Following birth, bilirubin is conjugated in the baby's liver, which is still adapting to extrauterine

life. Although this has been described as the liver having limited ability to take up, transport and excrete bilirubin, this is now considered normal for babies who are full term and have no additional risk factors for jaundice.

Physiological jaundice may also be exacerbated by additional factors within the baby—such as bruising, bleeding and birth trauma—but delayed cord clamping is not believed to have an effect (see Chapter 5) (Mercer et al., 2017; Carvalho et al., 2018).

Newborn Jaundice as an Adaptive Process

Evidence supporting the theory of newborn jaundice as an adaptive process is beginning to be understood and explored with developments in genetic research and scientific understanding (Sedlak and Snyder, 2004).

Bilirubin has previously been considered a waste product with limited biological activity or purpose, and jaundice a result of the fragile transition from in utero to ex utero life (Gazzin et al., 2016). Babies are born immunologically immature but are provided with physiological protective mechanisms (particularly against infection), including placental immunoglobulin transfer, breastfeeding, the gut microbiome and possibly bilirubin metabolism (Gazzin et al., 2016; Wagner et al., 2015).

Bilirubin has now been shown to have physiological roles which include:

- Being the main antioxidant in the serum, stronger than vitamin E (Wagner et al., 2015; McDonagh, 2010).
- Managing oxidative stress: neonates who have free radical–producing diseases such as circulatory failure, asphyxia, aspiration and sepsis had lower levels of bilirubin compared with controls (Gazzin et al., 2016; Sedlak and Snyder, 2004).
- A protective role at a cellular level (Gazzin et al., 2016).
- Antibiotic properties that have been shown to reduce the activity of Group B *Streptococcus* in vitro (Hansen et al., 2018).
- Antiinflammatory properties: There is emerging evidence of the complex role of bilirubin metabolism and its effect as an antiinflammatory. It has been proposed that this process could be fundamental to health but further research is required (Gazzin et al., 2016).

Bilirubinomics is a term that has been coined for the study of the role bilirubin has in determining disease resistance. The observed association of mild jaundice with a reduction in cardiovascular disease, inflammatory metabolic syndrome, diabetes, bowel cancer and

Crohn's disease, neurodegenerative diseases such as Alzheimer's, dementia and multiple sclerosis, cerebral infarctions and autoimmunity is supported by the fact that infants with Gilbert syndrome (who often have higher levels of bilirubin) are protected from cardiovascular disease, diabetes and cancer (Wagner et al., 2015).

When the Physiological Becomes Pathological

There are two main situations in which jaundice becomes a concern:

- When the level of jaundice exceeds the safe threshold of hyperbilirubinemia; this can lead to BIND and kernicterus (the associated long-term brain damage);
- When the jaundice is prolonged; this may point to an underlying serious diagnosis.

In either situation, the risks to the infant can be significant and include brain damage, liver failure and even death. The midwife has a pivotal role in minimizing the risk of a poor outcome by understanding the physiological and pathophysiological processes involved in hyperbilirubinaemia and providing appropriate information and support to each family.

Unconjugated Jaundice

The appearance of jaundice in the first 24 to 48 hours, or of high levels of bilirubin at any time, is of concern.

An unconjugated jaundice is the commonest type of jaundice seen in the first 2 weeks of life. Left untreated, the level of unconjugated bilirubin in the bloodstream can reach significantly elevated levels (hyperbilirubinaemia) and can result in BIND and kernicterus, which have a 10% and 70% morbidity respectively (Ip et al., 2004). Kernicterus has been estimated as occurring in 1 in 17 babies with a bilirubin above 340 μmol/l (Rennie et al., 2010). Although significant jaundice is often due to an underlying pathology (e.g., haemolysis), kernicterus has been demonstrated in newborn babies with no underlying diagnosis; this is particularly the case with the late preterm infant (Bhutani and Johnson, 2006). Analysis of cases in which preventable harm has occurred to the baby has shown this to be the result of system failures by multiple providers (Bhutani and Johnson, 2003).

General Considerations

As with any biological process, the normal physiological process of bilirubin metabolism relies on the complex interaction of genetics and environmental factors. A deviation from the expected 'normal' in any of these processes can result in bilirubin levels being markedly increased and these situations will be discussed later. The midwife needs to be aware of specific risk factors that may contribute to the development of hyperbilirubinaemia (see Tables 12.1 and 12.2).

TABLE 12.1 Factors That May Impact Lactation or the Establishment of Breastfeeds		
Antenatal	**Perinatal (Labour and Birth)**	**Postnatal**
Poor breast growth in pregnancy	Medications/drugs affecting baby's ability to breastfeed (e.g., opiates, antidepressants)	No early skin-to-skin with initiation of breastfeeding following birth
Medical conditions such as pre-eclampsia, diabetes, polycystic ovary syndrome	Overhydration of the mother in labour affecting breastfeeding	Inadequately resourced midwifery care in maternity units and community due to high workloads
Previous breast surgery	Retained placental products	Poor attachment to the breast leading to reduced milk transfer and decreased stimulation of milk supply
Previous breastfeeding history of concern	Delivery of preterm infant	Failure to regain birth weight by 10–14 days postnatally
Women who have experienced sexual or physical abuse impacting their psychological well-being	Baby unwell, requiring medical review and possible admission to neonatal unit	Congenital and physical anomalies such as cleft lip and/or palate

ROLE OF THE MIDWIFE

Midwives have an important role in assessing the well-being of the newborn, both within maternity units and at home. It is important to spend time with women, supporting them from birth through the postpartum period, and to individualize the level of care required in both settings.

Establishing Breastfeeds

Do not underestimate the impact that inadequate hydration secondary to ineffective milk transfer during breastfeeding has on the risk of the baby becoming pathologically jaundiced. Early initiation of skin-to-skin (Fig. 12.2) and breastfeeding, regardless of mode of birth, has been shown to minimize weight loss and ensure the early passage of meconium, which has a role in the excretion of bilirubin (Chen et al., 2011).

Women who have caesarean deliveries should also be encouraged and supported to have immediate skin-to-skin and early initiation of breastfeeding if the baby is stable and does not require any medical interventions (Fig. 12.3).

It has been shown that women who have continuity of midwifery care and ongoing community support have improved breastfeeding success (McFadden et al.,

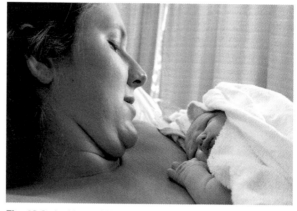

Fig. 12.2 Jackie and Her Baby Having Skin-to-Skin Immediately Following Birth.

2017). The midwife should be familiar with any clinical situations that may impact on lactation or breastfeeding (Table 12.1) and be alert to the need for closer observations and support of breastfeeding to reduce the risk of jaundice.

Together with skin-to-skin and early initiation of feeds, education about breastfeeding throughout the childbirth experience increases the likelihood of effective breastfeeding. This should ideally be delivered by

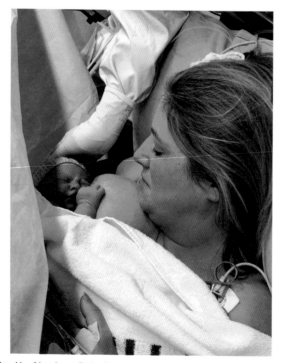

Fig. 12.3 Ruth Welcoming Her Newborn Baby Ruairi With Skin to Skin Shortly Before His First Breastfeeding.

TABLE 12.2 Clinical Situations to Alert the Midwife of a Higher Risk of Jaundice

Antenatal Factors

Genetic diagnosis	Some genetic conditions affecting the red blood cells make haemolysis more likely. These include G6PD deficiency (X-linked recessive), pyruvate kinase deficiency (autosomal recessive or autosomal dominant) and spherocytosis (autosomal dominant). There are also genetic conditions that affect the metabolism of bilirubin, such as Gilbert syndrome and Crigler–Najjar syndrome.
Genetic susceptibility (family history)	There may be changes in the genes associated with some of the above diagnoses that result in an increased susceptibility to jaundice without a specific diagnosis (Bartlett and Gourley, 2011; Azlin et al., 2011). A family history of jaundice in a newborn baby should alert the midwife to a likely increased risk of significant jaundice, even when the cause is unknown.
Growth restricted babies	An immature liver and lower glycogen stores increases the risk of hypoglycaemia and hypothermia (also see below) which places additional demands on the baby.
Haemolytic risk	Rhesus disease

Intrapartum Factors

Exposure to drugs that compete with albumin binding	Albumin is required to facilitate the transport of bilirubin; low levels of available albumin may increase the risk of free bilirubin which can cross into the brain.
Episodes of hypoxia in labour or at birth	Stressed babies in labour use more oxygen and glycogen stores which are also required for bilirubin processing. Compromised babies are at risk of hypoglycaemia and hypothermia.
Preterm delivery	A late preterm infant (34 weeks to 36+7) may not require admission to the neonatal unit but has an increased risk of complications that include poor feeding and jaundice secondary to: • immaturity of the liver • metabolic instability • reduced ability to maintain blood glucose and temperature.

Postnatal Factors

Bruising on baby from assisted birth	There is further red blood cell breakdown to occur in addition to the normal physiological changes.
Poor feeding and dehydration	This has been described in detail above.
Haemolytic disease	Newborn infection

health professionals in a continuity model (McFadden et al., 2017; Moore et al., 2016; Nilsson et al., 2017). The baby's urine and stool output should be routinely evaluated for frequency and colour, with the expectation that the stool will change from meconium to a loose yellow mustard colour by day 5 with effective breastfeeding. Once milk supply has established (often by day 5), a baby should have 6 to 8 wet nappies a day and the urine should be clear to pale. The average frequency of daily bowel motions should be three to six times daily in the first month (formula-fed babies one to four times daily) (Moretti et al., 2019).

The midwife should proactively assess the effectiveness of breastfeeding by asking the mother about breast fullness and how she feels feeding is going. Full breastfeeds should be observed to enable the midwife to assess the baby's latch and evaluate the coordination of suck and swallows which indicate milk transfer. Identification of concerns should prompt discussion with the woman and suggestions for potential courses of action. Good assessment of both mother and baby is imperative not only to prevent hyperbilirubinaemia, but also other complications of dehydration such as hypernatremia (increased blood sodium concentration), a serious and at times life-threatening problem (Moritz et al., 2005). Boer et al. (2016) suggest that weighing a baby at birth and then at days 2, 4 and 7 is the best frequency to identify a baby at risk of feeding inadequacy and reduces the outcome of hypernatraemia (Boer et al., 2016; MOH, 2012). If a baby has lost 7% of its weight following birth, proactive care and a plan with the mother are suggested to increase the milk supply; if over 10%, prompt consultation with a paediatrician is recommended (Lain et al., 2015). This can be a highly sensitive area to negotiate because feeding issues can impact on a woman's confidence in her breastfeeding abilities.

Monitoring in the Community

Early postnatal discharge (immediately after birth or within the first few days) is now accepted practice [18], but this can coincide with both the peak level of jaundice and the establishing of lactation. Research in Australia showed that 8% of discharged babies were re-admitted to hospital, of whom 91% had jaundice as the main reason for readmission (Lain et al., 2015). The risk factors for readmission included discharge before 48 hours, first time or young mothers (<18 years old), birth at 37–38 weeks' gestation, and breastfeeding.

Some of these readmissions may have been preventable with better feeding support; having intense individualized breastfeeding and midwifery support in the community has been shown to reduce hospital readmissions in the first week post-discharge, and is associated with less jaundice and better partner support (Nilsson et al., 2017). Other research shows that readmission has significant disempowering impacts on women, including broken expectations, shock or relief at being admitted, feelings of insecurity, the loss of a tranquil start at home, and a changed view of breastfeeding (Feenstra et al., 2018).

Risk Factors/Red Flags for Hyperbilirubinaemia

It is important that the midwife highlight the risk factors in each individual family that increase the chance of a baby becoming jaundiced. There are some conditions that require additional monitoring as they greatly increase the chance of hyperbilirubinaemia (see Table 12.2 and later sections of this chapter). An example is *haemolytic disease of the newborn*, the immune-mediated red cell breakdown which occurs in rhesus disease and ABO incompatibility (not to be confused with haemorrhagic disease of the newborn—vitamin K deficiency). In this condition, the mother has developed an immune response to specific blood group antigens expressed by the fetus. This 'immunization' occurs because of fetal blood cells passing into her circulation and most commonly occurs because of a previous pregnancy or after a blood transfusion, but can occur within the first pregnancy.

Rhesus D disease is a particular example where a significant unconjugated jaundice can develop rapidly. The role of the midwife can be considered in two possible situations:
- Recognizing the potential for isoimmunization in a woman who is rhesus negative and has suffered a miscarriage or a fetal/maternal bleed, or who has come to the end of a first pregnancy. Anti-D immunoglobulin can be given in these situations antenatally and/or postnatally to prevent the development of antibodies against the baby's blood group.
- Recognizing the risk of jaundice in a newborn infant of a mother who is rhesus D negative. Women and babies at risk can be identified by taking cord and maternal blood after the birth to determine the baby's blood group, and measuring the presence of fetal blood cells and antibodies in the maternal system.

All babies in whom risk factors have been identified need close observation and a lower tolerance for screening or accurate bilirubin assessments. Sharing information with the parents is important Parents need to be informed who to contact if they have any concerns about their baby; they should be made aware of the risk of their baby developing jaundice and why this is of concern, and how to recognize jaundice if they discharge from hospital early or have chosen to birth at home.

Supporting Women and Families

It is important to ensure that the parents or caregivers are given information both verbally and in a written format to help them understand jaundice and the decisions that need to be made, and that they are supported in these decisions (Amos et al., 2016) (see Chapter 15). Qualitative research has shown that when a woman has a baby who is jaundiced and/or requires treatment, the potential impacts include (Hannon et al., 2001; Brethauer and Carey, 2010):
- Mother–baby separation anxiety, including a loss of control and a sense of being unable to respond as they normally would when their baby shows breastfeeding cues or cries;
- Generalized increased levels of stress and anxiety associated with:
  - thoughts that they should have been able to prevent the jaundice
  - the stress of being admitted to a medical facility
  - receiving conflicting advice
  - observing blood samples being taken from their baby and the resulting reactions of the baby

- concern about the impact of the baby being in an incubator with lights for treatment and having to wear eye pads
- fear that if the bilirubin levels were to keep increasing, even with therapy, there may be long-term consequences
- fear for the baby's health even long after therapy has been discontinued, and feeling they needed to watch their baby constantly.

Women did perceive that jaundice was a serious condition and wished they had received further explanations about it. They expressed a preference for home treatment where possible, which would enable them to be in their own environment with family and avoid issues around, for example, the cost of transport to the hospital and childcare for other children.

Referral

Models of health and midwifery care within each country will affect the availability of community care, but community-based breastfeeding support groups should be considered for the mother and baby. Women need to be informed that they should contact their care provider if they notice:

- increasing levels of jaundice
- reduced urine output and urate crystals after day 3; dark yellow or concentrated urine
- meconium-like stools on day 4
- a sleepy baby who is not self-waking to feed at least every 4 hours. This is not normal behaviour in a well baby and prompt notification is important (Amos et al., 2017; Brethauer and Carey, 2010)
- the baby is 'fussy' on the breast (baby may be trying to communicate the insufficiency of milk flow) or unsettled after feeding, or who takes excessive amounts of time to feed
- signs of dehydration: clammy skin, dry lips and mucosa, delayed capillary refill, pale skin and a sunken fontanelle.

It is important to trust a mother's observations; previous research has identified that parents feel undervalued for their observations (Brethauer and Carey, 2010).

THE ASSESSMENT OF JAUNDICE

The assessment of jaundice involves performing a full clinical examination from head to feet with the baby undressed, except for a nappy, and should include an examination of the baby's eyes, gums and skin (jaundice progresses downwards), preferably in natural light (Rennie et al., 2010). The skin should be blanched by pressing gently to check for signs of jaundice. The absence of conjunctival jaundice is reassuring (Maisels et al., 2016). The Kramer tool (a visual assessment tool) has been found to have an accuracy of 86.27% (Aprillia et al., 2017); this method is particularly unreliable in babies with pigmented skin (Lancet, 2010). There has also been work using photographic imaging of the skin; the accuracy of this method is similar at 85% (Aydin et al., 2016), which indicates that cases of significant jaundice will be missed when undertaking assessment by either tool and reinforces the fact that visual assessment alone may not be sufficient.

A transcutaneous bilirubinometer (TcB) is a screening tool to aid decision-making about when to request a serum bilirubin (Maisels and Conrad, 1982; Allen et al., 2010; Maisels, 2015; Ercan and Özgün, 2018). A TcB is the recommended screening method for babies of greater than 35 weeks' gestation and over 24 hours of age, within hospital and the community and of any skin colour (Amos et al., 2017; Ercan and Özgün, 2018; Samiee-Zafarghandy et al., 2014). However, the TcB measures bilirubin in the extravascular tissue rather than the blood; the measurements are not reliable above 250 μmol/l and should not be used when a baby is receiving phototherapy. It is a tool to alert the midwife/doctor that further investigations are required and reduces the risk that a significantly raised total serum bilirubin will be missed (Maisels, 2015). If a bilirubinometer indicates a bilirubin of more than 250 μmol/l, a blood sample must be sent for serum bilirubin measurement.

The advantages of a TcB include:

- It is not painful for the baby and is less distressing for the parents (Hannon et al., 2001; Brethauer and Carey, 2010; McClean et al., 2018);
- It reduces the need to obtain a blood sample by 58%–79% (McClean et al., 2018);
- It reduces exposure to frequent heel incisions and their potential complications (pain, infection, behavioural aversion);
- It can be made available in the community;
- It reduces health care costs (McClean et al., 2018).

A safe level of unconjugated bilirubin has not been determined in either the term or preterm population and treatment guidelines are based on the current best evidence. If the TcB indicates higher than recommended bilirubin levels (refer to local policies or use the NICE 2016 guideline (Amos et al., 2017), a serum bilirubin level should be taken. Newer research methods of assessing jaundice include digital photography of the sclera which is highly sensitive (unlikely to miss significant jaundice) but not specific (may suggest significant jaundice when levels are actually within acceptable limits) which means that it has potential as a screening device to minimize unnecessary serum bilirubin measurements (Leung et al., 2015).

Serum Bilirubin

The measurement of total serum bilirubin (Figs 12.4 and 12.5) is the current gold standard for evaluating the risk of BIND but is likely to be replaced in the future by newer technologies that measure the free bilirubin or bilirubin binding capacity (Amin and Lamola, 2011; Ahlfors et al., 2018). The measurement of cord blood serum bilirubin in women of blood group O has been shown to be predictive for babies at an increased risk of significant jaundice secondary to haemolysis (Jones et al., 2017). In the newborn, serum tests require a blood sample to be taken, most commonly from the foot using capillary sampling; there are well-described techniques

to minimize the distress to the baby and parents as well as the complications (Shah et al., 2012; see also Chapter 14).

SPECIFIC DIAGNOSES

Some specific conditions can cause clinically significant jaundice in the early postnatal period; these usually do so because of their effect on red cell breakdown.

Haemolytic Disease of the Newborn

The two most common types of haemolytic disease to result in clinical concern are *rhesus disease* and *ABO incompatibility* (although less common, other red cell antigens such as Kell and Duffy can have a similar effect).

Rhesus Disease

Rhesus C, D and E antigens are expressed on red blood cells; it is the D antigen which is most commonly associated with rhesus disease. An individual who is 'rhesus negative' does not express the D antigen and has the genotype dd (Chapter 3). An individual who is 'rhesus positive' does express the D antigen; they can be heterozygous (Dd) or homozygous (DD) for the rhesus antigen D alleles. When a rhesus negative mother mounts

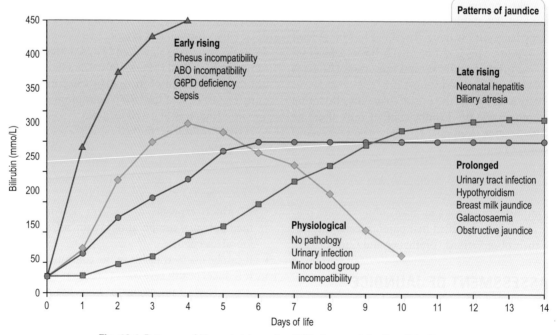

Fig. 12.4 Patterns of Neonatal Jaundice With Some of the Possible Causes.

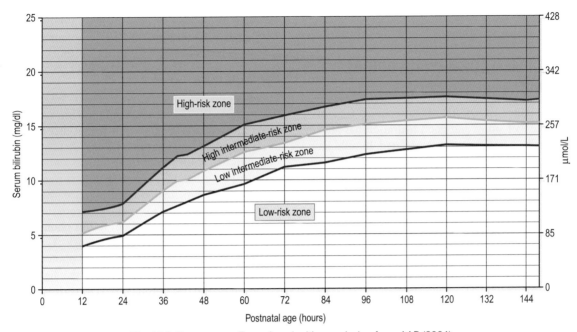

Fig. 12.5 Nomogram. Reproduced with permission from AAP (2004).

an immune response to the D antigen, she produces antibodies that are able to cross the placenta, resulting in the haemolysis of fetal blood cells. A similar process can happen with the rhesus C and E antigens. This can cause fetal anaemia and in some cases a need for intra-uterine blood transfusions to prevent the development of *hydrops fetalis* (severe anaemia associated with significant fetal oedema).

ABO Incompatibility

Severe haemolysis is less common with ABO incompatibility than with rhesus D incompatibility, but the principle of isoimmunization is similar. The ABO blood group refers to the pattern of expression of the A and B antigens on the red blood cells:

- Blood group O:
  - genotype homozygous OO (i.e., neither A nor B present)
  - most common cause of ABO incompatibility with antibodies against A and/or B antigen
- Blood group A:
  - genotype heterozygous AO or homozygous AA
  - may develop antibodies against the B antigen when exposed
- Blood group B:

- genotype heterozygous BO or homozygous BB
- may develop antibodies against the A antigen when exposed
- Blood group AB:
  - always heterozygous AB
  - will not develop antibodies against A or B antigens.

Maternal antibodies can remain in the infant's blood for some months after birth; the haemolysis of the red blood cells can become chronic, resulting in a persistent low level of jaundice and an accompanying anaemia. Symptoms include lethargy, pallor and poor feeding history. Folate and iron may be prescribed to encourage red blood cell production in the bone marrow, but it is not unusual for a baby to develop severe anaemia requiring blood transfusion.

Other Causes of Haemolysis

Biochemical or structural abnormalities of red cells may lead to a shortened cell lifespan with an associated increased risk of jaundice. Infection may also result in haemolysis (Berkowitz, 1991). Examples of inherited defects of red cells are:

- Gilbert syndrome
- G6PD (glucose-6-phosphate dehydrogenase) deficiency
- spherocytosis

- pyruvate kinase deficiency
- Crigler–Najjar syndrome.

MANAGEMENT OF PHYSIOLOGICAL JAUNDICE

The importance of effective breastfeeding to ensure early passage of stools and good hydration has already been described, but cannot be overstated. In mild jaundice there may also be a place for baby abdominal massage, which has been shown to increase the frequency of meconium stools and can be combined with phototherapy when the bilirubin is above the phototherapy line (Eghbalian et al., 2017). Filtered sunlight is recommended in some low- to middle-income countries (Colbourn and Mwansambo, 2018) but unfiltered sunlight is not generally recommended due to the associated risk of skin damage.

Guidelines

National or local guidelines should be consulted when planning the management of a jaundiced neonate. The NICE guidelines (Amos, 2017) (https://www.nice.org.uk/guidance/cg98) contain interactive nomograms with treatment thresholds for phototherapy and/or exchange transfusion based on the baby's gestation. These guidelines also highlight the importance of some factors that increase the likelihood of physiological jaundice becoming pathological: gestational age less than 38 weeks, family history of newborn jaundice, breastfeeding, and appearance of jaundice before 24 hours of age.

The American Academy of Pediatrics highlights additional risk factors: G6PD deficiency, haemolytic disease, hypoxia, infection, lethargy, and temperature instability. The AAP nomograms consider thresholds for treatment in three groups (American Academy of Pediatrics Subcommittee on Hyperbilirubinaemia, 2004):

- low risk: well infants >38 weeks
- medium risk: well infants 35 to 37+6 weeks, or infants >38 weeks with risk factors
- higher risk: infants 35 to 37+6 weeks with risk factors.

The antenatal and postnatal assessment of potential risk factors for jaundice are important aspects of management and it has been suggested that a bilirubin measurement should be performed prior to early hospital discharge to identify infants who have a greater chance of developing jaundice (Lease and Whalen, 2010). There are several smartphone applications that utilize predictive nomograms to identify those babies (Bhutani et al., 1999; AAP Subcommittee on Hyperbilirubinemia, 2004; Longhurst et al., 2009).

Phototherapy

Phototherapy remains the mainstay of treatment for unconjugated hyperbilirubinaemia and can be delivered using conventional or fibre-optic light sources (Hansen, 2011; Woodgate and Jardine, 2015). Remember that unconjugated bilirubin is lipid soluble and not water soluble; phototherapy converts it into a water-soluble isomer, lumirubin, that can be excreted through the kidneys. The most effective light spectrum for converting the yellow bilirubin pigment to this photoisomer is blue light, in the 425 to 475 nm range (Lamola and Russo, 2014). The effectiveness of any phototherapy is influenced by the characteristics of the light source (wavelength, energy output, prescribed distance from baby) and the way in which it is used (Stokowski, 2011). Each light source will only be effective on the exposed area of skin and so the baby should have a significant surface area exposed. There are now a wide variety of phototherapy delivery devices, from those for use in critical situations to those that enable more holistic care; for babies with critical levels, there are phototherapy units able to deliver 360° exposure. If these are not available, the baby can lie on a fibre-optic blanket with a standard phototherapy unit being used from above (Fig. 12.6) (Mills and Tudehope, 2001). It is important in these situations—where the bilirubin is increasing rapidly or approaching the exchange level—to limit the amount of time for which the infant is removed from the light source; some newer phototherapy devices enable the baby to have continuing therapy while having cuddles and being breastfed. It is possible to deliver phototherapy in the community in nonhaemolytic jaundice where the baby is not at immediate risk of kernicterus or requiring an exchange transfusion, as long as there is midwifery/nurse community care and medical follow-up (Walls et al., 2004; Malwade and Jardine, 2014).

Once phototherapy has been instituted, the level of jaundice can no longer be assessed visually or with the TcB because the skin that has been exposed to phototherapy will have been bleached. There need to be clear guidelines about when serum bilirubin testing needs to be repeated and when the phototherapy can be stopped. There is often a slight rebound in unconjugated bilirubin

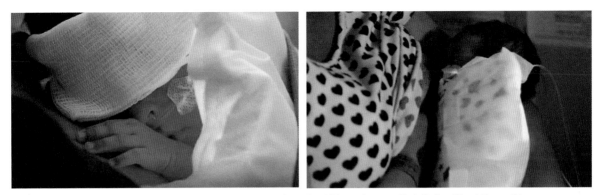

Fig. 12.6 Baby in a Fibre-Optic Blanket With a Standard Phototherapy Unit Being Used From Above.

following the cessation of phototherapy, which needs to be anticipated.

Disadvantages of phototherapy can include:

- May disrupt normal mother–baby interaction (Bili-Blanket may be less disruptive).
- Disruption of temperature regulation: baby's temperature must be regularly monitored.
- Significant increase in fluid loss from loose stools because of a decreased intestinal transit time. Stool colour may be dark due to excretion of bilirubin.
- Disruption of nutrition and hydration: it is important to continue to establish demand feeding and to prevent dehydration. Extra fluids do not need to be routinely prescribed but the baby should be regularly assessed for signs of dehydration.
- Need for eye protection: the eyes must be shielded as a precaution against possible damage. This can be disconcerting for parents.
- Maternal anxiety: it is important to ensure the mother understands the reasons for her baby's treatment and its basic principles; often, the mother's confidence and enjoyment of early mothering are impacted upon (Brethauer and Carey, 2010).
- Oxidative stress (Kale et al., 2013).
- DNA damage: there is some recent evidence that phototherapy has the potential to damage DNA, although the clinical significance of this has not been determined (Ramy et al., 2016).

Intravenous Immunoglobulin (IVIG)

The NICE guidelines (Amos, 2017) recommend intravenous immunoglobulin (IVIG) in addition to phototherapy in rhesus or ABO incompatibility when the

bilirubin is continuing to rise significantly. The theory is that the immunoglobulin binds to the antibodies causing the haemolysis and prevents them being available to bind to red blood cells.

Exchange Transfusion

Exchange transfusion is no longer a commonly performed procedure in high-resource countries, partly because of increasingly effective phototherapy devices and partly because of the administration of Anti-D to prevent rhesus isoimmunization. Exchange transfusion is a procedure that involves removing the baby's blood, complete with maternal antibodies and bilirubin, and replacing it with fresh rhesus negative blood. This requires the baby to have been admitted to a neonatal or paediatric intensive care unit. An exchange transfusion should only be performed in a baby who is at significant risk of BIND and kernicterus, in whom the benefits of transfusion outweigh the risks of complications (Ahlfors, 1994).

The removal of the maternal antibodies following an exchange transfusion in haemolytic disease minimizes the risk of the baby requiring a blood transfusion at a few weeks of age, which remains a risk with phototherapy treatment.

COMPLICATIONS OF SIGNIFICANT UNCONJUGATED JAUNDICE

Pathological jaundice with severe hyperbilirubinaemia can put the baby at risk of long-term morbidity and even death due to acute BIND or bilirubin encephalopathy (Usman et al., 2018). *Acute bilirubin encephalopathy* occurs because unbound, fat-soluble bilirubin can cross the blood–brain barrier to cause neuronal damage, primarily in the basal ganglia, central and peripheral pathways and the brainstem nuclei (Usman et al., 2018). The total serum measurement is not an accurate predictor of BIND risk or long-term complications such as deafness (Amin et al., 2016; Amin et al., 2017). The risk of deafness, in particular, has been shown to correlate better with measurements of unbound or free bilirubin than with the total serum bilirubin or the bilirubin to albumin ratio (Amin et al., 2016; Amin et al., 2017); work is ongoing to transform this laboratory research into an effective bedside test (Amin and Lamola, 2011; Ahlfors et al., 2018). Babies who suffer acute bilirubin encephalopathy have a 5% to 10% risk of mortality and a 70% to 90% risk of long-term sequelae (Beath, 2003; Ip et al., 2004; Bhutani and Johnson, 2006; Moritz et al., 2005; Maimburg et al., 2010; Wei et al., 2015). The term *kernicterus* is used to describe the brain damage that occurs following BIND with deposition of bilirubin in parts of the brain including the basal ganglia, leading to choreoathetoid cerebral palsy (movement disorder), deafness, visuo-cortical abnormalities (Hou et al., 2014) and dental enamel dysplasia (Rammal et al., 2013). There is also a possible increased incidence of autism and attention-deficit hyperactivity disorder (ADHD) (Maimburg et al., 2010; Wei et al., 2015).

PROLONGED JAUNDICE

Prolonged jaundice refers to jaundice that is visible after 2 weeks of age in a term baby, or after 3 weeks in a preterm baby. There have been attempts to quantify this in terms of bilirubin level; however—unlike the situation with early jaundice—in most cases the absolute level of bilirubin is not as relevant as the reason for the persistent jaundice. Current advice is to perform screening tests (as described later in the chapter) if jaundice is visible.

Conjugated or Unconjugated?

There are two types of prolonged jaundice: unconjugated and conjugated. The first line of investigations aims to differentiate between these two types, but it is also important to identify common treatable causes such as hypothyroidism (Andre and Day, 2016).

The first-line or screening tests needed for a baby with prolonged jaundice are blood tests and include:
- direct and indirect bilirubin (also known as conjugated and unconjugated)
- full blood count
- thyroid function tests.

Infection should also be considered and the baby should be reviewed. Further investigations and management will depend on whether the jaundice is conjugated or unconjugated.

Midwifery Role

The midwife has a role in identifying a baby who requires further investigation, and in supporting families by communicating well and providing education to help them make decisions about investigations and treatment for their baby (Paul et al., 2012). The midwife should recognize that pale stool and dark urine in a baby who is persistently jaundiced are highly suggestive of a conjugated jaundice, which needs urgent paediatric evaluation. There is now a wide selection of resources including the NICE leaflet (Amos et al., 2017) and locally produced information, as well as family support groups (locally and via social media), to help health care professionals communicate what can be quite complex information to families.

Conjugated Hyperbilirubinaemia

The term conjugated hyperbilirubinaemia is often misunderstood as meaning that the majority of bilirubin is in the conjugated form, but this is incorrect. The correct definition is that there is *more conjugated bilirubin than there should be*; that is, a situation where over 15% of the total bilirubin (or more than 25 mmol/l) is in the conjugated or 'direct reacting' form (Chiou et al., 2017). An increase in the conjugated proportion of bilirubin occurs because of obstruction to the flow (*cholestasis*) of bilirubin diglucuronide, produced by the liver, into the gut (Ananth, 2018). This leads to a decrease in *stercobilinogen* in the faeces and consequently pale stools. As the concentration of bilirubin diglucuronide within the liver cells (hepatocytes) increases, it diffuses into the bloodstream where, as a water-soluble molecule, it travels to the kidney to be excreted (darkening the urine). The presence of pale stools and dark urine together with persistent jaundice are highly suggestive of a conjugated jaundice. The importance of making this diagnosis is that the outcome from extrahepatic biliary atresia (discussed later) is much better if surgery is performed before the age of 6 weeks.

The main causes of a conjugated jaundice are:
- bile duct abnormality (biliary atresia):
  - intrahepatic (within the liver), (e.g., Alagille syndrome, an autosomal dominant genetic condition that also includes pulmonary stenosis)
  - extrahepatic (outside the liver), (e.g., extrahepatic biliary atresia)
- hepatitis with cholestasis
- congenital infection (e.g., cytomegalovirus, toxoplasmosis, rubella)
- hypopituitarism or primary adrenal insufficiency (associated with hypoglycaemia) (Braslavsky et al., 2012)
- metabolic disease (e.g., alpha-1 antitrypsin deficiency, galactosaemia, lysosomal storage disease (Niemann–Pick), Gaucher disease)
- prolonged parenteral nutrition
- bacterial infection (particularly gram negative).

Assessment of Conjugated Hyperbilirubinaemia

First-line investigations should include blood glucose, liver function tests and clotting studies. Early advice should be sought from a paediatric hepatologist so that the most appropriate investigations and subsequent management can be arranged (Fawaz et al., 2017). It is likely that improvements in the efficiency of gene sequencing may facilitate genetic diagnoses in the future (Chen et al., 2019).

Treatment

The treatment of conjugated jaundice is specific to the underlying disease. There is no requirement for phototherapy or exchange transfusion in conjugated jaundice; the inappropriate use of phototherapy may lead to the 'bronzed baby' syndrome, in which the baby's skin takes on a bronzed appearance.

Complications

Unlike unconjugated bilirubin, direct (conjugated) bilirubin is not lipid soluble and so will not cause kernicterus. Any complications may be general or specific complications of the underlying disease itself, rather than direct complications of the jaundice (in contrast to early jaundice).

General complications include:
- petechiae, bruising and bleeding because of deranged clotting
- signs secondary to liver issues
- hepatomegaly (large liver)
- hypoglycaemia (because the liver is responsible for responding to low glucose levels)
- reduced absorption of fat-soluble vitamins, including vitamins A, D and K; may require IV/IM vitamin K and appropriate vitamin preparations.

Complications specific to the underlying disease include:
- septicaemia
- cataracts in galactosaemia
- microcephaly in congenital infection.

Unconjugated Hyperbilirubinaemia

Once a conjugated hyperbilirubinaemia has been excluded, the differential diagnosis of an unconjugated hyperbilirubinaemia includes:
- breast milk jaundice
- hypothyroidism
- genetic diagnosis including G6PD deficiency, Gilbert syndrome, and Crigler–Najaar syndrome
- urinary tract infection (less likely if baby has no additional clinical signs).

Breast Milk Jaundice

Prolonged unconjugated jaundice has been noted in 10% of breastfed infants at 1 month of age (Rennie et al., 2010). It is nearly 60 years since an association was reported between breastfeeding and extended jaundice in healthy babies (Bratton and Stern, 2019). The recommended treatment of the day was to cease all breastfeeding, which resolved the jaundice within 48 hours. This method was often used to 'diagnose' breast milk jaundice but is now not recommended (Amos et al., 2017; Soldi et al., 2011). Prolonged jaundice is now recognized to be normal in babies who are well and healthy, although the cause and reason for it remains unknown; previously held ideas have been shown to be incorrect (Preer and Philipp, 2011). Babies who develop breast milk jaundice will usually become visibly jaundiced after their 5th day, or following normal physiological jaundice. The jaundice can last for weeks or even months. If it remains persistently visible or becomes worse—and particularly if the baby develops pale stools and dark urine, or there are other concerns such as poor weight gain—this suggests an aetiology other than breast milk jaundice. In this situation the midwife should consult with medical colleagues or advise the parents to seek medical advice.

FOLLOW-UP

The need for review will be determined by both the type and severity of jaundice. All babies who have had significant *early unconjugated* hyperbilirubinaemia should be reviewed at least once following their discharge or transfer. This enables test results to be reviewed, further investigations to be arranged if appropriate, and the baby's clinical condition to be reassessed. Due to the risk of hearing loss in these babies, referral to audiology needs to be considered and advice can be sought from the Newborn Hearing Screening Programme. These infants should be followed up by specialist paediatricians in view of the underlying diagnosis.

CONCLUSION

With increasing knowledge about the function and benefits of jaundice, this is an exciting time of learning for health professionals. It is now known that women having spontaneous nonmedicalized births and babies being allowed a gentle transition to extrauterine life with breastfeeding and early skin-to-skin contact will reduce the number of babies experiencing exaggerated physiological jaundice. It is the skill of the professionals in recognizing those babies who are a greater risk of hyperbilirubinaemia, and acting accordingly with appropriate and timely referrals, that reduces the risk of a baby progressing to severe hyperbilirubinaemia and its associated morbidities. By providing education and individualized support for mothers and babies—both in maternity units and the community, and ideally for longer than the first week after birth—we can expect better outcomes for both mother and baby with regard to breastfeeding success and a reduced risk of jaundice.

PARENTS' STORY

Hannah and Josh's story

My son Josh was born in the small country hospital close to my house—he was my second baby, so I felt confident to birth there. Josh became slightly jaundiced soon after birth, but it didn't worry me as my daughter had had the same—I thought he would just need lots of feeding. The first night went well, he was breastfeeding and sleeping well but, during the following night, I was feeding almost constantly and I got very little sleep. My nipples had become very sore, but I thought that was normal and told the midwives I was breastfeeding just fine. I just thought the more he fed the better off he would be, and I was quite happy to be up all night if it meant I could go home to my little girl and my husband. However, when his jaundice worsened, a heel prick showed his levels were serious enough to require phototherapy. The midwife told me I had to transfer to the main hospital in town as they didn't have a paediatrician out here. We were transferred by ambulance, which was quite scary as I didn't think he was that sick.

I was so exhausted and so disappointed that I wasn't going home that I broke down in tears. I'd been so confident that this time I would be able to go home within a couple of days, as I had a 5-day hospital stay with my first child.

I had to zip Josh into a bright blue blanket that had sleeves for his arms which was then secured onto the BiliBed. He only had his nappy on as the lights underneath him kept him warm, so every time I needed to feed him, I would have to wrap him up in lots of blankets to keep him warm. Managing a newborn is hard enough, let alone one with only a nappy on and wrapped in blankets! I tried to feed him in the blanket, but it was so awkward I gave up. After feeding, Josh would often need more burping, so I would have just put him back onto the blanket and secured him when I'd have to try to get him off it again so he could burp. That morning, I saw a lactation consultant who watched me feed Josh, and she said that 'he could be a little more deeply latched'. She helped me for about half an hour and I couldn't believe how different feeding felt. It didn't hurt and I could hear Josh drinking more! I was so grateful for her help. I did feel a little embarrassed—I thought I should have known how to breastfeed as this was my second baby—but I should have got the midwives to watch me feed!

Being in the BiliBed meant his arms and legs were free to move around, so at times it would take him a while to settle to sleep. It was really hard for me not to be able to put him in his little baby clothes or to simply hold him and

Hannah and Josh's story

cuddle him. Josh's jaundice levels seemed to improve by the end of the first day, but his levels showed he needed to stay under the lights. I felt so awful that Josh had to go through all of this, and I was so disappointed for my little girl that we wouldn't be coming home yet. He was only a few days old and his heels were full of little holes from all the heel pricks. He couldn't even be cuddled for comfort very often and he seemed so detached from me. It was even harder for him to settle to sleep, so I'd let him fall asleep on me after feeds before putting him back inside—at least this way I got to cuddle him a little more. The lights were very bright and it was very hard for me to get any sleep at night, because the whole room was alight!

After almost 2 days, he was finally allowed out of the BiliBed. With each day, his tolerance levels increased and his body was able to cope better with the bilirubin. After 4 days in hospital, we were finally allowed home.

I was very lucky I wasn't sent home without Joshua. I don't know how I would have coped had that been the case.

It was really hard to be away from my daughter and husband and I only saw them for an hour or so a day as they had to travel an hour to visit me. It was hard for my husband only to see his son for such a short time, and he couldn't hold him for long because he had to be under the lights as much as possible. We also spent a small fortune on parking meters and petrol! One very positive outcome from my long stay in hospital was that it gave my husband lots of one-on-one time with our daughter, and it was very evident that she became much more attached to her daddy after that. I also knew what a good latch was on the breast and Josh continued to breastfeed really well.

It was such a relief finally to be home again and it was great to be with my husband and daughter again.

KEY POINTS

- Jaundice and mild hyperbilirubinaemia have many physiological benefits and are a normal part of the baby's adaptive transitioning following birth.
- Physiological jaundice usually occurs after 48 hours following birth; jaundice prior to that time is considered a risk for pathological jaundice requiring appropriate assessment and possible treatment.
- It is important for midwives to know possible increased antenatal, labour, birth and postnatal risk factors for hyperbilirubinaemia, and to monitor appropriately.
- The midwife has a responsibility to discuss and educate the mother and family about jaundice and to plan care of the baby together to ensure informed choice and consent.
- Promoting normal birth, early skin-to-skin and successful breastfeeding outcomes reduces the risk of hyperbilirubinaemia.
- Transcutaneous bilirubin monitoring is a screening tool that is less invasive for the baby and reduces the amount of painful blood sampling. Use of this in the community is also advantageous.
- The presence of pale stools and/or dark urine in an infant who is jaundiced at 2 weeks is indicative

of a conjugated jaundice that requires immediate investigation.
- Early appropriate referral to paediatric care can reduce the risk of the baby experiencing severe hyperbilirubinaemia and its associated morbidities.
- Health care professionals need to collaborate in developing robust systems of practice that minimize preventable harm (e.g., significant jaundice).

REFERENCES

Ahlfors, C.E., 1994. Criteria for exchange transfusion in jaundiced newborns. Pediatrics 93 (3), 488–494.

Ahlfors, C.E., Bhutani, V.K., Wong, R.J., Stevenson, D.K., 2018. Bilirubin binding in jaundiced newborns: from bench to bedside? Pediatr. Res. 84 (4), 494–498.

Allen, N.M., O'Donnell, S.M., White, M.J., Corcoran, J.D., 2010. Initial assessment of jaundice in otherwise healthy infants—a comparison of methods in two postnatal units. Ir. Med. J. 103 (10), 310–313.

Amin, S.B., Lamola, A.A., 2011. Newborn jaundice technologies: unbound bilirubin and bilirubin binding capacity in neonates. Semin. Perinatol. 35 (3), 134–140.

Amin, S.B., Saluja, S., Saili, A., Laroia, N., Orlando, M., Wang, H., et al., 2017. Auditory toxicity in late preterm and term neonates with severe jaundice. Dev. Med. Child Neurol. 59 (3), 297–303.

Amin, S.B., Wang, H., Laroia, N., Orlando, M., 2016. Unbound bilirubin and auditory neuropathy spectrum disorder in late preterm and term infants with severe jaundice. J. Pediatr. 173, 84–89.

Amos, R.C., Jacob, H., Leith, W., 2017. Jaundice in newborn babies under 28 days: NICE guideline 2016 (CG98). Arch. Dis. Child. Educ. Pract. Ed. 102 (4), 207–209.

Ananth, R., 2018. Neonatal cholestasis: a primer of selected etiologies. Pediatr. Ann. 47 (11), e433–e439.

Andre, M., Day, A.S., 2016. Causes of prolonged jaundice in infancy: 3-year experience in a tertiary paediatric centre. N. Z. Med. J. 129 (1429), 14–21.

Aprillia, Z., Gayatri, D., Waluyanti, F.T., 2017. Sensitivity, specificity, and accuracy of kramer examination of neonatal jaundice: comparison with total bilirubin serum. Compr. Child Adolesc. Nurs. 40 (Suppl. 1), 88–94.

Askin, D.F., Diehl-Jones, W.L., 2003. The neonatal liver: Part III: pathophysiology of liver dysfunction. Neonatal Netw. 22 (3), 5–15.

Aydin, M., Hardalaç, F., Ural, B., Karap, S., 2016. Neonatal jaundice detection system. J. Med. Syst. 40 (7), 166.

Azad, M.B., Konya, T., Persaud, R.R., Guttman, D.S., Chari, R.S., Field, C.J., et al., 2016. Impact of maternal intrapartum antibiotics, method of birth and breastfeeding on gut microbiota during the first year of life: a prospective cohort study. Brit. J. Obstet. Gynaecol. 123 (6), 983–993.

Azlin, I., Wong, F.L., Ezham, M., Hafiza, A., Ainoon, O., 2011. Prevalence of uridine glucuronosyl transferase 1A1 (UGT1A1) mutations in Malay neonates with severe jaundice. Malays. J. Pathol. 33 (2), 95–100.

B.N., 2005. Adaptation to extrauterine life. In: Stables, D., Rankin, J. (Eds.), Physiology in Childbearing. Elsevier, Edinburgh UK, pp. 607–622.

Bartlett, M.G., Gourley, G.R., 2011. Assessment of UGT polymorphisms and neonatal jaundice. Semin. Perinatol. 35 (3), 127–133.

Beath, S.V., 2003. Hepatic function and physiology in the newborn. Semin. Neonatol. 8 (5), 337–346.

Berkowitz, F.E., 1991. Hemolysis and infection: categories and mechanisms of their interrelationship. Rev. Infect. Dis. 13 (6), 1151–1162.

Bhutani, V.K., Johnson L.H., 2003. Newborn jaundice and kernicterus – health and societal perspectives. Indian J. Pediatr. 70 (5), 407–416.

Bhutani, V.K., Johnson, L., 2006. Kernicterus in late preterm infants cared for as term healthy infants. Semin. Perinatol. 30 (2), 89–97.

Bhutani, V.K., Johnson, L., Sivieri, E.M., 1999. Predictive ability of a predischarge hour-specific serum bilirubin for subsequent significant hyperbilirubinemia in healthy term and near-term newborns. Pediatrics 103 (1), 6–14.

Boer, S., Unal, S., van Wouwe, J.P., van Dommelen, P., 2016. Evidence based weighing policy during the first week to prevent neonatal hypernatremic dehydration while breastfeeding. PLoS ONE 11 (12), e0167313.

Boskabadi, H., Zakerihamidi, M., Moradi, A., Bakhshaee, M., 2018. Risk factors for sensorineural hearing loss in neonatal hyperbilirubinemia. Iran. J. Otorhinolaryngol. 30 (99), 195–202.

Braslavsky, D., Keselman, A., Chiesa, A., Bergadá, I., 2012. Diagnóstico de endocrinopatía congénita en neonatos con ictericia prolongada e hipoglucemia (Diagnosis of congenital endocrinological disease in newborns with prolonged jaundice and hypoglycaemia). An. Pediatr. (Barc). 76 (3), 120–126 (in Spanish).

Bratton, S., Stern, M., 2019. Breast Milk Jaundice. In: StatPearls, Treasure Island, FL.

Brethauer, M., Carey, L., 2010. Maternal experience with neonatal jaundice. MCN Am. J. Matern. Child. Nurs. 35 (1), 8–14; quiz 15–16.

Carvalho, O.M.C., Augusto, M.C.C., Medeiros, M.Q., Lima, H.M.P., Viana Junior, A.B., Araujo Júnior, E., et al., 2018. Late umbilical cord clamping does not increase rates of jaundice and the need for phototherapy in pregnancies at normal risk. J. Matern. Fetal. Neonatal Med. 1–6.

Chen, C.F., Hsu, M.C., Shen, C.H., Wang, C.L., Chang, S.C., Wu, K.G., et al., 2011. Influence of breast-feeding on weight loss, jaundice, and waste elimination in neonates. Pediatr. Neonatol. 52 (2), 85–92.

Chen, H.L., Li, H.Y., Wu, J.F., Wu, S.H., Chen, H.L., Yang, Y.H., et al., 2019. Panel-based next-generation sequencing for the diagnosis of cholestatic genetic liver diseases: clinical utility and challenges. J. Pediatr. 205, 153–159.e6.

Chiou, F.K., Ong, C., Phua, K.B., Chedid, F., Kader, A., 2017. Conjugated hyperbilirubinemia presenting in first fourteen days in term neonates. World J. Hepatol. 9 (26), 1108–1114.

Colbourn, T., Mwansambo, C., 2018. Sunlight phototherapy for neonatal jaundice-time for its day in the sun? Lancet Glob. Health 6 (10), e1052–e1053.

Dennery, P.A., Weng, Y.H., Stevenson, D.K., Yang, G., 2001. The biology of bilirubin production. J. Perinatol. 21 (Suppl. 1), S17–S20, discussion S35–S39.

Ding, T., Schloss, P.D., 2014. Dynamics and associations of microbial community types across the human body. Nature 509 (7500), 357–360.

Dong, T., Chen, T., White, R.A., III., Wang, X., Hu, W., Liang, Y., et al., 2018. Meconium microbiome associates with the development of neonatal jaundice, Clin. Transl. Gastroenterol. 9 (9), 182.

Eghbalian, F., Rafienezhad, H., Farmal, J., 2017. The lowering of bilirubin levels in patients with neonatal jaundice using massage therapy: a randomized, double-blind clinical trial. Infant Behav. Dev. 49, 31–36.

Ercan, Ş., Özgün, G., 2018. The accuracy of transcutaneous bilirubinometer measurements to identify the hyperbilirubinemia in outpatient newborn population. Clin. Biochem. 55, 69–74.

Fawaz, R., Baumann, U., Ekong, U., Fischler, B., Hadzic, N., Mack, C.L., et al., 2017. Guideline for the evaluation of cholestatic jaundice in infants: joint recommendations of the North American Society for pediatric gastroenterology, hepatology, and nutrition and the European Society for pediatric gastroenterology, hepatology, and nutrition. J. Pediatr. Gastroenterol. Nutr. 64 (1), 154–168.

Feenstra, M.M., Jørgine Kirkeby, M., Thygesen, M., Danbjørg, D.B., Kronborg, H., 2018. Early breastfeeding problems: A mixed method study of mothers' experiences. Sex. Reprod. Healthc. 16, 167–174.

Gazzin, S., Vitek, L., Watchko, J., Shapiro, S.M., Tribelli, C., 2016. A novel perspective on the biology of bilirubin in health and disease. Trends Mol. Med. 22 (9), 758–768.

Gensollen, T., Iyer, S.S., Kasper, D.L., Blumberg, R.S., 2016. How colonization by microbiota in early life shapes the immune system. Science 352 (6285), 539–544.

Hannon, P.R., Willis, S.K., Scrimshaw, S.C., 2001. Persistence of maternal concerns surrounding neonatal jaundice: an exploratory study. Arch. Pediatr. Adolesc. Med. 155 (12), 1357–1363.

Hansen, R., Gibson, S., De Paiva Alves, E., Goddard, M., MacLaren, A., Karcher, A.M., et al., 2018. Adaptive response of neonatal sepsis-derived Group B Streptococcus to bilirubin. Sci. Rep. 8 (1), 6470.

Hansen, T.W., 2011. The role of phototherapy in the crash-cart approach to extreme neonatal jaundice. Semin. Perinatol. 35 (3), 171–174.

Hanson, L.A., 2007. Session 1: Feeding and infant development breast-feeding and immune function. Proc. Nutr. Soc. 66 (3), 384–396.

Hermansson, H., Kumar, H., Collado, M.C., Salminen, S., Isolauri, E., Rautava, S., et al., 2019. Breast milk microbiota is shaped by mode of delivery and intrapartum antibiotic exposure. Front. Nutr. 6, 4.

Ho, N.T., Li, F., Lee-Sarwar, K.A., Tun, H.M., Brown, B.P., Pannaraj, P.S., et al., 2018. Meta-analysis of effects of exclusive breastfeeding on infant gut microbiota across populations. Nat. Commun. 9 (1), 4169.

Hou, C., Norcia, A.M., Madan, A., Good, W.V., 2014. Visuocortical function in infants with a history of neonatal jaundice. Invest. Ophthalmol. Vis. Sci. 55 (10), 6443–6449.

Hyperbilirubinemia, A.S.O., 2004. Clinical practice guideline: management of hyperbilirubinemia in the newborn infant 35 or more weeks of gestation. Pediatrics.

Ip, S., Chung, M., Kulig, J., O'Brien, R., Sege, R., Glicken, S., et al., 2004. An evidence-based review of important issues concerning neonatal hyperbilirubinemia. Pediatrics 114 (1), e130–e153.

Jones, K.D.J., Grossman, S.E., Kumaranayakam, D., Rao, A., Fegan, G., Aladangady, N., 2017. Umbilical cord bilirubin as a predictor of neonatal jaundice: a retrospective cohort study. BMC Pediatr. 17 (1), 186.

Juretschke, L.J., 2005. Kernicterus: still a concern. Neonatal Netw. 24 (2), 7–19.

Kale, Y., Aydemir, O., Celik, Ü., Kavurt, S., Isikoglu, S., Bas, A.Y., et al., 2013. Effects of phototherapy using different light sources on oxidant and antioxidant status of neonates with jaundice. Early Hum. Dev. 89 (12), 957–960.

Lain, S.J., Roberts, C.L., Bowen, J.R., Nassar, N., 2015. Early discharge of infants and risk of readmission for jaundice. Pediatrics 135 (2), 314–321.

Lamola, A.A., Russo, M., 2014. Fluorescence excitation spectrum of bilirubin in blood: a model for the action spectrum for phototherapy of neonatal jaundice. Photochem. Photobiol. 90 (2), 294–296.

Lancet (editorial), 2010. Detection and treatment of neonatal jaundice. Lancet 375 (9729), 1845.

Lawrence, R.M., Lawrence, R.A., 2011. Breastfeeding: more than just good nutrition. Pediatr. Rev. 32 (7), 267–280.

Lease, M., Whalen, B., 2010. Assessing jaundice in infants of 35-week gestation and greater. Curr. Opin. Pediatr. 22 (3), 352–365.

Leung, T.S., Kapur, K., Guilliam, A., Okell, J., Lim, B., MacDonald, L.W., et al., 2015. Screening neonatal jaundice based on the sclera color of the eye using digital photography. Biomed. Opt. Express 6 (11), 4529–4538.

Longhurst, C., Turner, S., Burgos, A.E., 2009. Development of a web-based decision support tool to increase use of neonatal hyperbilirubinemia guidelines. Jt. Comm. Qual. Patient Saf. 35 (5), 256–262.

Maimburg, R.D., Bech, B.H., Vaeth, M., Møller-Madsen, B., Olsen, J., 2010. Neonatal jaundice, autism, and other disorders of psychological development. Pediatrics 126 (5), 872–878.

Maisels, M.J., 2015. Transcutaneous bilirubin measurement: does it work in the real world? Pediatrics, 135 (2), 364–366.

Maisels, M.J., Coffey, M.P., Gendelman, B., Smyth, M., Kendall, A., Clune, S., et al., 2016. Diagnosing jaundice by eye-outpatient assessment of conjunctival icterus in the newborn. J. Pediatr. 172, 212–214.e1.

Maisels, M.J., Conrad, S., 1982. Transcutaneous bilirubin measurements in full-term infants. Pediatrics 70 (3), 464–467.

Malwade, U.S., Jardine, L.A. 2014. Home- versus hospital-based phototherapy for the treatment of non-haemolytic jaundice in infants at more than 37 weeks' gestation. Cochrane Database Syst. Rev. (6), CD010212.

McClean, S., Baerg K., Smith-Fehr, J., Szafron, M., 2018. Cost savings with transcutaneous screening versus total serum bilirubin measurement for newborn jaundice in hospital and community settings: a cost-minimization analysis. CMAJ Open 6 (3), E285–E291.

McDonagh, A.F., 2010. The biliverdin-bilirubin antioxidant cycle of cellular protection: Missing a wheel? Free Radic. Biol. Med. 49 (5), 814–820.

McFadden, A., Gavine, A., Renfrew, M.J., Wade, A., Buchanan, P., Taylor, J.L., et al., 2017. Support for healthy breastfeeding mothers with healthy term babies. Cochrane Database Syst. Rev. 2, CD001141.

Mercer, J.S., Erickson-Owens, D.A., Collins, J., Barcelos, M.O., Parker, A.B., Padbury, J.F., 2017. Effects of delayed cord clamping on residual placental blood volume, hemoglobin and bilirubin levels in term infants: a randomized controlled trial. J. Perinatol. 37 (3), 260–264.

Mills, J.F., Tudehope, D., 2001. Fibreoptic phototherapy for neonatal jaundice. Cochrane Database Syst. Rev. (1), CD002060.

Ministry of Health (MOH), 2012. Guidelines for consultation with obstetric and related medical services. Ministry of Health, Wellington.

Moore, E.R., Bergman, N., Anderson, G.C., Medley, N., 2016. Early skin-to-skin contact for mothers and their healthy newborn infants. Cochrane Database Syst. Rev. 11, CD003519.

Moossavi, S., Sepehri, S., Robertson, B., Bode, L., Goruk, S., Field, C.J., et al., 2019. Composition and variation of the human milk microbiota are influenced by maternal and early-life factors. Cell Host Microbe 25 (2), 324–335.e4.

Moreno, I., Franasiak, J.M., 2017. Endometrial microbiota-new player in town. Fertil. Steril. 108 (1), 32–39.

Moretti, E., Rakza, T., Mestdagh, B., Labreuche, J., Turck, D., 2019. The bowel movement characteristics of exclusively breastfed and exclusively formula fed infants differ during the first three months of life. Acta Paediatr. 108 (5), 877–881.

Moritz, M.L., Manole, M.D., Bogen, D.L., Ayus, J.C., 2005. Breastfeeding-associated hypernatremia: are we missing the diagnosis? Pediatrics 116 (3), e343–e347.

Nilsson, I.M.S., Strandberg-Larsen, K., Knight, C.H., Hansen, A.V., Kronborg, H., 2017. Focused breastfeeding counselling improves short- and long-term success in an early-discharge setting: a cluster-randomized study. Matern. Child Nutr. 13 (4).

Pannaraj, P.S., Li, F., Cerini, C., Bender, J.M., Yang, S., Rollie, A., et al., 2017. Association between breast milk bacterial communities and establishment and development of the infant gut microbiome. JAMA Pediatr. 171 (7), 647–654.

Paul, S.P., Hall, V., Taylor, T.M., 2012. Prolonged jaundice in neonates. Pract. Midwife 15 (6), 14–17.

Peters, L.L., Thornton, C., de Jonge, A., Khashan, A., Tracy, M., Downe, S., et al., 2018. The effect of medical and operative birth interventions on child health outcomes in the first 28 days and up to 5 years of age: a linked data population-based cohort study. Birth 45 (4), 347–357.

Preer, G.L., Philipp, B.L., 2011. Understanding and managing breast milk jaundice. Arch. Dis. Child Fetal Neonatal Ed. 96 (6), F461–F466.

Rammal, M., Meador, M., Rodriguez, M., Lish, B., 2013. Green teeth in a premature infant following hemolytic jaundice. Gen. Dent. 61 (4), 28–29.

Ramy, N., Ghany, E.A., Alsharany, W., Nada, A., Darwish, R.K., Rabie, W.A., et al., 2016. Jaundice, phototherapy and DNA damage in full-term neonates. J. Perinatol. 36 (2), 132–136.

Rennie, J., Burman-Roy, S., Murphy, M.S., 2010. Neonatal jaundice: summary of NICE guidance. BMJ 340, c2409.

Ruiz, L., Espinosa-Martos, I., García-Carral, C., Manzano, S., McGuire, M.K., Meehan, C.L., et al., 2017. What's normal? Immune profiling of human milk from healthy women living in different geographical and socioeconomic settings. Front. Immunol. 8, 696.

Sally Tracy Interventions in pregnancy, labour and birth. In: Pairman, S., Pincombe, J., Thorogood, C., et al., (Eds.), Midwifery PrepAration for Practice. p. 890–942.

Samiee-Zafarghandy, S., et al., 2014. Influence of skin colour on diagnostic accuracy of the jaundice meter JM 103 in newborns. Arch. Dis. Child Fetal Neonatal Ed. 99 (6), F480–F484.

Sedlak, T.W., Snyder, S.H., 2004. Bilirubin benefits: cellular protection by a biliverdin reductase antioxidant cycle. Pediatrics 113 (6), 1776–1782.

Shah, P.S., Herbozo, C., Aliwalas, L.L., Shah, V.S., 2012. Breastfeeding or breast milk for procedural pain in neonates. Cochrane Database Syst. Rev. 12, CD004950.

Soldi, A., Tonetto, P., Varalda, A., Bertino, E., 2011. Neonatal jaundice and human milk. J. Matern. Fetal. Neonatal Med. 24 (Suppl. 1), 85–87.

Stokowski, L.A., 2011. Fundamentals of phototherapy for neonatal jaundice. Adv. Neonatal Care 11 (Suppl. 5), S10–S21.

Usman, F., Diala, U.M., Shapiro, S.M., Le Pichon, J.B., Slusher, T.M., 2018. Acute bilirubin encephalopathy and its progression to kernicterus: current perspectives. Res. Rep. Neonatol. 8, 33–44.

Vitek, L., 2005. Impact of serum bilirubin on human diseases. Pediatrics 115 (5), 1411–1412.

Wagner, K.H., Wallner, M., Mölzer, C., Gazzin, S., Bulmer, A.C., Tiribelli, C., et al., 2015. Looking to the horizon: the role of bilirubin in the development and prevention of age-related chronic diseases. Clin. Sci. (Lond). 129 (1), 1–25.

Walls, M., Wright, A., Fowlie, P., Irvine, L., Hume, R., 2004. Home phototherapy in the United Kingdom. Arch. Dis. Child Fetal Neonatal Ed. 89 (3), F282.

Wei, C.C., Chang, C.H., Lin, C.L., Chang, S.N., Li, T.C., Kao, C.H., 2015. Neonatal jaundice and increased risk of attention-deficit hyperactivity disorder: a population-based cohort study. J. Child Psychol. Psychiatry 56 (4), 460–467.

Weiss, A.K., Vora, P.V., 2018. Conjugated hyperbilirubinemia in the neonate and young infant. Pediatr. Emerg. Care 34 (4), 280–283.

Widström, A.M., Brimdyr, K., Svensson, K., Cadwell, K., Nissen, E., 2019. Skin-to-skin contact the first hour after birth, underlying implications and clinical practice. Acta Paediatr. 108 (7), 1192–1204.

Woodgate, P., Jardine, L.A., 2015. Neonatal jaundice: phototherapy. BMJ Clin. Evid. 2015, 0319.

13

Neonatal Skincare and Cord Care: Implications for Practice

Sharon Trotter

CHAPTER CONTENTS

INTRODUCTION

The skin is the largest organ and it plays an important role in maintaining our bodies and our health. It functions as a barrier against infection, protects the internal organs, prevents evaporation of essential fluid content from the body, and serves as a sensor to detect pain, irritation and changes in the external environment. In Chapter 2, where the practical newborn infant physical examination (NIPE) is discussed in more depth, we noted the importance of observing and monitoring the baby's skin, and we considered a number of common skin variations, abnormalities and birthmarks. In this chapter, the specific features and requirements of the neonate's skin will be explored in relation to common minor noninfective rashes, cord care and the effects of skin care products.

Rashes are very common in the first months of life and particularly in the first 4 weeks of life. Most of these are transient and benign, but more serious skin conditions including *pemphigus neonatorum* (staphylococcal infection), *paronychia* (infection of the nail bed) and *omphalitis* (infection of the umbilical cord), all of which

can lead to septicaemia, may occur; care should be taken to identify more serious conditions including candida, viral and bacterial infections during the NIPE. The occurrence of such conditions can be ameliorated by allowing the skin to maintain its essential protective barrier. Additionally, even common minor noninfective rashes including erythema toxicum neonatorum (normal neonatal rash), miliaria (heat rash) and milia (milk spots) that result primarily from the immaturity of skin structures may be reduced by using an evidence-based approach to skin care and by avoiding certain practices such as the premature introduction of baby toiletry products following birth.

Fashions in health care influence not only how women birth their babies, but also how babies' skin is cared for. Parents and professionals assume that baby products are safe and even beneficial, but this may not be the case. Comments like 'we used this product on all our babies' and 'they smell nice' are hard to challenge. It takes courage and conviction to question what has become the socially accepted norm. We are all influenced socially, psychologically, physically and culturally. We must keep this in mind when trying to bring about change and to communicate new ideas. Good communication is at the heart of this process.

Society has become de-centred as a result of globalization, and technology has allowed the world to shrink. Multinational organizations use the power of large-scale branding and marketing to persuade people around the globe to forego their valuable, tried and tested, traditional methods in favour of industry-driven values and beliefs. This can be seen clearly in the context of baby products, especially infant formula and baby skincare items. Parents buy into an 'ideal' of family life, as portrayed through advertising that has somehow become synonymous with modern life. This process can be so subtle that parents and professionals alike are unaware of its effect. Additionally, habits and practices which lack credibility may be adopted and can prove hard to break (Davies, 2011).

Midwives, health visitors and other health professionals in many Western settings are autonomous practitioners, responsible for their own actions. It is vital that their practice is based on the best available evidence. This ability is compromised when, for example, hospitals and maternity units continue to supply free baby products when there is no evidence to support their use on newborn babies. It is important to remember that anything placed on, in or around the neonate has the capacity to harm, and this is particularly applicable to products used for skincare and cord care (Trotter, 2004; 2013).

Before discussing appropriate guidelines for neonatal skincare and cord care, it is important that we consider the structure and the physiological role of the skin as a protective organ, and reflect on the natural process of cord separation in the neonate.

SKIN STRUCTURE

The skin of the newborn baby has the same structure as adult skin, with three layers (*epidermis*, *dermis* and *subcutaneous*), but is thinner and therefore does not provide the same level of immunologic, thermoregulatory or sensory protection. The epidermis, or outer layer of the skin (0.01–0.05 mm thick), consists of the *stratum corneum* (the inert top layer—dead cells which are constantly shed and replaced) and three living layers: *stratum granulosum*, *stratum spinosum* and *stratum basale*. *Melanocytes*, the cells that create skin colour by producing the pigment melanin, are also located in the epidermis.

The stratum corneum is made up of 10 to 20 microscopic layers in both the adult and the term infant. In premature infants, however, this number decreases to between 2 and 3. In extremely premature infants (<23 weeks), the stratum corneum may be virtually nonexistent (Visscher et al., 2015; Nikolovski et al., 2008). Consequently, the risk to these babies is even higher.

Babies are born with an alkaline skin surface which has an average pH of 6.34 (Kutlubay, 2017). However, within days, the pH falls to about 4.95, forming what is known as the *acid mantle*, a very fine film that rests on the surface of the skin and acts as a protector. The gestational age at birth does not affect the timing of this development, suggesting that it probably occurs as a direct result of the skin's exposure to air (Coughlin and Taïeb, 2014).

The stratum basale is at the junction of the epidermis and dermis, and is where the basal cells (*keratinocytes*) are renewed through constant cell division. The granules in the keratinocytes of the stratum granulosum are full of newly synthesized and stored lipids. These will be released before the cell dies and are processed enzymatically to form the lipid barrier. These lipids surround the lifeless keratin disc formed by a keratinocyte after its death and now called a *corneocyte*. These can be thought of as the bricks in a wall, with the mortar made up of lipid molecules. This whole structure forms the skin barrier and is situated in the stratum corneum, the most superficial layer of skin. When intact, this 'wall' regulates temperature, acts as a barrier to infection, balances water and electrolytes, stores fat and insulates against the cold. The skin is also a large tactile area used for the interpretation of stimuli.

The structure and function of this delicate layer are easily damaged, leading to a wide spectrum of inflammatory symptoms. The two main causes are the destruction of the skin's barrier (delipidization) within the stratum corneum and the stimulation of an inflammatory immune response which, in turn, compromises the skin's barrier (Kownatzki, 2003).

Beneath the epidermis lies the *dermis*, consisting of fibrous and elastic tissues (giving strength and elasticity), sebaceous and sweat glands (to maintain body temperature), hair shafts, blood vessels and cutaneous nerves; these nerves facilitate the sensations of pain, touch and temperature. The third layer is made of fat and connective tissue. This deeper subcutaneous tissue (*hypodermis*) protects internal organs and provides insulation and calorie storage; it is less developed in

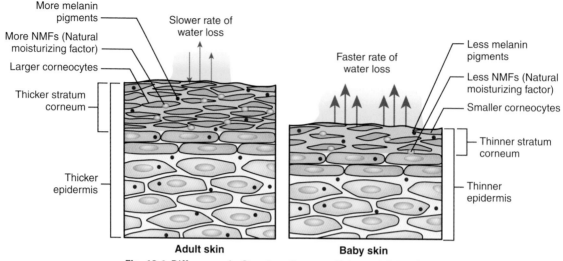

Fig. 13.1 Differences in Structure Between Baby and Adult Skin.

preterm and low birth weight babies (Visscher et al., 2015) (Fig. 13.1).

Vernix Caseosa

At birth, a baby's skin is covered with vernix caseosa, which gives added protection over the first few days of life. The thickness of this layer varies depending on the gestational age of the infant. Vernix is a highly sophisticated biofilm consisting of antimicrobial peptides and proteins and fatty acids. These combine to form a barrier that is antibacterial and antifungal. A study by Tollin et al. (2005) states that vernix caseosa helps to maintain an intact epidermal barrier.

Meanwhile, the skin becomes colonized with microorganisms and develops its own stable microbiota (Oranges et al., 2015). The transitional environment, from alkaline to acid (the acid mantle described in the previous section) further adds to the protective barrier. Its delicate balance must be maintained if the skin is to achieve an optimum level of protection. There is no evidence that the acid mantle exists beyond this point, so acidic pH detergents are not thought to provide any protection (Oranges et al., 2015).

'Epidermal lipids play a key role in maintaining the skin's barrier, integrity and health' (Ertel, 2003). This statement is backed up by evidence that individuals suffering from atopic eczema have reduced levels of epidermal lipids (Agrawal et al., 2014). As the epidermis continually sheds, it is vital for the lipid seal around each keratinocyte to be left undisturbed. This protective layer ensures that the skin does not dry out; this can only be achieved in the presence of certain enzymes and the right lipid precursors (Kownatzki, 2003). This barrier cannot be reproduced by artificial means. Great care must therefore be employed to avoid its destruction and delipidization by the chemicals used in manufactured personal care products.

Once damaged, the epidermis is more prone to transepidermal water loss, which leads to dry skin. This in turn increases the likelihood of sensitization by foreign materials such as microorganisms and allergens, and the damaging effects of chemical irritants (Kownatzki, 2003).

Interaction with keratinocyte surface molecules or membrane lipids leads to cell activation; cytokines are released and send signals to blood vessels and white blood cells. Activation of Langerhans cells initiates an immune response which is particularly effective when a foreign substance is encountered repeatedly. Once a certain level of response has been exceeded, inflammatory symptoms (e.g., skin irritation and eczema) become evident (Boer et al., 2016).

Delipidization

Delipidization is the selective removal of lipid (fat) components from the stratum corneum. Many studies on the damaging effects of surfactants (detergents) on the skin have been carried out, highlighting changes to the skin's pH, the drying effects of hand cleaners and the associated swelling of the stratum corneum (Ertel, 2003; Kownatzki, 2003). All have agreed that every method employed to clean the skin affects its surface fat content, thereby reducing the effectiveness of its barrier against irritants, allergens and microorganisms.

In adults, washing removes lipid- and water-soluble substances, as well as natural antibacterial agents. This could lead to increased bacterial growth that negates the original skin-cleansing technique.

It is interesting to note that the damage to the lipid barrier caused by overhydration as a result of using latex gloves actually recovers quickly due to evaporation—in stark contrast with the many days necessary for the barrier to recover from detergent damage. The kinetics of damage and repair, and epidemiological evidence, suggest that modern synthetic detergents (as used in foaming liquid cleansers) cause the most damage (Kownatzki, 2003). Although these disturbing findings relate primarily to adult skin, the implications for neonatal skincare are obvious.

The Microbiome and Skin

As discussed in Chapter 6, the microbiome plays a significant role in boosting the immune system and this has as much bearing on the skin as on any other organ or system. That is why skin-to-skin is such an important part of the birthing sequence and why maintaining skin integrity by delaying bathing of the baby is significant (Harman and Wakeford, 2016).

Immediate skin-to-skin contact following birth is important because it encourages nonpathogenic colonization from mother to baby (UNICEF, 2019). It is also known to encourage bonding, attachment and successful breastfeeding and to stabilize the baby's heart rate and temperature (Ludington-Hoe et al., 2006) (Chapter 5). Baby massage follows on naturally from this and is now widely practised. Twenty-four-hour rooming-in is common practice in hospitals worldwide; this is important because it cuts down the risks of cross-infection and nosocomial (hospital-acquired) infection (Shrivastava et al., 2013) As the mother is the sole carer, there is less chance of health care workers spreading infections from one baby to another.

SKINCARE

The Nursing and Midwifery Council (NMC, 2019) states that practitioners should: 'make sure that any

information or advice given is evidence based including information relating to using any health and care products or services'.

Evidence-based guidelines for neonatal skincare and cord care are pivotal in order to ensure consistency. Based on an understanding of neonatal skin physiology and the available evidence, the following guidelines for neonatal skincare are recommended.

Bath Care

- Before and after carrying out any baby care, especially cord care, it is very important to wash your hands thoroughly in order to avoid any cross-infection.
- Following birth, the healthy term neonate, once stabilized, should be bathed in plain water. This will help to protect the delicate skin while it is vulnerable to germs, chemicals and water loss.
- Wash cloths should be avoided because they can be harsh. Washing using cotton wool or a natural sponge is gentler. A baby comb can be used to gently remove any debris from thick hair after delivery.
- The purpose of washing newborn skin is to clean it without removing the lipid barrier that is essential to the surface ecosystem. Few studies to date have demonstrated the benefits of emollient use on healthy, full-term infants (Telofski et al., 2012).
- After the first bath, neonates should not be immersed in water until separation of the umbilical cord. This will allow the natural process of cord separation to continue unhindered, while avoiding disruption to the delicate colonization of flora at the base of the cord (Trotter, 2003).
- Bathing in plain water *only* (Fig. 13.2) should continue for at least the first month before *gradually* introducing baby products (optional but not necessary). By this time, the skin's natural barrier will be better developed. Baby products should be free from sodium lauryl sulphate (SLS), sodium laureth sulphate (SLES), colours and strong perfumes.
- All cleansing agents—even tap water—influence the skin's fat content to some degree. However, the dissolution of fat molecules in the upper epidermis by synthetic detergents is not only worrying but avoidable. It should be considered that even short-term effects, when repeated several times a day, can disturb the acid mantle and its protective function, leading to dry and squamous skin in some infants

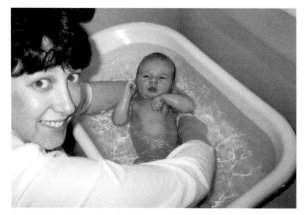

Fig. 13.2 Author With Her Son Using Water Only for Bathing.

(Coughlin and Taïeb, 2014) Daily baths can dry the skin; 2 or 3 baths a week are sufficient.

- It is best to leave the delicate area around the eyes untouched; the ears and nose should also be left alone, and cotton buds should be avoided. Sticky eyes can be safely treated with drops of fresh colostrum or breastmilk (Verd, 2007).
- Washing baby's genital region: girls should be cleaned from front to back to prevent the transfer of bacteria from the perianal region to the vagina or urethra which could introduce infection; boys should be cleaned carefully around their testicles and penis.
- It is safer to file nails with a soft nail file rather than using scissors (which can leave sharp edges, in addition to the risk of cutting the baby's skin which is attached under the nails). Nails that have started to come away can be peeled off gently.
- Vernix caseosa should be left undisturbed. As discussed in the previous section, this is nature's own moisturizer and gives added protection against infection in the first few days (Visscher and Narendran, 2014).
- If a baby is overdue, its skin may well be dry and cracked. This is to be expected, as the protective vernix has mostly been absorbed. Don't be tempted to use any oils, creams or lotions—they may do more harm than good. The top layer of skin will peel off over the next few days, leaving perfect skin underneath.Baby wipes should also be avoided for at least the first month.
- Petroleum-based oils with perfumes and essential oils should not be used.

- If there is a history of nut allergies in the immediate family, nut-based oils should also be avoided.
- Even some vegetable oils are not ideal for delicate baby skin. For example, olive oil is high in oleic acid, which can have the same effect on the skin as detergents, stripping away the delicate barrier that protects baby's skin. This can dry the skin and make it more prone to eczema (Danby et al., 2013).
- It is safer to use oils that are lower in oleic acid and higher in linoleic acid—for example, sunflower, sesame seed, evening primrose or pomegranate oil—and organic is always best (Danby et al., 2013).
- Products should never be used on broken skin.
- Shampoo is not necessary for babies under a year old. Once baby bath products have been introduced, baby's hair can simply be rinsed in the bath water. If used, shampoo should also be free from sulphates (SLS and SLES—see later in the chapter).
- A thin layer of barrier cream can be used on the nappy area. The ideal cream should be free from preservatives, colours, perfumes, antiseptics, and clinically proven as an effective treatment for nappy rash (Atherton and Mills, 2004).
- If, after a few weeks, a moisturizer is required, preparations that are emollient based should be used. These will not dry out the skin but can give some protection.
- When laundering baby clothes and bedding, do not overload the machine. This ensures thorough rinsing.
- Fabric conditioners, if used, should be mild and free from colours and strong perfumes.
- Cloth nappies are as efficient as disposable ones and do not present a higher risk of nappy rash.

Baby Products: What to Avoid

Due to the myriad of potentially toxic ingredients used in products today, it would seem sensible for the manufacturers of baby products to remove any chemicals that have been shown to cause irritant or sensitizing reactions. With this in mind, the following ingredients should always be avoided.

Sodium Lauryl Sulphate (SLS)

Sodium lauryl sulphate (SLS, also known as sodium dodecyl sulphate) is a harsh industrial degreasant found in many personal care products (Day, 2005). It is known to strip away the lipid barrier and erode the skin, leaving it rough and pitted. It can stay in the tissues for days and is also known to strip the skin of moisture, cause cracking and severe inflammation of the epidermis, separate and inflame skin layers. It is routinely used in clinical trials as a standard irritant for skin (Vance, 1999). It is intended for 'discontinuous' use. However, when added to other ingredients, such as triclosan (which is now common in antibacterial preparations), it has the potential to stay next to the skin for many hours, increasing the likelihood of damage to the skin's natural protective barrier. There are two main reasons for the use of SLS in products: it is cheap, and when added to salt, it thickens, making a product appear more concentrated.

Sodium Laureth Sulphate (SLES) and Ammonium Laureth Sulphate (ALES)

When SLS is ethoxylated (a chemical process that increases molecular size and is thought to produce a milder formulation, with potentially less risk of skin irritation) to enhance its foaming properties, it becomes sodium laureth sulphate (SLES).

This is commonly used as a foaming agent in toothpastes, bath gels, bubble baths and degreasants. It dissolves proteins and can lead to mouth ulcers. Sodium laureth sulphate and ammonium laureth sulphate (ALES) stay in the tissues for up to 5 days and can form nitrates and nitrosamines, which are carcinogens; they can lead the body to absorb nitrates at higher levels and this may be linked to the development of cancers (Vance, 1999). During the ethoxylation process, the extremely harmful compound 1,4-dioxane is created. This is one of the principal components of the chemical defoliant Agent Orange.

Parabens (Methylparaben, Propylparaben, Ethylparaben and Butylparaben)

These are synthetic preservatives used in cosmetics and personal care products—especially baby wipes, baby lotions and shampoos. They are also used as food preservatives. They have been found to act like the hormone oestrogen in laboratory experiments, although activity was weak. They may cause dermatitis, rashes or allergic skin conditions (Breast Cancer UK).

Are There Safe Alternatives?

By shopping around and reading the labels before buying, it is possible to find safe alternatives to the above ingredients. Business revolves around the ethos of supply and demand; if parents and professionals demand safer products, manufacturers are more likely to deliver. Ethical consumerism has increased the demand for products without additives in recent years and an increasing number of products are filling the niche that has been created. These are not only safer for babies (over 1 month of age) and children, but are more likely to be environmentally friendly.

CORD CARE

Physiology of Umbilical Cord Separation

The umbilical cord is a unique tissue consisting of two arteries and one vein covered by a mucoid connective tissue known as Wharton's jelly, which is in turn covered by a thin layer of mucous membrane (a continuation of the amnion). During pregnancy, the placenta provides all the nutrients for fetal growth and removes waste products simultaneously through the umbilical cord.

Following delivery, the cord quickly starts to dry out, harden and turn black (a process called dry gangrene). This is helped by exposure to the air. The umbilical vessels remain patent for several days, so the risk of infection remains high until separation (Fig. 13.3).

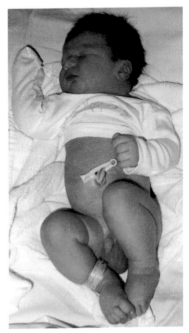

Fig. 13.3 Umbilical Cord Clamped.

Colonization of the area begins within hours of birth as a result of nonpathogenic organisms passing from mother to baby via skin-to-skin contact. Harmful bacteria can be spread by bad hygiene, poor hand washing techniques and especially cross-infection by health care workers.

Separation of the umbilical cord continues at the junction of the cord and the abdominal skin, with leucocyte infiltration and subsequent digestion of the cord. During this normal process, small amounts of cloudy mucoid material may collect at the junction; this may unwittingly be interpreted as pus. A moist and/or sticky cord may present, but this too is part of the normal physiological process. Separation should be complete within 5 to 15 days, although it can take longer. The main reasons for prolonged separation include the use of antiseptics and infection.

Antiseptics appear to reduce the number of normal nonpathogenic flora around the umbilicus. This reduction in leucocytes prolongs the healing process and hinders cord separation (Zupan et al., 2004).

After the cord has separated, a small amount of mucoid material is still present until complete healing takes place, a few days later. This means that there is still a risk of infection, although this is not as great as in the first few days.

The Evidence

Many studies and reviews have been carried out to compare differing treatments and their effects on infection rates, colonization and length of time for cord separation (McConnell et al., 2004; Pezzati et al., 2002; Golombek, 2002). Overall, they have concluded that the more the cord is treated, the longer it will take to separate. Prolonged cord separation rates are also associated with reduced colonization levels.

This would suggest that a certain level of colonization is actually a healthy sign and not necessarily a precursor to infection. This is why 24-hour rooming-in is such an important factor in the care of the newborn. It not only avoids cross-infection by health care workers, but also encourages the early colonization of nonpathogenic organisms which, in turn, promotes faster healing (Rush, 1987).

Maybe Barr (1984) was right when she postulated that: 'Wharton's jelly may possess an, as yet, unknown factor, that is essential to the natural healing process'. It certainly seems to be true that the use of treatments on the umbilical cord appears to interrupt and prolong the natural process of cord separation.

As there is no evidence to recommend the widespread use of topical treatments for cord care, further studies would be helpful, especially in developing countries where neonates are at higher risk of contracting infections. However, for the healthy term infant 'open cord care' using no topical treatments continues to be the safest and most cost-effective advice.

While in most parts of the UK and other parts of the world the cord clamp is now routinely used to 'clamp' the cord, in many other countries (including New Zealand), there has been much discussion about what should be used to tie off the cord. Many women opt for sterile cotton ties. Some Maori women choose to use flax ties, which has cultural significance (Simmonds, 2017).

Guidelines for Cord Care

The following guidelines are based on the WHO (1998) review of the evidence and the Cochrane Database systematic review (Zupan et al., 2004) on topical umbilical cord care at birth.

Cord Care for the Healthy Term Baby

- Keep the cord area clean and dry. The best way to achieve this is to leave it alone (this practice is also known as 'open cord care').
- After the first bath in plain water, pat dry with a clean towel. Fold the nappy down to expose the cord at each nappy change, until the cord has separated.
- Parents should be advised to avoid bathing their baby while the cord is in situ. Instead, they should be advised to 'top and tail' their baby until the cord has separated naturally.
- Never use dry cotton wool as it may leave filaments behind.
- Wet cotton wool can be used if the area becomes soiled with urine or faeces.
- There is no need for routine use of antiseptic wipes or powders.
- The cord clamp may or may not be removed, depending on hospital policy.
- If the cord or surrounding area becomes red, inflamed or has an offensive odour, a swab may need to be sent for culture.

Cord Care for the Sick or Premature Baby

- Where infants cannot benefit from 24-hour rooming-in, it may be necessary to use a topical antiseptic for the first few days.
- This can be followed by open cord care when the cord has become dry and hard.
- The reasons for these extra precautions include the higher risk of nosocomial infection, the increased number of carers, and the infant's compromised immune system.

Observe for Signs of Umbilical Cord Infection (Omphalitis)

- Symptoms include redness, erythema, oedema and tenderness.
- Infection is known to prolong the patency of the umbilical vessels, leading to bleeding from the cord.
- Purulent discharge may also be present.
- Pyrexia, lethargy and poor feeding alongside the signs of infection point to systemic involvement.
- Complications of the above include septicaemia and peritonitis.
- Broad-spectrum antibiotic cover is the treatment of choice, although with increasing antibiotic resistance this needs to be used judiciously. If a microbiology swab result is available, targeted antibiotics can be used.
- The prevalence of a moist and/or sticky cord base, which may or may not be smelly, is not necessarily a positive sign of infection. If the baby is alert, feeding well and afebrile, then the chances of infection remain low. Observation is the only treatment required in this instance.

Future Research

Although open cord care is common practice throughout the world, more research may be beneficial to persuade health professionals who still advocate unnecessary treatments. For instance, does leaving the cord clamp in situ have an effect on infection or separation rates? Studies into the care of sick and premature infants using the updated cord care guidelines would be useful. It would also be interesting to compare the efficiency of natural plant and herb treatments with that of conventional antiseptics. Natural treatments include breast milk and colostrum, which are known to possess antimicrobial properties (Stanway and Stanway, 1996).

Ironically, it may be that the very practice of cleaning the cord has the potential to cause cross-infection. Left untouched, the cord is more likely to separate without problems. This not only saves money on antiseptic preparations—which have, in any case, yet to be proven effective—but also has the potential to save midwifery time. The most expensive commodities in the care of mother and baby are the health care professionals. Further research into the microbiome is ongoing and this will hopefully result in the development of new protocols. Such research also has the potential to help boost the immune systems of the next generation of babies so they can reduce their risk of developing the autoimmune diseases that have become all too common (Finlay and Arrieta, 2016).

CONCLUSION

Health care professionals' duty of care includes alerting parents to the risks associated with the early overuse of manufactured baby products, and advising them about safe alternatives.

Manufacturers must play their part by reevaluating formulations in light of the growing evidence against the use of synthetic detergents, ingredients which are likely to have contributed to the rise in skin-related conditions in recent years. The increased and widespread use of baby products is coincident with this statistic (Cork et al. 2002).

Fundamentally, midwives want and need good evidence in order to develop clear guidelines for practice. This is provided by a range of stakeholders, including manufacturers. As independent practitioners, midwives should consider the doctrine of their medical colleagues: 'Primum non nocere' ('First do no harm'). This is critical for neonatal skincare. We have yet to see data to support the claims made by some manufacturers that their baby skincare products 'do no harm', 'have no long-term effects on the development of immune system sensitization', or actually offer a benefit over and above using water alone.

By raising the profile of neonatal skincare, I want health care professionals to start reviewing and updating existing policies in line with the latest NICE guidelines. As well as leading to the standardization of best practice throughout the UK, this should also, I hope, encourage manufacturers to stop promoting their baby skincare products for neonatal use.

Jacqueline's story

Eczema

When we brought our baby daughter home from hospital, she had beautiful soft skin. As a gift, we had been given some natural bath products, so for the first few months we bathed her in those. When they ran out, we changed to use a well-known commercial brand of shampoo and bubble bath. Within 2 weeks, we noticed some small red patches appear on her leg. Over the next few days the patches got bigger and, while our daughter wasn't bothered by them, we were—so we changed to another well-known brand. It didn't get any better, so we decided to take her to see our GP.

Our GP took a quick glance at our daughter's legs and told us she had childhood eczema. We said we weren't sure it was eczema as she wasn't bothered by it. However, still convinced, the GP gave us a prescription and told us to come back if it didn't clear up.

At this point, we decided to do some research of our own and, on speaking to a friend about the problem, she gave us the contact details of Sharon Trotter and told us to e-mail her as she may be able to help. We e-mailed her and outlined what had gone on. We made it clear that the dry patches weren't irritating our daughter and said that

the problem had only flared up since we started using the commercial brands in her bath. Sharon told us the problem was probably being caused by the SLS in the products we were using—we should stop using them and bathe our daughter in plain water. That night, we did as she asked, and continued to do so for the next few weeks. Within that time, we noticed a marked difference, and within 8 weeks the patches had gone completely.

This continued to be the case until one day we noticed the patches were starting to come back on her lower legs. I noticed that the patches were in the shape of my fingers and that they were exactly where I held her legs while changing her nappy. We looked at the ingredients on the liquid soap we used to wash our hands prior to changing our daughters' nappies and found that it contained SLS. These patches have cleared up since we found soap that had no SLS. We've been amazed at the adverse reaction our daughter has had to it.

Sixteen months down the line, we still bathe her in plain water and we've never had any further problems.

KEY POINTS

- The objective of washing newborn skin is to clean without removing the lipid barrier that is essential to the surface ecosystem.
- The development of more serious skin conditions may be avoided by refraining from using baby skincare products, thereby allowing the skin to maintain its essential protective barrier.
- Vernix caseosa forms a barrier of protection for the newborn baby's skin that is not only antibacterial but also antifungal.
- Babies should be bathed in plain water for at least the first month, and baby products should be introduced gradually.
- Separation of the umbilical cord should be complete within 5 to 15 days, although it can take longer.
- It may be that the more the cord is treated, the longer it will take to separate.

REFERENCES

Agrawal, R., Woodfolk, J.A., 2014. Skin barrier defects in atopic dermatitis. Curr. Allergy Asthma Rep. 14 (5), 433. doi:10.1007/s11882-014-0433-9.

American Academy of Pediatrics (AAP), American College of Obstetricians and Gynecologists, 2012. Guidelines for Perinatal Care, seventh ed. American Academy of Pediatrics, Elk Grove Village, IL; American College of Obstetricians and Gynecologists, Washington, DC.

Atherton, D., Mills, K., 2004. What can be done to keep babies' skin healthy? RCM Midwives 7 (7), 288–290.

Barr, J., 1984. The umbilical cord: to treat or not to treat? Midwives Chron. and Nurs. Notes. 97 (1159), 224–226.

Boer, M., Duchnik, E., Maleszka, R., Marchlewicz, M., 2016. Structural and biophysical characteristics of human skin in maintaining proper epidermal barrier function. Postepy. Dermatol. Alergol. 33 (1), 1–5. doi:10.5114/pdia.2015.48037.

Breast Cancer UK online: https://www.breastcanceruk.org.uk/science-and-research/background-briefings/parabens/

Cork, M.J., Murphy, R., Carr, J., et al., 2002. The rising prevalence of atopic eczema and environmental trauma to the skin. Dermatology in Practice. 10 (3), 22–26.

Coughlin, C.C., Taïeb, A., 2014. Evolving concepts of neonatal skin. Pediatr. Dermatol. 31, 5–8. doi:10.1111/pde.12499.

Danby, S.G., AlEnezi, T., Sultan, A., Lavender, T., Chittock, J., Brown, K., et al., 2013. Effect of olive and sunflower seed oil on the adult skin barrier: implications for neonatal skin care. Pediatr. Dermatol. 30 (1), 42–50.

Davies, L., 2011. Parents as consumers. In: Davies, L., Daellenbach, R., Kensington, M. (Eds.), Sustainability, Midwifery, and Birth. Routledge, London.

Day, P., 2005. Cancer—Why We're Still Dying to Know the Truth. Credence Publications, USA.

Ertel, K., 2003. Bathing the term newborn: personal cleanser considerations. In: Maibach, H.I., Boisits, E.K. (Eds.), Neonatal Skin: Structure and Function. Marcel Decker, New York, pp. 211–238.

Finlay, B., Arrieta, M.C., 2016. Let Them Eat Dirt: Saving Your Child from an Oversanitized World. Alonquin Books, New York, NY.

Golombek, S.G., Brill, P.E., Salice, A.L., 2002. Randomized trial of alcohol versus triple dye for umbilical cord care. Clin. Pediatr. 41 (6), 419–423. Available from: https://doi.org/10.1177/000992280204100607.

Harman, T., Wakeford, A., 2016. The Microbiome Effect: how your baby's birth affects their future health. London: Pinter & Martin

Kownatzki, E., 2003. Hand hygiene and skin health. J. Hosp. Infect. 55, 239–245.

Kutlubay, Z., Tanakol, A., Engýn, B., Onel, C., Sýmse, E., Serdaroglu, S., et al., 2017. Newborn skin: common skin problems. Maedica (Buchar) 12 (1), 42–47.

Ludington-Hoe, S.M., Lewis, T., Morgan, K., Cong, X., Anderson, L., Reese, S., 2006. Breast and infant temperatures with twins during shared kangaroo care. J. Obstet. Gynecol. Neonatal Nurs. 35, 223–231.

McConnell, T.P., Lee, C.W., Couillard, M., Sherrill, W.W., 2004. Trends in umbilical cord care: Scientific evidence for practice. Newborn Infant Nurs. Rev. 4 (4), 211–222.

Nikolovski, J., Stamatas, G.N., Kollias, N., Wiegand, B.C., 2008. Barrier function and water-holding and transport properties of infant stratum corneum are different from adult and continue to develop through the first year of life. J. Invest. Dermatol. 128, 1728–1736.

Nursing and Midwifery Council (NMC), 2019. The Code: Professional Standards of Practice and Behaviour for Nurses, Midwives and Nursing Associates. NMC, London, p. 93.

Oranges, T., Dini, V., Romanelli, M., 2015. Skin physiology of the neonate and infant: clinical implications. Adv. Wound Care (New Rochelle) 4 (10), 587–595. doi:10.1089/wound.2015.0642.

Pezzati, M., Biagioli, E.C., Martelli, E., Gambi, B., Biagiotti, R., Rubaltelli, F.F., 2002. Umbilical cord care: the effect of eight different cord-care regimens on cord separation time and other outcomes. Biol. Neonate 81, 38–44.

Rush, J.P., 1987. Rooming-in and visiting on the ward: effects on newborn colonization rates. Infect. Control 2 (Suppl. 3), 10–15.

Shrivastava, S.R., Shrivastava, P.S., Ramasamy, J., 2013. Fostering the practice of rooming-in in newborn care. J. Health Sci. 3 (2), 177–178.

Simmonds, N., 2011. Mana wahine: Decolonising politics. Women's Studies Journal. 25 (2), 11–25.

Stanway, A., Stanway, P., 1996. Breast is Best: A Common-Sense Approach to Breastfeeding. Pan Books, London, pp. 44–50.

Telofski, L.S., Morello, A.P., Mack Correa, M.C., Stamatas, G.N., 2012. The infant skin barrier: can we preserve, protect, and enhance the barrier? Dermatol Res. Pract. 2012, 198789. doi:10.1155/2012/198789.

Tollin, M., Bergsson, G., Kai-Larsen, Y., Lengqvist, J., Sjövall, J., Griffiths, W., et al., 2005. Vernix caseosa as a multi-component defence system based on polypeptides, lipids and their interactions. Cell Mol. Life Sci. 62 (19-20), 2390–2399.

Trotter, S., 2003. Management of the umbilical cord—a guide to best care. RCM Midwives 6 (7), 308–311.

Trotter, S., 2004. Care of the newborn: proposed new guidelines. BJM 12 (3), 152–157.

Trotter, S., 2013. Why no baby skincare product should be advertised or promoted as 'suitable for newborn skin'. Midirs Midwifery Digest. 23 (2), 217–221.

UNICEF, 2019. Skin-to-skin contact. Available from: https://www.unicef.org.uk/babyfriendly/baby-friendly-resources/implementing-standards-resources/skin-to-skin-contact/.

Vance, J., 1999. Beauty to die for: the cosmetic consequence. Available from: www.iuniverse.com.

Verd, S., 2007. Switch from antibiotic eye drops to instillation of mother's milk drops as a treatment of infant epiphora. J. Trop. Pediatr. 53 (1), 68–69.

Visscher, M.O., Adam, R., Brink, S., Odio, M., 2015. Newborn infant skin: physiology, development, and care. Clin. Dermatol. 33(3), 271–280. Available from: https://www.sciencedirect.com/science/article/pii/S0738081X14003022#!

Visscher, M.O., Narendran, V., 2014. Vernix caseosa: formation and functions. Newborn Infant Nurs. Rev. 14 (4), 142–146.

World Health Organization (WHO), 1998. Care of the Umbilical Cord: A Review of the Evidence. Reproductive Health (Technical Support), Maternal and Newborn Health/safe motherhood. WHO, Geneva.

Zupan, J., Garner, P., Omari, A.A., 2004. Topical umbilical cord care at birth. Cochrane Database Syst. Rev. (3), CD001057. doi:10.1002/14651858.CD001057.pub2.

14

Newborn Screening and Immunization

Sharon McDonald and Lindsey Rose

CHAPTER CONTENTS

The term *newborn screening* refers to a series of screening opportunities in the early weeks of life and is offered almost universally in some form or other. The screening mechanisms generally include the newborn blood spot test (metabolic screening of the newborn), newborn hearing screen and the newborn infant physical examination (NIPE). In the UK, the NIPE is undertaken up to 72 hours after birth and again by 8 weeks after birth, at which time commencement of the immunization programme is recommended (NHS, 2019a; PHE, 2017a; PHE, 2017b). In other countries, this schedule may vary.

This chapter focuses predominantly on the blood spot screening tests, but also encompasses the options for newborn hearing screening and screening for developmental dysplasia of the hips (DDH). The newborn screening options are offered to parents of newborn babies as part of the antenatal and newborn screening timeline identified by the UK National Screening Committee (UK NSC) (PHE, 2019) which was discussed in

Chapter 4 and is similar to pathways adopted in other countries. The examination of the hips as a component of the NIPE was discussed at length in Chapter 2, but is addressed further in this chapter because there has been considerable debate regarding the efficacy of screening methods and treatment of DDH.

BLOOD SPOT SCREENING (NEWBORN METABOLIC SCREENING)

The first newborn blood spot screening test was introduced in the United States in 1961 by Dr Robert Guthrie, who formulated the idea of using filter paper to collect drops of blood from a baby's heel. This method of using a specimen of dried blood was almost universally adopted and is now used for metabolic screening of the newborn throughout the world. Dr Guthrie went on to further the screening process by introducing the bacterial inhibition assay for phenylketonuria (PKU) which was used in all programmes in the first decades of newborn screening. The term *Guthrie test* has now been replaced by *blood spot* in the UK and some other countries, although the terms 'Guthrie' and 'heel prick' continue to be used by some practitioners and women alike.

The scope of the screening tool has changed dramatically in the intervening years. With the introduction of tandem mass spectrometry in the early 1980s, mass screening for metabolic conditions from single blood spots became possible. The range of conditions or disorders that can be detected from blood samples like those collected in the Newborn Screening Programme has increased exponentially; as we witness further advances in technology, we will see increasing potential for the screening of asymptomatic babies to identify other severe disorders (Bhattacharya et al., 2014).

Screening strategies for metabolic disorders vary markedly between countries, with some disorders proving to be more prevalent among certain ethnic groups and populations. Table 14.1 highlights the various screening options available in the UK and Australasia (the standard tests which are offered universally are denoted as such).

Since 2015, all babies in the United Kingdom have been offered the blood spot (cystic fibrosis screening has been universally offered since early 2007). It screens for nine conditions which, although rare, can be serious if early treatment does not commence. These are:

- sickle cell disease
- cystic fibrosis (CF)

- congenital hypothyroidism (CHT)
- six further inherited metabolic diseases (IMDs):
  - phenylketonuria (PKU)
  - medium chain acyl-CoA dehydrogenase deficiency (MCADD)
  - maple syrup urine disease (MSUD)
  - isovaleric acidaemia (IVA)
  - glutaric aciduria type 1 (GA1)
  - homocystinuria (pyridoxine unresponsive) (HCU).

In Australia, each state and territory is responsible for funding and operating their own program; universally, newborn blood spot screening includes PKU, CF and CHT; in a policy statement, the Human Genetics Society of Australia (O'Leary and Maxwell, 2015) argued in favour of incorporating screening for CF, congenital adrenal hyperplasia (CAH) and galactosaemia. In New Zealand, the number of tests routinely offered was extended in December 2006 to include 28 metabolic disorders, including PKU, biotinadase deficiency, CAH, CF, galactosaemia, MSUD and hypothyroidism (New Zealand Ministry of Health, 2020).

Newborn screening is discussed with parents by health professionals every day, and it is important that they understand the reasons why screening is offered, To refer back to the health literacy principles introduced in Chapter 11: it is easy for this discussion to become a 'routine' event for health professionals, but it is essential that the issues are discussed in detail with both sensitivity and awareness of cultural diversity (Table 14.2). Health professionals should have

TABLE 14.1 Screening Options Available in the UK and Australasia

Disorder	UK	Australasia
Phenylketonuria (PKU)	Universal	Universal
Congenital hypothyroidism (CHT)	Universal	Universal
Cystic fibrosis (CF)	Universal	Universal
Sickle cell disorders (SCD)	Universal	
Medium chain acyl-CoA dehydrogenase deficiency (MCADD)	Universal	
Galactosaemia		
Congenital adrenal hyperplasia (CAH)		
Hearing	Universal	Some states

TABLE 14.2 Some Reasons why Screening is Offered

- To enable early detection of presymptomatic newborns
- To ensure appropriate early treatment of newborns
- To ensure newborns born with congenital metabolic disorders have their development potential impacted as little as possible by the disease
- To inform the community of all aspects of newborn screening including advantages and outcomes
- To facilitate early diagnosis, appropriate treatment and continuous monitoring of specific metabolic diseases
- To facilitate continuous quality improvement through the development of a quality assurance, reporting and strategic planning framework
- To provide educational resources to parents and their families.

(PHE, 2019a)

accurate, up-to-date knowledge and understanding of the screening tests available, which will enable parents to make an informed choice. They need to be able to discuss fully with parents any concerns or queries they may have. The discussion should include the advantages and any risks of the tests, and establish whether the parents have offered explicit consent or wish to decline the tests; a summary of the discussion and the parents' final decision should be documented in the maternal notes (paper and/or electronic). The results of screening tests can have a huge impact on families and their significance should not be underestimated. It is essential that parents embark on their screening journey as fully prepared as possible for what may lie ahead. To facilitate parental discussion, health professionals should ensure parents are given adequate information; in the United Kingdom, the booklet *Screening Tests for You and Your Baby* is routinely distributed to women (PHE, 2017a).

Numerous support groups are available to help parents. It is impossible to list all of these; however, Antenatal Results and Choices (ARC) is an excellent resource for both health professionals and parents. It provides individualized information for parents during antenatal screening and offers longer-term help and support including forums and links to other parents, in addition to a range of publications for parents and professionals (ARC, 2019).

GUIDELINES FOR PRACTICE

In the United Kingdom, the blood spot screening procedure is carried out on day 5 (the day of birth being day 0) of life, regardless of gestation, medical condition or feeding status (PHE, 2016a), although this is not the same in other parts of the world; practitioners in New Zealand, for example, take the sample within 72 hours of birth. The UK guidelines for newborn blood spot sampling (PHE, 2016a) recommend that midwives ensure parents have been given the information leaflet, *Blood Spot Tests: an Easy Guide to Screening Tests for Your New Baby* (PHE, 2017c) a minimum of 24 hours before the test but, as discussed previously, ideally the leaflet should have been given in the third trimester of pregnancy to allow the parents time to absorb and digest the information.

All cards should be completed legibly and accurately. Where parents decline the test, this observation should be marked on the card, which is then sent to the laboratory as usual (PHE, 2016a). Midwives are required to advise parents that they may be contacted regarding further research into screening. However, parents can opt out of this; if so, the midwife must record this decision on the blood spot card. Antenatal and newborn screening quality assurance procedures, programme guidelines and literature are available online for practitioners and parents, in a number of languages. A summary is given in Table 14.3.

TABLE 14.3   **Guidelines for Newborn Blood Spot Sampling: Quick Reference Guide**
To take a newborn blood spot sample you will need: • NHS Screening Programme booklet *Screening Tests for You and Your Baby* • baby's NHS number (use of a bar-coded label is recommended) • blood spot card and glassine envelope • personal child health record (PCHR, Red Book) and maternity/professional record • water for cleansing • nonsterile protective gloves • age-appropriate automated incision device • sharps box • cotton wool/gauze • hypoallergenic spot plaster (if required) • prepaid/stamped addressed envelope (first class) if not using a courier.
Collecting the Blood Spot Sample:
• Sample takers should check that consent for screening has been obtained and recorded.
• Recommend comfort measures for the baby.
• Ensure the baby is cuddled and in a secure position; suggest breastfeeding.
• Clean the heel by washing thoroughly with plain water and cotton wool/gauze. The water should not be heated and the baby's foot should not be immersed. Do not use alcohol or alcohol wipes.
• Allow the heel to dry completely.
• Wash hands and apply gloves.
• Ensure the baby is warm and comfortable. Warming of the foot is not required.

TABLE 14.3 Guidelines for Newborn Blood Spot Sampling: Quick Reference Guide—cont'd

- Obtain the sample using an age-appropriate automated incision device (manual lancets must not be used). An arched-shaped incision device is recommended. (Fig. 14.1 show preferred puncture sites).
- Avoid posterior curvature of the heel.
- Allow the heel to hang down to assist blood flow.
- Before activation, place the automated incision device against the heel in accordance with the manufacturer's instructions.

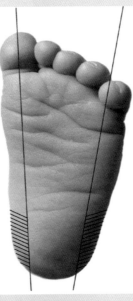

Fig. 14.1 Heel punch areas for full-term and preterm infants

If blood flow ceases, the congealed blood should be wiped away firmly with cotton wool or gauze. Gently massage the foot (avoid squeezing) and drop the blood onto the card. If the baby is not bleeding, perform a second puncture on a different part of the same foot or on the other foot.

When sample collection is complete, wipe excess blood from the heel and apply gentle pressure to the wound with cotton wool or gauze. Apply a hypoallergenic spot plaster if required, and remind parents to remove it in a few hours.

Allow blood spots to air-dry away from direct sunlight or heat before placing in the glassine envelope—take care to avoid contamination. If not using a courier, despatch the blood spot card in the prepaid/stamped addressed envelope (first class) on the same day. If not possible, despatch within 24 hours. Despatch should not be delayed in order to batch blood spot cards together for postage. If a post box is used, ensure it is emptied daily (Monday to Saturday). Before sending the sample to the laboratory, there should be no additional checking that would cause delay. Record that the sample has been taken in the PCHR and maternity/professional record, complying with local protocols. If the baby is in hospital, record and notify the baby's screening status on discharge/transfer notifications. Inform parents that they will receive the results within 6 weeks, or sooner if the baby screens positive for a condition. Ensure that parents know to contact their health visitor if results are not received within 6 weeks.

Continued

TABLE 14.3   Guidelines for Newborn Blood Spot Sampling: Quick Reference Guide—cont'd

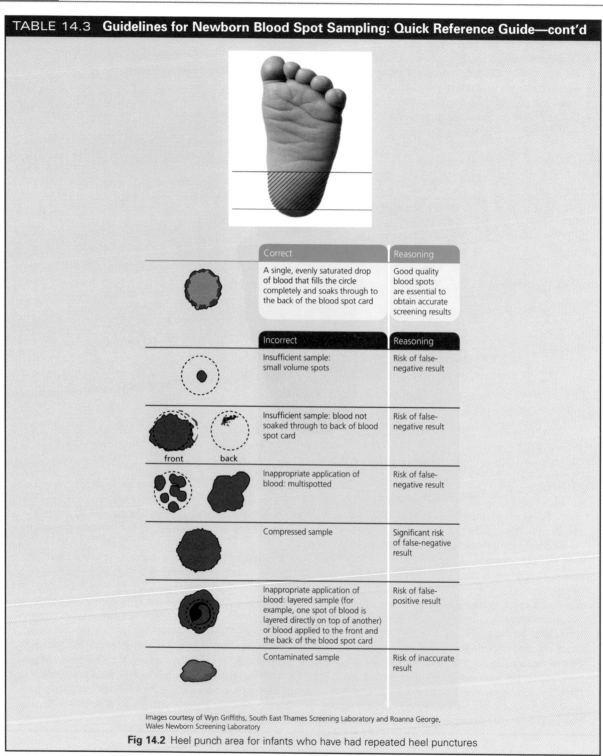

Correct		Reasoning
	A single, evenly saturated drop of blood that fills the circle completely and soaks through to the back of the blood spot card	Good quality blood spots are essential to obtain accurate screening results

Incorrect		Reasoning
	Insufficient sample: small volume spots	Risk of false-negative result
front back	Insufficient sample: blood not soaked through to back of blood spot card	Risk of false-negative result
	Inappropriate application of blood: multispotted	Risk of false-negative result
	Compressed sample	Significant risk of false-negative result
	Inappropriate application of blood: layered sample (for example, one spot of blood is layered directly on top of another) or blood applied to the front and the back of the blood spot card	Risk of false-positive result
	Contaminated sample	Risk of inaccurate result

Images courtesy of Wyn Griffiths, South East Thames Screening Laboratory and Roanna George, Wales Newborn Screening Laboratory

Fig 14.2 Heel punch area for infants who have had repeated heel punctures

After Taking the Blood Sample

It is important that the laboratory receives the blood sample promptly to ensure that babies screening positive for any of the conditions are referred quickly. In most cases, the results will be available by 8 weeks, unless a problem is identified earlier.

CURRENT TESTS IN THE UK AND OTHER COUNTRIES

We will now look at the metabolic conditions that are currently tested for in the United Kingdom, and some of the other disorders commonly screened for in Australasia and other parts of the world. *Metabolic disorders* are inherited genetic conditions caused by enzyme abnormalities or deficiencies. These abnormalities cause an interruption in the metabolic pathway, resulting in an increase or decrease in the level of one or more chemicals necessary for normal functioning. Early detection of these disorders allows early and effective treatment of the symptoms and the prevention of long-term effects, such as irreversible brain damage and intellectual disabilities within the first few months of life; however, it is important to note that there is no 'cure' for these disorders. There are dozens of metabolic disorders, and they are identified either by the substance which cannot be metabolized properly or by the part of the metabolic pathway in which the problem occurs.

Phenylketonuria (PKU)

Phenylketonuria (PKU) is an autosomal recessive metabolic disorder that affects an individual's ability to metabolize phenylalanine, an amino acid present in many foods that is converted into tyrosine, which is essential for tissue growth and brain development. The incidence of PKU varies widely between ethnic groups and different populations. However, in the United Kingdom, European populations and Australasia the estimated incidence is 1:10,000 births. In African American populations, PKU is extremely rare.

PKU was identified in 1934 by Ivar Asbjørn Følling, who noticed that there was a link between hyperphenylalaninaemia and irreversible brain damage. Følling found that a diet that restricted phenylalanine-rich foods improved the cognitive function of affected patients, and this remains the course of treatment for those affected by PKU today. Phenylalanine-rich foods

include milk, eggs and other dairy products, including formula and breast milk, and artificial sweeteners such as aspartame. Babies born with PKU present as normal at birth, however, if the condition is left untreated, affected infants will initially fail to reach their developmental milestones. They can develop an eczema-type rash and lighter colouring of the hair, skin and eyes. Some babies will become cerebrally impaired; this can present as hyperactivity, microcephaly and seizures.

Hyperphenylalaninaemia can result from causes other than PKU, but PKU is the most widely recognized cause.

Congenital Hypothyroidism (CHT)

Congenital hypothyroidism (CHT) is the inadequate production of thyroid hormones in the newborn and can be due to a number of reasons; it may result from an absent or nonfunctioning thyroid gland. The cause is often genetic, but many cases are sporadic and a cause is not identified. Primarily, CHT is seen in geographical areas where there are low levels of iodine, resulting in endemic congenital hypothyroidism. This has been overcome in affected Western countries by the addition of iodine to foods including salt, milk and bread. The incidence of CHT in the United Kingdom is reported as 1:3000 births (Morgan and Pylypiw, 2015) and varies worldwide from 1:2500 to 1:5500; incidences as high as 1:1570 have been reported in the United Arab Emirates. This is due to the variation in levels of endemic CHT; isolated parts of Bangladesh, Chad, China, Indonesia, Nepal, Peru and Zaire still have endemic CHT today. African populations are thought to have a lower risk, while individuals from Indian, Pakistani and Bangladeshi origin are at greater risk of CHT (Bagcchi, 2014).

Untreated severe CHT in newborn infants can result in failure to grow appropriately and moderate to severe cognitive impairment. Infants born with CHT present initially as normal babies; prior to the introduction of screening, CHT was usually only diagnosed when symptoms of brain impairment presented. Where CHT is diagnosed at an early stage through the blood spot test, it can be successfully and simply treated with a daily dose of oral thyroxine.

Sickle Cell Disorders (SCD)

Screening for sickle cell disorders is an integral part of the newborn blood spot screening programme in the United Kingdom, and the test will detect a large number of haemoglobin variants. Some of the variant haemoglobin has no clinical significance and the detection of these variants is not the primary aim of the screening programme; however, it is important that parents are made aware of this possibility before they consent to the screening test (PHE 2018a). See Chapter 4 for information about haemoglobinopathies.

Where only one copy of the sickle haemoglobin chain gene has been inherited along with one normal haemoglobin gene, the individual is a carrier for sickle cell disease and can pass the gene on. This carrier status is also known as sickle cell trait. Carriers are not affected by crises, but may need extra care during general anaesthetics.

Other Inherited Metabolic Diseases

The following four inherited metabolic diseases are rare; however, all babies in the United Kingdom are screened for these conditions (PHE, 2016a).

Glutaric Aciduria Type 1 (GA1)

This condition affects 1:110,000 babies worldwide. It is caused by a difficulty in breaking down the amino acids hydroxy lysine and tryptophan.

Maple Syrup Urine Disease (MSUD)

Maple syrup urine disease (MSUD) affects 1:116,000 babies in the United Kingdom. It is caused by a difficulty in breaking down the amino acids leucine, isoleucin and valine.

Homocystinuria (Pyridoxine Unresponsive) (HCU)

Homocystinuria (HCU) affects 1:144,000 babies in the United Kingdom. It prevents the breakdown of the amino acid methionine, causing a build-up of methionine and another chemical called homocysteine. It can be harmful if left untreated.

Isovaleric Acidaemia (IVA)

The incidence worldwide is unknown. Babies with IVA do not have the enzyme that breaks down the amino acid leucine into isovaleric acid, which is then converted into energy. This leads to harmful high levels of isovaleric acid in the baby's system.

Cystic Fibrosis (CF)

Cystic fibrosis (CF) is an inherited genetic condition that affects an estimated 100,000 people globally. In the United Kingdom, it is the commonest life-threatening inherited disease, affecting 1:2500 babies; approximately 1:20 people carry a CF mutation. Cystic fibrosis is an autosomal recessive condition caused by a range of mutations of the same gene; however, the mutation ΔF508 is responsible for 90% to 95% of cases in the United Kingdom. Cystic fibrosis affects mainly populations of European origin. (PHE, 2016a).

Cystic fibrosis affects the infant's lungs and bowel due to the production of thicker mucoid secretions, which make affected individuals prone to chest infections, lung damage and malabsorption of their food. In the longer term, there may be fertility issues. The screening test in babies is only reliable up to 8 weeks of age (56 days). Early diagnosis allows for prompt treatment, diet modification and physiotherapy; today, with significant improvements in treatment, life expectancy for affected individuals has improved—more than half of individuals now live beyond 47 years of age. Due to the advances in treatment and understanding of the condition, it is anticipated that the life expectancy of babies born now will be even further improved (Cystic Fibrosis Trust, 2019).

Medium Chain acyl-CoA Dehydrogenase Deficiency (MCADD)

Medium chain acyl-CoA dehydrogenase deficiency (MCADD) is a deficiency in one of the enzymes used to break down fats and make energy for the body; it is an inborn error of metabolism. It affects approximately 1:10,000 babies born in the United Kingdom.

If diagnosed early, MCADD can be managed effectively; affected children develop normally through regular meals and modification of their diet. Symptoms of MCADD can be poor feeding, drowsiness, vomiting and seizures. Untreated MCADD may lead to serious illness or sometimes death (NHS, 2019b).

Galactosaemia

Galactosaemia is an inherited condition which is routinely screened for in the United States and New Zealand as part of the newborn blood spot screen, but is not part of routine screening in the United Kingdom. It is a metabolic disorder with a varied incidence of live births worldwide between 1:20,000 and 1:47,000 (Welling et al., 2017; Tidy and Bonsall, 2015).

Galactosaemia is caused by the inability of the body to digest galactose properly. Galactose is a by-product of the metabolism of lactose, which is present in dairy products and breast milk (Frye, 2007). There are several different types of galactosaemia which are caused by deficiencies of different enzymes. Classic galactosaemia is caused by a deficiency in galactose-1-phosphate uridyl transferase (GALT). If not identified through screening, this condition presents as vomiting, liver enlargement and jaundice within the first few days of ingesting lactose. Liver, kidney, eye and brain damage may occur if it is left untreated. The only treatment for galactosemia is to eliminate lactose from the diet.

Congenital Adrenal Hyperplasia (CAH)

At the time of writing, congenital adrenal hyperplasia (CAH) is not universally screened for in the UK. This condition has a number of genetic causes, but all lead to a defect in the synthesis of cortisol from cholesterol in the adrenal glands, which in turn affects the production of hormones governing the development of sexual characteristics (Rull and Bonsall, 2018). Classical CAH occurs in 1:18,000 births in the United Kingdom. Non-classical CAH occurs in between 1:100 and 1:1000 births, depending of the ethnic origin of the population; there is a higher prevalence in Ashkenazi Jews (1:27), Hispanic populations (1:40) and Italians (1:300). Classical CAH may result in adrenal failure and salt wasting. Affected individuals can be treated with appropriate medication such as glucocorticoids (Cares Foundation, 2019).

HEARING SCREENING

A newborn hearing screening programme (NHSP) was introduced in the United Kingdom in 2006 and in New Zealand in 2009 (NSU, 2016); other countries also introduced programmes around the same time. The introduction of screening was a significant development in improving the lives both of babies born with a hearing loss and of their families (NSU, 2016). Hearing screening aims to identify moderate, severe and profound hearing loss in newborn babies in one or both ears (AAP, 2007). There are many screening pathways around the world using different technologies and varying protocols; hence it is important for midwives to be familiar with their local pathways for both well babies and those who receive NICU care (PHE, 2017a; NSU, 2016; NHS, 2015).

It is estimated that each year, up to 2 babies per 1000 are born with a permanent hearing loss in one or both ears (PHE, 2016b). Of those, more than half will have had no previously identified risk factors (PHE, 2016b); in the United Kingdom, that equates to approximately 1000 babies each year. Prior to the screening programmes, over a quarter of babies born with a hearing loss were not identified until they were at least 3{1/2} years old, which led to significant developmental and communication delays (JICH, 2007). The benefits of early identification in newborns include improved language skills and significantly improved speech, better social and emotional development, and improved educational and employment opportunities. If hearing loss is identified early and interventions put in place, the baby will develop communication skills equal to those of their hearing peers (Yoshinaga-Itano, 2014; Ching et al., 2018).

Hearing screening should be undertaken early in the postnatal period and ideally by 1 month of age; the most common goal of international programmes is to complete hearing screening by 1 month, so that an audiology diagnosis can occur by 3 months and interventions can be put in place by 6 months. Meeting these goals ensures the best possible outcomes for the baby, because the first 6 to 12 months are critical for communication and speech development (PHE, 2016b).

The hearing screening test takes a few minutes and is painless. It is a cost-effective, reliable, quick and simple screening mechanism and is, importantly, acceptable to most parents. The screening tests can identify if a baby has a higher risk of having hearing loss and requires further diagnostic testing by audiology; it is important to note that hearing screening cannot identify hearing loss, only those who have a greater risk of having it. Two screening tests are available and in common use: automated otoacoustic emissions (AOAE) and automated auditory brainstem response (AABR). There are different pathways in different countries that determine whether a baby will have an AOAE once or twice and then an AABR before being referred to audiology. Some countries only use AABR screening, and a baby has two opportunities to pass the screen before being referred to audiology (NSU, 2016).

For the AOAE screen (Fig. 14.3A), a small, soft earpiece is placed in the baby's ear canal and soft clicking sounds are played to stimulate the outer hair cells of the cochlea. These cells produce sound in response to the stimulus, and this sound is picked up by a microphone in the earpiece; the machine decodes the sound and registers a 'pass' or a 'refer' result. In the United Kingdom, if a clear response is not achieved in both ears (possible causes include amniotic fluid, temporary blockage in the ear, and hearing loss) from this first screen, the hearing screener will repeat the test a minimum of one hour later. If no clear response is achieved at the second attempt, an AABR screen is carried out (once only). An AABR screen takes slightly longer. Again a soft clicking stimulus is utilized, but this time via ear muffs and sensors which are placed on the baby's head and neck (Fig. 14.3B). These sensors detect the electrical response when the sound is transmitted from the inner ear via the inner hair cells of the cochlea and the auditory nerve. This is a more sensitive and specific test.

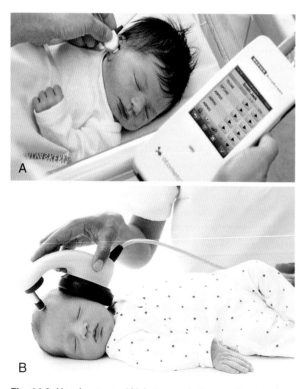

Fig. 14.3 Hearing tests. **(A)** Automated otoacoustic emissions (AOAE) hearing test (UK). **(B)** Automated auditory brainstem response (AABR) hearing test (NZ).

If the baby does not pass either test or a clear response cannot be obtained, this could indicate a possible hearing loss, so a referral is made to the appropriate audiology department for diagnostic testing.

Risk Factors for Hearing Loss

Babies who have one or more identified risk factors for hearing loss following a passed hearing screen require further follow-up in early childhood so as to detect any progressive hearing loss. One of the more common risk factors is a *family history* of permanent congenital hearing loss. In some countries, even if the baby passes the screen, they will be offered another screen before 18 months of age; other countries do not offer this rescreen. *Cytomegalovirus* (CMV) is the other significant risk factor for hearing loss and is the most common noninherited cause. Even if a baby with confirmed CMV passes the hearing screen, they will commonly be clinically assessed until the age of 5 because there is a significant risk of developing progressive hearing loss (Dumanch, 2017). For this reason, it is very important that midwives pass on information to hearing screening programmes and/or screeners about confirmed CMV infections in pregnancy (especially primary infections). Hearing screeners should also be informed about women who have had toxoplasmosis and rubella in pregnancy because these infections also increase the risk of hearing loss in the baby.

Sharing Information with the Woman and Family

It is important that informed consent is obtained prior to screening. Information brochures are available and should be provided in different languages. Information is also shared verbally by the newborn hearing screeners and any questions answered. As with all screening tests, the way in which practitioners communicate news about the test and subsequent screening or referral can have a significant impact on parents' perceptions and feelings, especially in the early postnatal period. Additional information and videos are available from the NHS website (NHS, 2018a) and the New Zealand National Screening Unit websites. Families whose baby is diagnosed with a hearing loss will receive care from a range of different health professionals and services including audiologists, hearing aid technicians, ear, nose and throat specialists, cochlear implant services, advisors on deaf children and genetics services. Ideally, families will be offered local community support groups; in the United Kingdom, these include the National Deaf Children's Society and Hearing Link.

DEVELOPMENTAL DYSPLASIA OF THE HIP (DDH)

The hip is a ball (femoral head) and socket (acetabulum) joint composed chiefly of cartilage, which is relatively soft in the newborn. Developmental dysplasia of the hip (DDH) is an abnormal formation of the hip joint in which the acetabulum is insufficiently formed, leading to instability or complete dislocation. Deviations may have occurred during the embryonic period or may develop in infancy. Developmental dysplasia of the hip should not be confused with congenital dislocation of the hip (CDH), which was the term previously used to describe any condition associated with hip anomalies. It was previously thought that the problem originated in utero and was present at birth; however, it is now understood and recognized that a hip may appear normal at birth and become dysplastic or malformed later.

The cause of DDH is not fully known, though the condition is thought to be multifactorial and dependent on geographical, ethnic and familial influences (Jones, 1998; Sahin et al., 2004). An estimated 1–2 per 1000 babies have a hip problem that requires treatment. However, the incidence is difficult to determine fully, because many hips which were unstable in the newborn spontaneously resolve within the first 2 to 4 weeks of birth; it is reported that as many as 1 in 80 hips have some instability at birth, and by 6 weeks 60–80% will have resolved without intervention (Taperro and Honeyfield, 2019). It is believed that this high level of false positive screening occurs because of maternal hormones circulating in the infant's bloodstream; as the levels diminish, the hip muscles will tighten up and stabilize. However, delayed diagnosis can result in abnormal growth of the acetabulum and contraction of the muscles around the hips; the consequent reduction in leg length can result in chronic pain.

Screening for DDH is essential for the early detection of this condition. Following a 2019 review of the DDH pathway, the most up-to-date UK guidance is available at https://www.gov.uk/topic/population-screening-programmes/newborn-infant-physical-examination. Practice and clinical opinion vary within the UK and Australasia—specifically in relation to which manoeuvre to undertake first—but what is consistent is the practice of performing two manoeuvres: the Ortolani (to determine if the hip is dislocated) and the Barlow (to determine if the hip is dislocatable). These two manoeuvres are described in detail in Chapter 2. If there is neonatal hip instability, this is described as a *positive Ortolani or Barlow sign*. The evidence suggests that the practitioner's skill and ability to detect and diagnose the condition early on results in better outcomes for the newborn thanks to prompt treatment (NHS, 2018b; PHE, 2018b).

Diagnosis and Screening

By gathering a family history, practitioners will be alerted to the reported risk factors associated with DDH; these are outlined in Table 14.4 (Sahin et al., 2004, Gill and O'Brien, 2007). The Ortolani and Barlow manoeuvres are an effective and well-established way of identifying the possible presence of DDH in many cases.

The following points are important to remember:
- Undertake both the Ortolani and Barlow manoeuvres on each hip separately.
- The Ortolani manoeuvre is used to screen for a dislocated hip.
- The Barlow manoeuvre is used to screen for a dislocatable hip.
- Do not perform the Barlow manoeuvre if there is a positive Ortolani.

Screen Negative

If no abnormality is detected, the baby will continue on to the usual route for well child provision. However, parents should be advised to contact their midwife, GP or health visitor if they have concerns about their baby's hips. In particular, they should note if:
- There is a difference in the deep skin creases of the thighs between the two legs;
- One leg cannot be moved out sideways as far as the other when changing the nappy;
- One leg seems to be longer than the other;
- A click can be felt or heard in one or both hips;
- One leg drags when their baby starts crawling;
- Their child walks with a limp or has a 'waddling' gait.

Screen Positive

This should be assumed when the assessor finds some or all of the following:
- Difficulty in abducting the hip to 90 degrees;
- A difference in leg length;

TABLE 14.4 **Risk Factors for Developmental Dysplasia of the Hips (DDH)**	
Family history (first-degree relative)	A genetic predisposition to DDH has been shown in a number of studies (i.e., inherited joint or ligament laxity or malformation of the acetabulum) (Jones, 1998).
Female infants	Females are up to 8 times more at risk than male infants. A reaction to the maternal hormone oestrogen causes ligaments surrounding the hip to become lax. Male infants produce androgens which provide a degree of protection against the maternal hormones.
First-born infants	Fetal movements may be restricted due to an unstretched uterus and tight abdominal muscles. Seen in oligohydramnios.
Breech presentation	Increased risk is associated with babies with a history of transient breech or breech position at delivery. The relationship is believed to be a mechanical one whereby the breech position results in increased flexion of the hip and therefore decreased movement. The ligaments surrounding the hips will become lax, causing the femur to dislocate from the acetabulum. Infants in the frank breech position are considered to be more at risk because there is adduction of the hips and hyperextension of the knees.
Multiple gestation	Fetal movements are restricted.
Oligohydramnios	Fetal movements are restricted.
Large for gestational age (LGA) babies	Fetal movements are restricted.
DDH presenting in the newborn period occurs three times more often on the left than on the right.	This is thought to be due to the left occiput anterior position of most newborns who lie in the vertex position, placing the left hip posteriorly against the mother's spine. This position may limit movement of the left leg and contribute to DDH.
Musculoskeletal deformity	Increased incidence in babies with positional talipes and other postural deformities.

- The knees are at different levels when the hips and knees are bilaterally flexed (Allis sign);
- Asymmetry of groin skin folds when the baby is in ventral suspension;
- A palpable *clunk* when undertaking either the Ortolani or Barlow manoeuvres.

Babies who are found to have dislocated or dislocatable hips should be referred for ultrasound of the hip within two weeks of birth.

Screen Negative Examination With Risk Factors

If babies have additional risk factors (see Table 14.4) but have a normal outcome (i.e., are screen negative) on the hip assessment, they should be referred for ultrasound of the hip within 6 weeks of birth.

Screen Positive Following 6- to 8-week Infant Examination

The effectiveness of the Ortolani and Barlow manoeuvres is reduced by 6 to 8 weeks, which has implications for practitioners carrying out the ongoing assessment at that time. This is because, as the hips continue to develop and muscle tone improves, if the hip is already dislocated, the manoeuvres are not necessarily conclusive. When examining the older infant, practitioners are encouraged not to perform the Ortolani manoeuvre but to look closely for unequal leg length, asymmetrical skin folds and limited hip abduction; GPs and health visitors should be monitoring for DDH until a child is walking. Parents should also be given information and advice related to the condition, and be made aware of the risks of late treatment. If the baby is screen positive, an urgent referral should be made to an orthopaedic surgeon for expert opinion, and the baby should be seen by age 10 weeks.

A plan of care is based on the findings of the examination and will vary from country to country; in the United Kingdom, ultrasound screening of the hips prior to discharge (or within 6 weeks) is the recommended screening method for babies with identified risk factors.

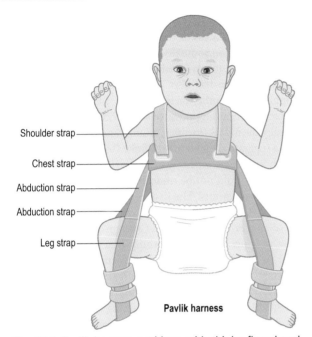

Fig. 14.4 Pavlik harness positions with thighs flexed and abducted. (Adapted from Cooperman DR, Thompson GH (2002) Neonatal Orthpedics. In: Fanaroff AA, Maris R J (eds) Neonatal-perinatal medicine: diseases of the fetus and newborn, 7th edn, pp. 1603–1632 with permission from Mosby, St Louis).

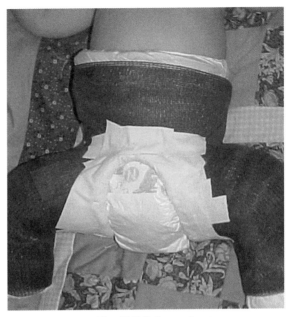

Fig. 14.5 Spica cast.

Additionally, suspicions raised by the presence of asymmetrical gluteal folds, increased femur length or joint laxity should alert the practitioner to the possible value of further screening (PHE, 2018b).

If treatment is required, the baby is usually placed in a Pavlik harness (Fig. 14.4) for about 4 months. This treatment stabilizes the hip joint by promoting hip flexion and abduction and preventing hip extension or adduction. It is important to note that this noninvasive treatment does not mean further treatment will not be required; such treatment could involve traction or closed reduction of the hip (surgery in which the physician, guided by x-ray, manipulates the hip and relocates it), followed by the application of a Spica cast (Fig. 14.5). The Pavlik harness, which positions the baby with thighs flexed and abducted, is not advised after 6 months of age. The use of x-rays is not recommended until an infant is 3 months old and ultrasound is not effective after 6 to 8 months because the hip will have become ossified. The use of double or triple nappies as a form of treatment is now contraindicated.

TESTES

The UK National Screening Committee emphasizes the importance of detecting the presence of testes in the newborn period, and the need for prompt referral if testes remain undescended or nonpalpable in the scrotal sac at the 6- to 8-week check (PHE, 2018b). However, this part of the NIPE has not been discussed to any great extent in the literature. A detailed description of the practical examination of the testes is included in Chapter 2.

The term *undescended testes*, also called *cryptorchidism*, refers to 'a testis or testes that assumes an extrascrotal location'. At 28 weeks, the testes are located in the abdominal cavity, hence cryptorchidism is much more common in preterm infants. By term, more than 95% of testes will be fully descended and should be palpable in the scrotum (Tappero and Honeyfield, 2019).

Undescended testicles may descend without intervention within the first 3 months of life. If the testicle remains undescended after this time, the cryptorchidism should be corrected because undescended testicles are associated with inguinal hernia, infertility, testicular torsion and testicular tumour (Tappero and Honeyfield, 2019).

Treatment options include surgical correction and hormonal therapy. Although treatment aims to reduce the risks of infertility and testicular cancer, this cannot be guaranteed in the long term. Surgery for undescended testes is therefore the recommended treatment of choice. Ideally, surgery is performed before the infant is 2 years old, with the best outcomes when done within the first year. Due to the potential serious sequelae of undescended testes as identified above, the 6- to 8-week check and subsequent developmental checks provide general practitioners and health visitors with an ideal opportunity to discuss and reiterate the importance of testicular self-examination for future health.

IMMUNIZATION

Immunization aims to protect individuals and to prevent disease spreading, both to those children who are too ill to be immunized and to the general population (WHO, 2014). It is estimated that 2.5 million deaths per year globally are prevented as a result of immunization programmes.

Live vaccines contain small amounts of the virus or bacterium that causes a specific disease; these stimulate the immune system to produce antibodies against that microorganism and protect the individual from possible future infection. However, children who are immunosuppressed should not be given a live vaccine; furthermore, if the child is hypersensitive, unwell or has an infection—for example, of the gastrointestinal tract—then the vaccine may well be ineffective (WHO, 2014).

The vaccines in the immunization programme are free for all children and until the late 1990s, uptake was increasing steadily (WHO, 2014; Brewer et al., 2017). However, some areas of the United Kingdom have seen a recent increase in some diseases, mainly due to the popularity of travel to places where the disease may be more prevalent; there has also been an increase in transient populations. Another factor has been the concerns raised by parents regarding possible side effects of vaccines, specifically the MMR (measles, mumps and rubella) injection and a suggestion that it may be linked to autism—a link for which there is no scientific evidence (Hviid et al., 2019).

What should not be underestimated is the effect this has had on parents. The decline and/or delay in uptake of the MMR vaccine is almost certainly a reflection of these concerns; with the ever-increasing availability of new vaccines, this is something practitioners need to bear in mind when they are conveying information to parents (see Chapter 15). To address this, parents need to have the opportunity to discuss their concerns with the health professional administering the vaccine. They need to be informed, rather than morally cajoled, when presenting their offspring for what can feel like endless rounds of injections. The moral and ethical debate around the immunization programme and parents being given informed choice is beyond the remit of this chapter; the subject is emotive and not to be taken lightly. Up-to-date, detailed information about vaccines and their side effects is available for both practitioners and parents at www.immunisation.nhs.uk.

The UK immunization programme is based on up-to-date evidence and changes are made accordingly. The current NHS recommendations for routine childhood immuizations can be seen in Table 14.5.

TABLE 14.5 Childhood Immunizations for Babies Up to 18 Years of Age: Routine Childhood Immunization Programme

Each Vaccination Is Given as a Single Injection Into the Muscle of the Thigh or Upper Arm.

When to Immunize	Diseases Protected Against	Vaccine Given
2 months	Diphtheria, tetanus, pertussis (whooping cough), polio and *Haemophilus influenza* type b (Hib), pneumococcal infection	DTaP/IPV/Hib and pneumococcal conjugate vaccine (PCV)
3 months	Diphtheria, tetanus, pertussis, polio and *Haemophilus influenza* type b (Hib), meningitis C (meningococcal C)	DTaP/IPV/Hib and MenC
4 months	Diphtheria, tetanus, pertussis, polio and *Haemophilus influenza* type b (Hib), meningitis C, pneumococcal infection	DTaP/IPV/Hib, MenC and PCV

TABLE 14.5 Childhood Immunizations for Babies Up to 18 Years of Age: Routine Childhood Immunization Programme—Cont'd

Each Vaccination Is Given as a Single Injection Into the Muscle of the Thigh or Upper Arm.

When to Immunize	Diseases Protected Against	Vaccine Given
Around 12 months	*Haemophilus influenza* type b (Hib) and meningitis C	Hib/MenC
Around 13 months	Measles, mumps and rubella (German measles), pneumococcal infection	MMR and PCV
3 years 4 months to 5 years	Diphtheria, tetanus, pertussis and polio, measles, mumps and rubella	DTaP/IPV or dTaP/IPV and MMR
13 to 18 years	Tetanus, diphtheria and polio	Td/IPV

The BCG (Bacillus Calmette–Guérin) vaccine, which gives protection against tuberculosis (TB), is recommended for all babies born in areas of the UK where the rates of TB are high, or who have a parent or grandparent born in a country with a high rate of TB, or who will be travelling to a high risk area (NHS, 2016).

CONCLUSION

This chapter has explored a range of the newborn screening tests that are offered to families. Sensitivity and empathy are essential when discussing screening with parents and families; the first few days in the life of a newborn are exciting, but for many, may also contain anxiety and uncertainty. For this reason, discussion of the options for screening tests should ideally be introduced in the antenatal period.

Any health professional discussing screening has a responsibility to undertake relevant training and regular updates and to make themselves aware of the numerous resources available to support their practice and facilitate informed choice. This should enable them to give a full and frank discussion of the possible consequences of the screening tests which are currently available.

Dottie and Patsie's story

Development Dysplasia of the Hip

My first daughter, Dottie, was born in 2013. After a great pregnancy, I was told at my 34 weeks check that baby's head was already engaged, which was good to know. My contractions started when I was nearly 40 weeks—I stayed at home for as long as possible, finally going into hospital with my partner Mitch, where I was found to be 4 cm dilated. I had an epidural when I was about 5 cm, which was great and I felt a lot more comfortable. I was being monitored every so often by my midwife. I was there about 3 hours when the baby's heart rate kept slowing and so she examined me to see how I was dilating—it was at that point that my waters burst and she said I was 9 cm. With the waters came meconium, and the midwife realized it was the baby's bottom that was making my waters bulge and not the head. Baby was in a breech position. I was given the choice to continue to labour but after being told of the risks, we decided it was probably safer to have an emergency caesarean. Dottie was born soon after.

Fast forward 8 weeks and we went to the hospital for Dottie's 8-week hip check appointment. I was told it was just a routine hip check because she'd been breech. I remember being really anxious, not knowing if she was going to be OK and not really knowing what to expect, so I was shocked and got really upset when they said she would need a Pavlik harness. I had no idea what that was or what it would mean. She had to have the harness on for the next 6 weeks until her hip joints were correctly in the sockets. All her scans came back normal and she doesn't have any problems with her hips now.

My second daughter, Patsie, was born in 2017. This was a totally different experience labour-wise; I'd been to a VBAC (vaginal birth after caesarean) talk and opted to try for a normal birth after a scan confirmed she was head first. Again, I stayed at home as long as I could, finally going into hospital when I was 7 cm dilated. I only had gas and air and within 1½ hours my waters went—after two

Continued

Dottie and Patsie's story

really intense contractions, I wanted to push. Patsie was born vaginally following a very quick labour.

We received a scan appointment for Patsie for when she was 8 weeks old. She hadn't been breech and I went along assuming I would be in and out pretty quickly—I even said to Mitch, 'I can't imagine I'll be in there long, it's just a routine check' and we only got the appointment because Dottie had been breech, so he didn't come. In fact, the ultrasonographer said, 'you'd be surprised at how many people don't turn up for this scan'. When they said she would probably have to have the Pavlik Harness (Fig. 14.4) as both hips were out of the sockets, it was worse than it had been for Dottie! I think I was just in shock and remember thinking, I can't believe this—if it wasn't for Dottie, we would never have had the appointment and I wouldn't have known. I waited to see the consultant and he confirmed she needed the harness.

After 6 weeks, they said the harness needed to stay on for a further 6 weeks. They took the harness off after that, but at the routine appointment 4 weeks later, they said one side was still not in properly and the harness had to go back on—I was told it would probably resolve itself but it was safer to have it on. The harness was taken off when she was around 6 months old. I had to go back once she was walking, and thankfully everything was OK.

Looking back, Patsie was fine, but it was a really stressful time. The harness could only come off for 1 hour at a

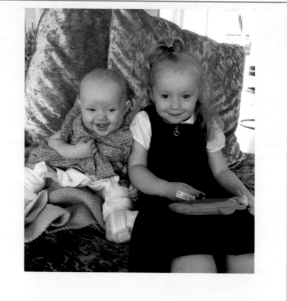

time when she had a bath, so for 23 hours a day it was on, it was really restricting and difficult changing her. I really didn't think she would have needed this and it was only because Dottie was breech we got it, but I really had no idea what to expect. There was no family history of hip problems in my family or Mitch's; although he did have irritable hip when he was younger, I was told that had nothing to do with it.

KEY POINTS

- Metabolic disorders are inherited genetic conditions caused by enzyme abnormalities or deficiencies.
- Audit data show that more than 99% of babies born in the United Kingdom are screened for some metabolic disorders.
- The blood spot screening procedure is carried out on day 5 of life regardless of gestation, medical condition or feeding status.
- It is important that the laboratory receives the blood sample promptly to ensure that babies screening positive for any of the conditions are seen quickly.
- It is estimated that each year, up to 2 babies per 1000 are born with some form of hearing loss (profound, severe or moderate).

- The benefits of early detection of hearing loss include improved communication skills and significantly improved speech, social and emotional development.
- Physical examinations by well-trained practitioners have been identified as the most important method by which to detect DDH.
- The effectiveness of the Barlow and Ortolani manoeuvres is reduced by 6 to 8 weeks.

REFERENCES

American Academy of Paediatrics (AAP), 2007. Position Statement: Principles and Guidelines for Early Hearing Detection and Intervention Programs. Joint Committee on Infant Hearing. www.pediatrics.org/cgi/doi/10.1542/peds.2007-2333

Antenatal Results and Choices (ARC), 2019. https://www.arc-uk.org/about-arc

Bagcchi, S, 2014. Hypothyroidism in India https://www.thelancet.com/pdfs/journals/landia/PIIS2213-8587(14)70208-6.pdf

Bhattacharya, K., Wotton, T., Wiley, V., 2014. The evolution of blood-spot newborn screening. Transl. Pediatr. 3(2), 63–70. https://www.ncbi.nlm.nih.gov/pmc/articles/PMC4729101/

Brewer, N.T., Chapman, G.B., Rothman, A.J., et al., 2018. Increasing vaccination: putting psychological science into action. Psychol. Sci. Public Interest 18(3), 149–207.

Cares Foundation, 2019. https://www.caresfoundation.org/

Ching, T.Y., Dillon, C.H., Leigh, G., Cupples, L., 2018. Learning from the Longitudinal Outcomes of Children with Hearing Impairment (LOCHI) study: summary of 5-year findings and implications. Int. J. Audiol. 57: sup2, S105-S111, doi: 10.1080/14992027.2017.1385865

Cystic Fibrosis Trust, 2019. www.cysticfibrosis.org.uk.

Dumanch, K.A., Holte, L., O'Hollearn, T., Walker, E., Clark, J., Oleson, J., 2017. High risk factors associated with early childhood hearing loss: A 3-year review. Am. J. Audiol. 26 (2), 129–142. doi:http://dx.doi.org.monash.idm.oclc.org/10.1044/2017_AJA-16-0116

Frye, A., 2007. Understanding diagnostic tests in childbearing year, seventh edition, Labrys Press, OR.

Gill, D., O'Brien, N., 2007. Paediatric Clinical Examination Made Easy, fifth edition. Churchill Livingstone, Edinburgh, UK.

Hviid, A., Hansen, J.V., Frisch, M., et al., 2019. Measles, mumps rubella vaccination and autism; a nationwide cohort study. Annals of Internal Medicine. https://www.acpjournals.org/doi/10.7326/M18-2101. Accessed August 2020.

Jones, D.A., 1998. Hip screening in the newborn: a practical guide. Butterworth-Heinemann, Oxford, UK.

Morgan, T., Pylypiw, L., 2015. Data collection and performance analysis report newborn blood spot screening in the UK, 2013–14. https://assets.publishing.service.gov.uk/government/uploads/system/uploads/attachment_data/file/512538/2013-14_Data_Collection_and_Performance_Analysis_report.pdf

New Zealand Ministry of Health, 2020. National Screening Unit https://www.nsu.govt.nz/. Accessed August 2020.

New Zealand National Screening Unit (NSU), 2016. Universal newborn hearing screening and early intervention programme national policy and quality standards. https://www.nsu.govt.nz/health-professionals/universal-newborn-hearing-screening-programme/procedures-guidelines-and-repor-0

NHS, 2015. Newborn hearing screening: care pathways. https://www.gov.uk/government/publications/newborn-hearing-screening-care-pathways

NHS, 2016. Vaccinations. Who should have the BCG (TB) vaccine? https://www.nhs.uk/conditions/vaccinations/when-is-bcg-tb-vaccine-needed/

NHS, 2018a. Newborn Hearing Screening. https://www.nhs.uk/video/Pages/newborn-hearing-screening.aspx

NHS, 2018b. Developmental dysplasia of the hips. https://www.nhs.uk/conditions/developmental-dysplasia-of-the-hip/

NHS, 2019a. Newborn bloodspot test. https://www.nhs.uk/conditions/pregnancy-and-baby/newborn-blood-spot-test/

NHS, 2019b. MCADD. https://www.nhs.uk/conditions/mcadd

O'Leary, P., Maxwell, S., 2015. Newborn bloodspot screening policy framework for Australia. Australias Medical Journal (9), 292–298. doi:10.4066/AMJ.2015.24822015. https://www.ncbi.nim.nih.gov/pmc/articles/PMC4592945/. Accessed August 2020.

Public Health England (PHE), 2016a. Guidelines for Newborn Blood Spot Sampling. PHE Screening, London. www.gov.uk/topic/population-screening-programmes.

Public Health England (PHE), 2016b. Newborn hearing screening: programme overview. https://www.gov.uk/guidance/newborn-hearing-screening-programme-overview.

Public Health England (PHE), 2017a. Screening tests for you and your baby. www.gov.uk

Public Health England (PHE), 2017b https://www.gov.uk/government/publications/uk-nsc-evidence-review-process/uk-nsc-evidence-review-process

Public Health England (PHE), 2017c. Blood spot tests: an easy guide to screening tests for your new baby. https://www.assets.publishing.service.gov.uk

Public Health England (PHE), 2018a. Sickle cell disease NHS sickle cell and thalassaemia screening programme. https://www.gov.uk/government/publications/health-professional-handbook-newborn-blood-spot-screening/7-conditions#sickle-cell-disease.

Public Health England, 2018b. Newborn and infant physical examination: programme handbook

Public Health England, 2019. Antenatal and newborn screening timeline. https://www.gov.uk/guidance/nhs-population-screening-education-and-training#screening-timeline

Rull, G., Bonsall, A., 2018. Congenital Adrenal Hyperplasia https://patient.info/health/congenital-adrenal-hyperplasia-leaflet

Sahin, F., Akturk, A., Beyazova, U., et al., 2004. Screening for developmental dysplasia of the hip: results of a 7 year follow-up study. Pediatrics International 46(2), 162–166.

Tappero, E., Honeyfield, M., 2019. Physical assessment of the newborn, sixth edn. NICU Ink, Santa Rosa, CA.

Tidy, C., Bonsall, A., 2015. Galactosaemia https://patient.info/doctor/galactosaemia-pro#nav-1

Welling, L., et al. (On behalf of the Galactosemia Network (GalNet)), 2017. Galactosemia Network (GalNet) International clinical guideline for the management of classical galactosemia: diagnosis, treatment, and follow-up. J. Inherited Metab. Dis. 40(3), 2, 171–176. https://link.springer.com/article/10.1007/s10545-016-9990-5

World Health Organization (WHO), 2014. Societal benefits of immunization http://www.euro.who.int/__data/assets/pdf_file/0009/339624/Sociatal-benefits.pdf?ua=1

Yoshinaga-Itano, C., 2014. Principles and guidelines for early intervention after confirmation that a child is deaf or hard of hearing. J. Deaf Stud. Deaf Educ. 19(2),143. https://search-proquest-com.monash.idm.oclc.org/docview/1510299548?accountid=48406

Support groups and useful websites

Antenatal Results and Choices (ARC): www.arc.org.uk

Hearing Link: https://www.hearinglink.org/connect/useful-hearing-loss-organisations/useful-organisations-uk/

Immunization: https://www.gov.uk/government/collections/immunisation#childhood-immunisation-schedules

MCADD: https://www.metabolicsupport.org

National Deaf Children: https://www.ndcs.org.uk/

National Society for Phenylketonuria: https://www.nspku

Sickle Cell Society: http://www.sicklecellsociety.org/

UK Thalassaemia Society: http://www.ukts.org/

15

Helping Parents Make Decisions

Elaine Jefford, Lorna Davies, Corinne Neville, Martina Donaghy and Sharon McDonald

CHAPTER CONTENTS

INTRODUCTION

The face of midwifery has changed significantly since the first version of this book was published. Nationally and globally, there has been an increase in medical intervention; for example, caesarean rates have risen to as high as 25% in the UK (Aref-Adib et al., 2018) and to an alarming 50% in China (Hellerstein et al., 2015). It is important to note that interventions like caesarean delivery have a place in lifesaving situations. Yet the medical lens of risk may at times distort the concept of normality, not only for midwives but also for the consumers of maternity services (Scamell, 2016). At the same time, research has shown that women being cared for by midwives practising within a continuity of care model experienced increased satisfaction and less intervention. Rates of adverse outcomes for these women and their infants were comparable with those for women who received other models of care (Sandall et al., 2015).

Trying to navigate this changing terrain of contemporary midwifery—where the lens should be woman-centred, including her emotional, social, environmental, cultural and spiritual wellbeing, with a focus on childbirth as a normal physiological event (ICM, 2008)—is complex and challenging for the midwife. Additionally, the midwife's role in facilitating women to feel empowered to make a choice and to be the final decision-makers about their own care and that of their babies (ICM, 2017) means it is important to revisit the midwife's role in decision-making.

DECISION-MAKING

The UK Nursing and Midwifery Council (NMC) is currently reviewing its Standards for Competence for Registered Midwives (2014). When the new standards are finalized and released, it is anticipated they will embrace some of the mandates from the International Confederation of Midwives' (ICM) key documents around professional responsibilities, accountability and clinical skills (ICM, 2010; 2014b; 2014c; 2017). In these documents, the ICM asserts that a midwife, as an autonomous practitioner, is professionally accountable for her/his clinical reasoning, decisions, resultant actions and any related outcomes (ICM, 2014a, 2017).

The NMC Standards for pre-registration midwifery education (2009) state that a student must be '*able to undertake critical decision-making*', yet how or when the necessary education occurs within a midwifery curriculum is not noted. Such an oversight of a fundamental skill is not limited only to the UK; the situation is the same in Australia (ANMAC, 2014) and in New Zealand (MCNZ, 2019). Nevertheless, upon registering with the professional regulators, a qualified midwife must be '*able to make critical decisions*' (NMC, 2014). Such decision-making, however, appears to be limited to supporting '*the appropriate referral of either the woman or baby to other health professionals or agencies when they recognise that normal processes have been adversely affected and compromised*'. (NMC, 2014). One then has to question whether midwifery is being constrained to align with a medical perspective, and therefore whether it is timely that the standards are being reviewed.

Decision-Making Models

The history of midwifery shows a dependence on other disciplines' decision-making theories, models and frameworks (Jefford, 2012; 2014), with two—medical clinical reasoning and the intuitive humanistic model—being the most utilized. The reason these two are used in contemporary midwifery is that, although they derived from medicine and nursing respectively, they each have something to offer midwives. Here, we will present a brief synopsis of each; they have been discussed in detail elsewhere (Benner, 1984; Dreyfus and Dreyfus, 1986; Elstein et al., 1978; Jefford, 2012; 2014; 2020; Jefford and Fahy, 2015).

Medical Clinical Reasoning

This approach derives from the dominant health sciences theory of hypothetico-deductivism. Medical Clinical Reasoning (MCR) is used particularly in medicine and is based on what Kahneman describes as analytical or slow thinking (Kahneman, 2011). Hypothetico-Deductive Theory is defined as:

> The standard research method of empirical science, in which hypotheses are formulated and tested by deducing predictions from them and then testing the predictions through controlled experiments, hypotheses that are falsified being rejected and replaced by new ones...
>
> *(Colman, 2006)*

The five senses are used to formulate deductions because they can be tested logically and rationally—in other words, we are testing what can be seen, heard, touched, smelled and tasted against what is known theoretically (Lawson, 2000). In medicine, this theoretical knowledge would be empirical data derived from such sources as a randomized controlled study or a Cochrane review.

MCR has been adapted over time (Chodzaza, 2018; Elstein et al., 1978; Elstein and Schwartz, 2000; Jefford et al., 2014; Jefford et al., 2014), and now consists of eight clear steps:

- cue acquistion
- cue clustering
- cue interpretation or hypothesis generation
- focused cue acquisition
- diagnosis
- evaluating treatment options
- implementing or prescribing treatment
- evaluating treatment outcomes.

The value midwifery can draw from the MCR model is that its steps actively show the influencing factors that were taken into consideration when a midwife made a decision (Elstein and Schwarz, 2002; Mong-Chue, 2000; Thompson and Dowding, 2009). Consensual checking of the reasoning behind a decision can, therefore, be undertaken should it be necessary (Elstein et al., 1978). The disadvantage with MCR, however, is that it does not take into consideration any of the cogent influences that can impact on the woman or neonate, including those of an emotional, social, environmental, cultural and spiritual quality.

Intuitive Humanistic Theory

This theory is derived from nursing—specifically, from the work of Dreyfus and Dreyfus (1977). This work was adapted and adopted by Benner (1984), resulting in her classification of five levels of experience and practice: novice, advanced beginner, competent, proficient and expert practitioner. She argued that as they gain experience, midwives move along the continuum from novice practitioner to expert practitioner, as a consequence of which their decisions move from slow to fast in what appears to be an almost spontaneous way. This theory thus embraces what Kahneman (2011) describes as nonanalytical (novice) or fast (expert) thinking. The expert midwife uses her/his intuition to rapidly select or reject options in order to make a decision.

Dreyfus and Dreyfus (1977) noted that intuition contains pattern and similarity recognition, common sense, a sense of salience, and deliberate rationality. For expert practitioners, knowing what to do in a particular situation usually depends on intuitive pattern-matching. Pattern-matching is defined by Mok and Stevens (2005, p. 59) as 'a process of making a judgement on the basis of a few critical pieces of information'. Berry and Dienes (1993) argued that part of this process can be referred to as automatic, whereby tacit nursing (midwifery) knowledge acquired through health care exposure and experience is subsequently forgotten. In other words, a midwife demonstrates embodied knowing and intuition. Embodied knowing is defined as 'personal understanding, sensory, psychomotor (practical), affective (emotional) and interpersonal skills associated with experience and intuition' (Standing, 2010).

The value midwifery can draw from the Intuitive Humanistic Theory is that it takes into consideration the cogent influences that can impact on the woman or the neonate, including those of an emotional, social, environmental, cultural and spiritual quality. It has been argued that intuition has a place within nursing and midwifery (Benner, 1984; Mong-Chue, 2000), yet caution is sounded as reliance on intuition alone is detrimental to the credibility of the individual midwife and the midwifery profession (Jefford, 2012; Jefford and Fahy, 2015; Jefford et al., 2014).

While MCR and the Intuitive Humanistic Theory have some elements to offer midwifery, neither model aligns with the midwifery philosophy of working in partnership with women, nor demonstrates the importance of shared decision-making where a midwife empowers women to make informed choices (ICM, 2005, 2014b; Miller and Bear, 2019; NMC, 2014). The following decision-making model may offer a solution.

Three-Talk Model for Shared Decision-Making

Although designed by medical practitioners for medical practitioners, the three-talk model for shared decision-making (Elwyn et al., 2017; Elwyn et al., 2012) is beginning to be embraced by midwives around the world. Elwyn and his fellow authors created this shared decision-making model in clinical practice; it consists of 'three talks' between (in the midwifery context) the woman and her midwife or other care provider: *team talk, option talk* and *decision talk*. These talks are intended to promote equal collaboration and exchange between the people involved in the decision-making process. All three talks may take place within one consultation if there is a time pressure; however, people often need more time to process information, so ideally more time should be allowed and the conversation spread over two or more consultations.

In midwifery, the value of the three-talk model is that it facilitates reciprocity. In such a partnership, the midwife and woman establish what matters, what is valued and why. The midwife gains a clear understanding of the influences on the woman and her individual understanding of the brand-new world of the neonate, including those of an emotional, social, environmental, cultural and spiritual quality. This is really important, because one approach does not fit everyone (Noseworthy et al., 2013). Care options are discussed within this framework, drawing on empirical knowledge (including MCR) and subjective or experience-based knowledge (intuitive humanistic theory) and considering what will be possible within the environment. The way in which this information is communicated is paramount to maintaining the philosophy of partnering with women and empowering them to feel confident in their decision-making (Miller and Bear, 2019).

TRANSLATING THEORY INTO PRACTICE

Having looked at some of the theory behind midwives' decision-making, we will now address the most important questions:
1. How do midwives and other health professionals help parents to use the skills and models above to assist them in making informed decisions about their baby?
2. How do midwives and other health professionals facilitate empowerment of parents so that they are able to make valid and informed decisions around subjects such as immunization and antenatal screening?

Firstly, it is important to remember that women's childbearing experience is an emotional, spiritual and social event (Downe et al., 2018; Olza et al., 2018). Secondly, during the life-defining period of childbearing, a woman may feel vulnerable and experience a loss of control; this may affect her ability to make decisions for herself and her baby in the way that she might at other times in her life (Declercq et al., 2013; Ebert et al., 2014; Vedam et al., 2017). This feeling of loss of control may be compounded by having a pregnancy with complications or by being in a highly medicalized, fragmented birthing environment and/or neonatal unit. Thirdly, it is at such times that a midwife with the required knowledge and skills acts to provide support, care and advice. In so doing, the midwife facilitates the woman's empowerment and enhances her self-confidence, enabling her to maintain a sense of control in order to make necessary and informed decisions (ICM, 2014b; 2014c; 2017).

Decision-Making Tools and Option Grids

These tools, developed and implemented in the United Kingdom, are designed to enhance the process of shared decision-making and can be used alongside decision-making theories. An example of when an option grid can be used is offered by Fay et al. (2015) in their study on neonatal circumcision. In essence, an option grid was designed consisting of common parental questions and concerns about circumcision, and the questions were answered using literature-based evidence. Giving the option grid to the parents removed the doctors' tendency to provide information in a 'rote' fashion; rather, it encouraged active engagement in the decision-making process, thus giving agency to the parents.

Decision-making aids are much like the option grids; they are educational tools that promote shared decision-making. In other words, they can act as a pathway to promote effective two-way communication. For example, an online decision aid tool was used in a study of parental decision-making in children with cancer (Allingham et al., 2018). The tool helped parents understand the possible outcomes of treatment and its risks and benefits using plain language. Like the grid option, it provided parental agency.

An example of a simple tool that can be used is the BRAN analysis (Box 15.1). BRAN is an acronym (benefits, risks, alternatives, nothing) that describes a framework for the sharing of information with parents, enabling a discussion of the decision to be made. The advantage of this tool is that it offers the opportunity to move beyond the physical aspects and to extend the discussion into a more holistic exploration of the treatment/intervention.

There are multiple examples of parental decision aids and the newer option grids working effectively with a variety of situations, but there are other areas where their implementation and effectiveness are limited, such as for childhood vaccinations (Corben and Leask, 2018).

BOX 15.1   BRAN Analysis

In order to demonstrate the usefulness of this tool, we will apply it to the discussion about frenectomy for tongue-tie.

B
- What are the **B**enefits?
  - What percentage of babies are able to feed more effectively following frenectomy?
  - Are there social or emotional benefits of the treatment?

R
- What are the **R**isks?
  - What are the physical risks and side effects of tongue-tie release?
  - Are there emotional or social risks?
  - Do the parents perceive risks that you do not?

A
- What are the **A**lternatives?
  - Are there other medical or alternative treatments that could be tried first?
  - If you are unaware of these, is there another practitioner who may be able to offer useful information?

N
- What if we do **N**othing?
  - Is there a timeframe in which it would not be harmful to the baby to 'wait and see'?

(Wickham, 2002)

CASE STUDIES

In order to further frame the questions posed above within the context of practice, we will now look at a series of case studies addressing specific public health issues and scenarios in which parents may need to consider a range of options. These include smoking cessation; consenting to a frenectomy; infant feeding choices; cosleeping and bed sharing; and the optional administration of vitamin K. It should be acknowledged that these represent a small number of the potential decision-making points for parents during the childbirth continuum; there are many other examples throughout the book, including vaccination, antenatal and newborn screening, and a host of birthing options relating directly to the baby. However, for the purposes of applying the decision-making theory we explored in the first half of the chapter, the scenarios outlined will be used to explore how the questions above may be used in any decision-making interaction between midwives and/or other health professionals and families.

Practical Application of the Three-Talk Model: Vitamin K Administration

In order to demonstrate how the three-talk model may be utilized, we will use the example of vitamin K administration (Case scenario 15.1).

The first step of the three-talk model for shared decision-making (Elwyn et al., 2017; Elwyn et al., 2012) is to agree on what the issue is that requires a decision—in other words, the agreement that a decision needs to be made, the time frame within which it needs to be made and the options available. It may be that this conversation occurs face-to-face, or it may take place over the telephone or online.

The second step is the exchange of evidence-informed information, and establishing and sharing what matters to the woman and her newborn baby—what is valued, and why. This important information should be framed within her sociocultural context, which will impact on her individual understanding of the brand-new world of the neonate and thus on her decision-making. The woman may have 'googled' vitamin K and read that it is needed for blood clotting and can prevent a rare but potentially fatal disease (NCT 2020), and that only one dose is required if given intramuscularly. In the same search, however, she may have seen that in 1992, one study linked vitamin K injections with an increased risk of childhood cancer (North Bristol NHS Trust), or that side effects include rash, itching, facial, tongue and throat swelling (WebMD, 2016), or that the injection is painful (BabyCentre, 2019). An alternative may be oral vitamin K. In her own sociocultural context, the woman may believe birth is a natural process and therefore that giving medicine, either orally or intramuscularly, sits outside the way she identifies herself.

Balancing all the evidence in case scenario 15.1 and considering it within the sociocultural context of a medically dominated environment, where the 'authority' figure makes the decisions, highlights the challenging terrain to be navigated by the midwife who works within this context. This step is vital if midwives and other health professionals are to facilitate the empowerment of parents to make valid and informed decisions around providing consent. Yet the midwife needs to take the time to create an environment where a woman feels safe and supported to share this information.

CASE SCENARIO 15.1   VITAMIN K

Lorna Davies

Juanita and Alec approach you to discuss the issue of vitamin K administration for their baby Tia, who was born at term after a normal pregnancy and physiological birth in water. They are both science teachers and, before deciding whether to consent, want to know why there is an expectation that all babies need vitamin K.

Vitamin K is necessary to synthesize the functional forms of coagulation factors II, VII, IX, and X in the liver. It is believed that poor placental transfer of vitamin K to the fetus leaves the newborn baby depleted of this necessary component in the clotting mechanism (Lippi and Franchini, 2011). This, combined with relatively limited growth of intestinal flora, is thought to place the newborn at risk of developing vitamin K deficiency bleeding (VKDB) (Rankin, 2017). The early prophylactic administration of vitamin K is commonly believed to prevent VKDB of the newborn (classical VKDB and late VKDB) and has become a common practice following birth (Table 15.1).

There is not a lot of evidence for this, although a 2017 study was carried out in Tennessee following the births of a small number of babies with VKDB in a relatively short time frame (Marcewicz et al., 2017). Parents who had declined the intervention for their newborn at the time were asked for their rationale; the most common reasons given were a belief that it was not necessary, and a desire to keep birth natural.

The midwife knows vitamin K is offered as a prophylactic measure to prevent early, classical and late VKDB (Blackburn, 2017). It is a rare disease, but the prevalence is rising, as is the rate of the corresponding adverse outcomes in such countries as New Zealand and the United Kingdom where mothers often decline vitamin K (Zurynski et al., 2018). The World Health Organization (2017) strongly recommends that all newborns are given vitamin K (1 mg intramuscularly) at 1 hour post birth. They go as far as to say that any neonate who requires surgery, has suffered a birth trauma, was born preterm, or has been exposed to any medication that may inhibit vitamin K in utero, *must* be administered this injection. The dosage is not standardized internationally, however, and different doses and preparations are prescribed in

Continued

CASE SCENARIO 15.1   VITAMIN K—cont'd

different countries (Coffey and Gerth-Guyette, 2018). Oral multidose vitamin K is a possibility, but the intramuscular route is generally favoured due to concerns around the reliability of administration and the efficacy when administered orally. Although it may seem as though the evidence around vitamin K administration is fairly unequivocal, there are a few factors which could create a slight sense of disquiet. The microbiome (see Chapter 6) may play an important part in the synthesizing of vitamin K in the newborn. Dominguez-Bello et al. (2010), who researched the microbiome extensively, ask whether the newborn's low levels of vitamin K hold adaptive value or are a maladaptation; if the former is the case, we may have been interfering with a natural process on a grand scale for the last 70 or so years. It may be that our lack of attention to the integrity of the gut environment has contributed to our prophylactic approach to what has become viewed as a deficit. Artificial formula is supplemented with vitamin K, which is believed to give bottle-fed babies a greater degree of protection; however, it may be that the low quantities of vitamin K in breast milk are related to microbiome development. As discussed in Chapter 6, some critics have suggested that premature clamping/cutting of the umbilical cord may be a contributing cause of VKDB, but there is no global consensus in the literature, midwifery practices, or international policies and procedures about the optimal time to clamp and cut the cord. What is known is that immediate post-birth cord clamping and cutting deprives a term baby of 20–30 mg/kg of iron. Delaying cord clamping for 3 minutes in term and preterm infants has been shown to significantly reduce infant anaemia at 8 and 12 months of age (Ashish et al., 2016; Ashish et al., 2017; McDonald et al., 2013). Could it be that, when a baby is allowed to receive a complete placental transfer, the coagulation factors are more likely to prevent haemorrhage?

It is also argued that other causes of VKDB are equally iatrogenic—for example, the use of instruments in assisted deliveries, which may cause bruising or internal bleeding which causes the depletion of the baby's clotting factors. The use of antibiotics is also believed to inhibit the generation of clotting factors in the newborn.

There is clearly a need for further research around the prophylactic administration of vitamin K to the newborn. In the meantime, some parents will, for whatever reason, opt not to give their baby vitamin K as either an intramuscular injection or an oral preparation, and midwives need to provide them with the information they need in order to monitor their baby for any signs or symptoms of VKDB. These would include:

- bleeding from the umbilicus, nose, mouth, ears or puncture site (such as from the blood spot test)
- blood in the baby's urine or stools; black, tarry stools after meconium has already been expelled
- any bruise not related to a known trauma
- pinpoint bruises (petechiae)
- black vomit
- bleeding longer than 6 minutes from a blood sampling site, even after pressure on the wound
- symptoms of intracranial bleeding including unusual-shaped fontanelles, paleness, glassy-eyed look, irritability or high-pitched crying, loss of appetite, vomiting, fever, prolonged jaundice.

Adapted from Enoch, J. (1996). Vitamin K: Is It Necessary? Midwifery Today Childbirth Education. Winter, 40 p28-30 and Wickham, S. (2017). Vitamin K and the Newborn (2nd Ed). Birthmoon Creations, UK. ISBN -13:978-1-9998064-0-8

TABLE 15.1   Vitamin K Deficiency Bleeding

Types of VKDB	
Early VKDB	Occurs in the first 24 hours of life. Usually related to medication taken by mother (e.g., warfarin, antiepileptic drugs, TB medication). The bleeds generally occur in the skin, brain and abdomen of the newborn.
Classical VKDB	Occurs in days 2–7 following birth. Origin unknown but believed to be associated with inadequate feeding, particularly breastfeeding. Bleeding takes place in GI system, skin, nose, and umbilicus.
Late VKDB	Occurs after first week of life and usually between weeks 3–8. Brain, skin and GI tract are most common sites. Can result from undiagnosed liver and gallbladder disease as well as cystic fibrosis, chronic diarrhoea and antibiotic use. Also associated with exclusively breastfed babies who have not received vitamin K prophylactically.

GI: gastrointestinal; TB: tuberculosis; VKDB: vitamin K deficiency bleeding.
(Adapted from Shearer, 2009.)

In a reciprocal relationship, the midwife can explore, learn and understand the concerns and issues that may be influencing the woman's behaviour and the subsequent decisions she makes. Misunderstandings can be clarified and parental fears can be discussed (some examples were noted earlier). It is important that midwives or health care professionals imparting information consider and accept the woman's own spiritual and sociocultural context. A New Zealand study (Miller et al., 2016) looked at the information offered by health practitioners such as midwives and doctors, as well as by Health Boards and other organizations. This work concluded that the attitudes of health professionals had a significant influence on parents' decisions, and that resources relating to vitamin K prophylaxis have subtle but significant differences in content which may also be impacting on those decisions.

Having engaged in an information exchange with the woman, clarified any misunderstandings or misinformation, and presented balanced evidence around vitamin K (case scenario 15.1), the final step of the three-talk model (Elwyn et al., 2017; Elwyn et al., 2012) can occur. This focus in this step is on the decision. The woman must feel confident in the decision she makes and must know that if she wishes to reconsider or change her decision, the midwife or other health professional will support her.

Tongue-Tie

The principles of the three-talk model can be applied to the decision-making scenarios that follow, as well as to other examples within the book. We would recommend that the reader uses these examples as a basis for reflection. The scenarios can also be used within a formal educational context for role-play around decision-making. The decision-making models referred to here can form the basis of supporting and empowering shared decision-making, and the decision aid tools and option grids can also be incorporated into this framework.

CASE SCENARIO 15.2   TONGUE-TIE

Corinne Neville

Alisha has recently given birth to Rory, who is now 7 days old and struggling with latching on during breastfeeding. You carry out a breastfeeding assessment and agree there is some difficulty. You note on assessment that Rory is having problems protruding his tongue and that it has a heart-shaped appearance.

What information might you provide in order to enable Alisha and her partner Don to make a decision about frenectomy?

Ankyloglossia is a congenital anomaly characterized by an abnormally short lingual frenulum, meaning that the tip of the tongue cannot protrude beyond the lower incisor teeth. It varies in degree from a mild form where the tongue is bound only by a thin mucous membrane on the very tip of the tongue to a severe form where the tongue is completely fused to the floor of the mouth. The global incidence of this condition is reported to range from 3% to 16%, with more boys than girls affected. Around half of these babies will have a problem with feeding which may be associated with having a restricted frenulum (Ingram, 2015).

Division of ankyloglossia (tongue-tie) is a technique that has been used for many years, primarily to improve the baby's ability to feed effectively by 'snipping' the frenulum. However, in the last 10 years controversy about the safety and efficacy of the procedure has led to considerable debate and policy development relating to the diagnosis and treatment of tongue-tie.

Many tongue-ties are asymptomatic and do not require treatment; some may resolve spontaneously over time. However, if the baby is unable to suckle effectively, this may result in sore nipples, poor weight gain and early cessation of breastfeeding (NICE, 2005b). Conservative approaches to addressing the problem include the provision of breastfeeding advice and counselling, massaging the frenulum and exercising the tongue. Further measures may include the surgical division of the frenulum by the procedure known as frenotomy (or frenulotomy or frenulectomy) which, if carried out as early as possible, may enable the baby to continue breastfeeding. If division of the tongue-tie is performed within a few weeks of birth (Fig. 15.1), it is usually achieved without anaesthesia, although local anaesthetic is sometimes used. The baby is swaddled and supported at the shoulders to stabilize the head and sharp, blunt-ended scissors are used to divide the lingual frenulum. There should be little or no blood loss, and feeding may be resumed immediately

Continued

CASE SCENARIO 15.2   TONGUE-TIE—cont'd

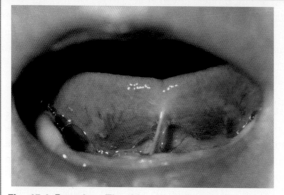

Fig. 15.1 Frenulum That May Need Tongue-Tie Division. (NHS sites 2005)

(NICE, 2005b). Current evidence suggests there are no major safety concerns about division of ankyloglossia, and there is some limited evidence that this procedure can improve breastfeeding (NICE, 2019).

Often a tongue-tie diagnosis is made without a comprehensive feeding assessment, which can give rise to an overdiagnosis of tongue-tie (Jin et al., 2018). Visible ankyloglossia is not, on its own, an indication that there is a problem with the tongue movement; if the baby is feeding effectively, a frenotomy should not be undertaken without serious consideration. A referral should only be considered if the health professional is satisfied that the restrictive tongue movement is affecting feeding (breast or bottle).

If tongue-tie is suspected, a full assessment—including feeding history, visual assessment and the observation of a full feed—should be undertaken before a diagnosis is proffered. It is not unusual to have a low-risk reluctant feeder in the first 48 hours, so it may not be accurate to diagnose a tongue-tie restriction until more evidence is obtained while the baby is awake and feeding.

For some mothers and babies, immediate relief may be experienced following frenulum release, and their breastfeeding journey will continue without further issue. However, it is often difficult to pinpoint whether the improvement in breastfeeding is due to the frenotomy, expert infant feeding advice given in a clinic, or a combination of both. Douglas and Geddes (2018) claims that after posterior tongue-tie divisions, breastfeeding outcomes often do not change but some mothers create a powerful placebo effect around the pain felt during breastfeeding. Data proving the efficacy of tongue-tie division are difficult to collect and quantify due to other external factors, such as a woman's confidence in her own ability to breastfeed, or the introduction of formula substantially reducing her milk supply which can affect the baby's ability to breastfeed responsively (Kapoor et al., 2018).

Some parents have reported health professionals telling them their baby needs a frenotomy to prevent speech problems (Muldoon et al., 2017). Once parents hear this, they may feel that tongue-tie division is the best and only option for the baby, even if the tongue is subsequently examined and no abnormalities of tongue movement are found. Parents should be advised that it is impossible to predict whether a tongue-tie will definitely have an effect on their child's speech.

Frenotomy for ankyloglossia seems to be on the increase at a global level. One Australian study found that tongue-tie surgery rates have risen by 3.71% between 2006 and 2016 (Kapoor et al., 2018). Canada recorded an 89% increase between 2004 and 2013 (Kinnilburth et al., 2016), and in the United States a 300% increase was recorded between 1997 and 2012 (Walsh, 2017). It is therefore important that a full and thorough assessment is carried out before any diagnosis is made, and that the practitioner is fully aware of the effect any findings may have on parents in terms of their decision-making. This may be particularly pertinent when the baby is breastfed; ensure that appropriate support is provided by a lactation specialist if necessary.

CASE SCENARIO 15.3   INFANT FEEDING

Martina Donaghy

Maria is 28 weeks pregnant with her second baby. She bottle-fed her last baby after struggling with positioning and attaching the baby onto the breast for the first 2 weeks. She is anxious about attempting breastfeeding this time, although she really wants to give it a go, as her mother has just passed away from breast cancer.

Helping Parents Make Decisions About Infant Feeding

How women make decisions about infant feeding is complex and sculpted by sociocultural influences, peer and family pressure, self-efficacy, their own values and beliefs, previous vicarious experience, social support, personal motivation, expectations, knowledge and lifestyle considerations (Edwards et al., 2018; Roll and Cheater, 2016). As a consequence, health professionals have a challenging role to play in facilitating parents' decisions, particularly when those decisions have been made pre-pregnancy and formalized during the antenatal period. In contrast, feeding decisions made postnatally are directly influenced by the woman's feeding experience and the level of support she receives during this time (Robinson, 2017).

Of course, for any health professional to facilitate a woman's choice in infant feeding, they must have knowledge and understanding of the importance of breastfeeding, in terms of its implications for future infant health. There is increasing evidence that an infant's early development has a long-term impact on health outcomes. Research has highlighted the public health importance of promoting breastfeeding as a key component of life programming (Binns, 2016).

Empirical evidence has repeatedly shown the strong association between exclusive breastfeeding and reduced infant morbidity and mortality, coupled with reducing maternal morbidity (Kramer et al., 2001; Quigley et al., 2006; Renfrew et al., 2006; Rollins et al, 2016). These benefits span every population, race and creed irrespective of socioeconomic status (Victora et al., 2016). As previously mentioned in Chapter 5, the health benefits of breastfeeding have recently been given further credence, with a focus on the role of breastmilk in supporting the development of a robust infant microbiome and immune system, which can improve the health of future generations through epigenetic changes (Tow, 2014).

Women appear to acknowledge the importance of breastfeeding, seeing it as a reflection of their maternal role (Roll and Cheater, 2016). This is reflected in the overall high initiation rates in most westernized countries. However, although an intention to breastfeed is predictive of initiation, the duration appears to be influenced by levels of support (Rollins et al., 2016). This is borne out by the current picture of breastfeeding in the UK: initiation rates are 81%, with exclusive rates falling to 24% at 6 weeks and 1% at 6 months (ONS, 2012). This fall in breastfeeding duration is caused by various factors, including difficulties with feeding, a lack of professional support, feeling uncomfortable feeding in public places, and anxiety about returning to work (McAndrew et al., 2012).

Changing the Conversations Around Infant Feeding

Success in breastfeeding is not the sole responsibility of a woman—the promotion of breastfeeding is a collective societal responsibility.

(Rollins, 2016)

The recent publication of three major studies by the Gates Foundation (Rollins et al., 2016; Victora et al., 2016; Acta Paediatrica, 2015) resoundingly confirms the previous evidence that breastfeeding saves infant and maternal lives, improves global health and cuts costs to all countries. It is hoped that this research will prompt a shift in policy thinking and in public beliefs and attitudes around breastfeeding. These papers have already precipitated a change in the United Kingdom, with UNICEF Baby Friendly incorporating practical communication steps for all professionals around 'Having antenatal and breastfeeding conversations' (UNICEF, 2018).

Communicating With Mothers in the Antenatal and Postnatal Periods

It is worth noting that pregnant women and new mothers have greater right-brain dominance (intuitive, subjective) than left-brain (analytical, objective), which increases their sensitivity to nonverbal forms of communication. They are less able to process large volumes of information and hence they benefit from information-sharing conversations (UNICEF, 2018).

Antenatal Conversations

Historically, health professionals have directed antenatal conversations about infant feeding, promoting the notion that 'breast is best' and suggesting this feeding method was the preferred one, endorsed by the professional, irrespective of the mother's thoughts (Tricky, 2016). As a result of this approach, women often felt obliged to 'give it a go' despite reservations because they feared being judged.

Women have suggested they want professionals to talk about the realities of breastfeeding, how to overcome difficulties, how breastfeeding will fit into their life situation and where to find support (Sheehan et al., 2013). It has been suggested that women could use a 'pros and cons' list or a mind map, or ideally that they should have the opportunity to meet other breastfeeding women through parent education classes.

Those women who choose to feed their infants with artificial formula are entitled to have the same open conversations about their feeding goals. These women need time to discuss how to increase their responsiveness and infant contact during feeds. Interventions—such as paced bottle feeding to reduce the risk of childhood obesity, recommended formula appropriate for the infant's age, and correct preparation and storage of feeds—need to be discussed with women to ensure their infants' safety (UNICEF, 2019).

Continued

CASE SCENARIO 15.3   INFANT FEEDING—cont'd

Postnatal Conversations

It is recognized that knowledge and interpersonal communication skills are important when supporting women with breastfeeding difficulties. However, it has been suggested that generic practical support (help with positioning and attachment of the baby at the breast) is not effective; women want meaningful, relevant and effective support tailored to their own personal breastfeeding experience and life circumstances (Robinson, 2017). As hospital stays grow shorter and postnatal contact more limited, it is important to make every conversation meaningful and tailored to the woman's needs (UNICEF, 2016).

When a woman's breastfeeding journey fails to go according to plan, she wants advice and guidance to understand the options that will work best for her, considering her initial feeding goals (Box 15.2). Professionals need to acknowledge women's disappointment, and encourage and praise them for their efforts. Hoddinott and Pill (2000) suggest that continuity of carer, in which a woman could form a relationship with a health professional who could reassure, praise and encourage her, was a key factor to women's satisfaction with infant feeding.

CASE SCENARIO 15.4   SAFE-SLEEPING, COSLEEPING AND BED SHARING

Martina Donaghy

You visit Fiona on day 8 to provide some breastfeeding support. When you ask about feeding, Fiona becomes tearful and upset. She divulges to you that she fell asleep on the sofa last night with baby Ruby. She was worried and anxious about it, as she knew it was dangerous, but because her 2-year-old son was still getting into bed with her and her husband, she thought she would have more room on the sofa. You discuss the risk factors of cosleeping and bed sharing with Fiona. Fiona then also reveals that her husband is a smoker and occasionally goes out drinking at the weekend.

The key to improving care around safe infant sleep for all new parents is that health professionals engage in an exploratory conversation with them, discussing safe sleeping practices and night-time parenting, the risks associated with unintentional bed sharing, and how to minimize the potential risks that may arise with bed sharing. Ideally, this conversation should be held in the antenatal period to address any risk factors such as smoking, alcohol and drug use (Ball et al. 2016). Health professionals should take every opportunity in the postnatal period to ascertain parents' understanding of the risks, enquiring about their personal circumstances, viewing their sleeping arrangements and providing up-to-date information and practical advice (see links at the end of this section). Box 15.3 outlines current recommendations relating to safe sleeping and potential risk factors, with a focus (though not exclusively) on babies who are placed in their own sleeping spaces.

Cosleeping and Bed Sharing: What's the Difference?

Cosleeping and bed sharing have been associated with sudden infant death syndrome (SIDS) and this has resulted in strong resistance to the practice on the part of some health care systems. It is clearly necessary to consider the cultural context when cosleeping is contemplated, and there are inevitably issues to address to ensure that the practice is carried out as safely as possible. Cosleeping has been linked with SIDS and, although this link has been contested by some researchers, it would be in the interests of the family to aim to ensure that the environment provided is as safe as it can be. Further discussion of the link between SIDS and cosleeping is addressed later in this topic review.

Defining Cosleeping and Bed Sharing

Poor interpretation and consistency of the definitions of cosleeping and bed sharing has contributed to confusion and misunderstanding of the concept, and has also led to a lack of clarity between studies of the topic (Fetherston and Leach, 2012; McKenna and McDade, 2005). Mother–infant cosleeping has been defined as 'any situation in which a committed mother or caregiver sleeps within sensory range of an infant, on the same or a different surface' (Gettler and McKenna, 2011). Conversely, bed sharing is when an adult caregiver and an infant sleep together in the same adult bed. Hence bed sharing is only one form of cosleeping; cosleeping can include a different sleep surface such as a cot, crib, box, hammock or basket in the same room. 'Cosleeping' is a large umbrella term (McCoy et al., 2008).

Cosleeping confers multiple benefits for both the mother and infant; the main short-term benefits are summarized in Box 15.4.

Normal Infant Sleep and Infant Biology

It is normal for babies to wake at night. McKenna and McDade (2005) postulate it to be protective, especially if

CASE SCENARIO 15.4   SAFE-SLEEPING, COSLEEPING AND BED SHARING—cont'd

the mother is in close contact, because her presence has been shown to change the infant's physiology, regulating breathing patterns and heart rate, and easing excessive crying. The availability of close contact is of great importance to infant development and survival. The infant is reliant on its mother for a long period of time for physiological contact, system regulation and the delivery of long-chain polyunsaturated fatty acids (LCPs) via the breast milk to enhance the development of its central nervous system and encourage brain growth (Trevathan et al., 2008).

Maternal Instinct

Breastfeeding mothers protect their infants from hazards in the bed by adopting an instinctual position. This is sometimes called the breastfeeding 'cuddle curl' (Wiessinger et al., 2010). Breastfeeding mothers typically keep their babies away from pillows, place their infants on their backs, positioning them below their shoulders, with their arm raised above them. They also typically tuck their legs up and lie on their sides, facing the infant and protecting it from overlay and smothering by pillows or covers (Ball et al., 2012) (Fig. 15.2).

This close proximity, coupled with the baby's frequent waking, allows the infant to expel accumulating CO_2, while the mother's expiration of CO_2 over the baby's face will stimulate the breathing reflex and stimulate arousal (Trevathan et al., 2008).

Multiple studies (McKenna et al., 2007; Blair et al., 2006; Kendall-Tackett et al., 2010) have proven that breastfeeding

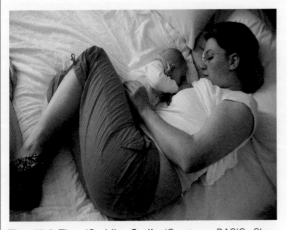

Fig. 15.2 The 'Cuddle Curl'. (Courtesy BASIS Sleep Information Service.)

mothers who bed share get more sleep overall than mothers who are bottle-feeding their infants. Often, women are unaware of the number of times they are waking for feeds.

Sudden Infant Death Syndrome (SIDS) and Bed Sharing

Breastfeeding has been shown in a meta-analysis to reduce the risk of SIDS by half (Hauck et al., 2011). McKenna et al. (2007) also suggested that practices which increase breastfeeding, such as bed sharing, may in fact be protective against SIDS.

The incidence of SIDS is higher in infants with: mothers who smoked during pregnancy, parents in low socioeconomic groups, parents who currently abuse alcohol or drugs, parents who sleep with their infant on a sofa, and young mothers with more than one child. The incidence is also increased in premature infants and those with low birth weight (UNICEF, 2016).

However, it must be noted that bed sharing has been proven to be safe in the absence of hazardous circumstances such as sofa sharing, alcohol consumption or smoking. In an analysis of two UK case–control studies on sleep location and SIDS, Blair et al. (2014) surprisingly found that bed sharing after 3 months was actually significantly protective. He noted that infants under 3 months of age are at greater risk if parents have consumed alcohol or are smokers.

Smoking

The link between smoking and SIDS was first discovered in New Zealand in the 1990s, within the Maori population. Recent research from New Zealand (Mitchel et al., 2017) states that the risk of SIDS among infants bed sharing with a mother who smokes is more than four times that for infants bed sharing with non-smoking mothers. In the United Kingdom, the risk of SIDS while sleeping with a regular smoker is 1 in 800 (Blair et al., 2014).

Alcohol

Consumption of alcohol is another significant risk factor for SIDS when bed sharing. Blair et al. (2014) suggested there is an 18-fold increase in the SIDS risk if an infant sleeps next to an adult who has drunk more than two units of alcohol, or with an adult on a sofa. In England and Wales the risk of SIDS while cosleeping with a parent who has consumed alcohol or drugs is 1:180 (UNICEF, 2016). Adults under the influence of alcohol are less likely to be aware of the infant's movements and have less ability to be roused, increasing the risk of overlaying.

Continued

CASE SCENARIO 15.4   SAFE-SLEEPING, COSLEEPING AND BED SHARING—cont'd

Sofa Sharing

As a consequence of public health messages portraying bed sharing as a high-risk practice for SIDS, we have seen a rise in parents sleeping with infants on sofas, with devastating results. The only practice that has seen a rise in SIDS deaths in the last 20 years is that of infants sleeping with an adult on a sofa (Marinelli et al., 2019).

Car Seat Safety

Car seats are essential for babies when travelling, but infants should not sleep in a car seat for long periods because they are at increased risk of adverse cardiorespiratory effects from being slumped over in the seat. If parents are going on longer journeys, advise them to have regular breaks during which they remove the baby from the seat. It is also advisable to have an adult sit with the baby in the back of the car, if possible.

Websites for Up-to-Date Accurate Advice
UNICEF: https://www.unicef.org.uk/babyfriendly/
Lullaby Trust: https://www.lullabytrust.org.uk
BASIS (Baby Sleep Info Source): https://www.basisonline.org.uk/about-us/
Infant Sleep Info App for parents: https://www.basisonline.org.uk/infant-sleep-info-app/

BOX 15.2   Infant Feeding Choices

Key Tips to Having Meaningful Conversations With Women

- **Agree an agenda**: find out what the woman wants to explore.
- **Ask open questions**: explore her feelings, thoughts and emotions.
- **Listen actively**: nod, smile and ensure you make eye contact.
- **Reflect back** a summary of the conversation to avoid misunderstandings.
- **Don't overload** with information, but build on what the woman knows.
- **Show empathy**: respect her concerns.
- **Don't collude**: keep the discussion evidence-based.
- **Remain neutral**: avoid being judgemental.
- **Present the evidence** for all options.

Adapted from UNICEF UK (2018) Having meaningful conversations with mothers: A guide to using the Baby-Friendly signature sheets.

BOX 15.3   Current Recommendations Relating to Safe-Sleeping

Environment

The baby should sleep in the same room as its parents for the first 6 months of life.

The room should be kept at an ambient temperature of 20°C.

The baby's environment should always be smoke-free (including e-cigarettes).

Alcohol or social drugs should not be used by the mother during pregnancy or after the baby is born.

Car seats and capsules should not be used in place of a cot, crib or bassinette.

It is never safe to sleep with a baby on a sofa or couch.

Parents should be advised not to use medication that causes them to sleep more heavily.

In a Cot or Bassinette

The baby should be placed on its back to keep the airway clear. Sleeping a baby on its front or side greatly increases the chance of SIDS.

The mattress should be firm and protected with a waterproof cover to keep it clean and dry.

There should be no gaps between the cot frame and the mattress that could trap or wedge the baby.

The baby should have its feet close to the end of the bed so it cannot burrow under the blankets.

There should be nothing in the cot that might cover the baby's face, lift its head or choke it (i.e., no pillows, toys, loose bedding, bumper pads or teething necklaces).

If parents choose to swaddle their baby, they should be advised to use thin materials and not to swaddle above the shoulders to allow some movement; the baby should not be wrapped too tightly.

BOX 15.4 Short-term Benefits of Cosleeping

Mother

More sleep and increased nightly satisfaction

Increased sensitization to infant's physiological status

Increased comfort and the ability to interpret infant's behavioural cues

Increased sucking behaviour of infant, ensures ongoing milk supply

Increased prolactin levels help to delay ovulation and menstruation, leading to a longer birth interval

Increased ability to monitor, physically manage and respond to infant's needs

Enhanced attachment and parental fulfilment

Infant

Increased breastfeeding: total minutes at the breast and number of night feeds

Increased sleep duration

Less crying time

Increased sensitivity to mother's communication

More light (stage 1–2) sleep, and less deep (stage 3–4) sleep, appropriate for age of infant

Increase in heart rate

Reduction in number of obstructive apnoeas in stage 3–4 sleep

Practice at arousing

Adapted from McKenna (2009).

CASE SCENARIO 15.5 SMOKING IN PREGNANCY

Sharon McDonald

Jaime is a 30-year-old mother of two. This is her third pregnancy and was unplanned, with a new partner. She is unemployed and lives in a one-bedroom rented flat with her two children; the elder son can be hyperactive. Initially, she declined any referral or support from smoking cessation services, but she is now 28 weeks pregnant, smoking eight cigarettes a day, and has asked for support to quit. She really wants to quit but is finding it difficult with so many other stresses in her life and knows she 'can't do it without support'.

The evidence for the damage caused to the fetus by maternal tobacco smoking during pregnancy is so comprehensive and so consistent that it is largely incontrovertible. Cigarette smoke contains a complex and potentially lethal cocktail of over 7000 toxic chemicals including nicotine, hydrogen cyanide, lead and arsenic. These are able to enter the maternal circulation—creating risks to the mother—and to cross the placenta, adversely affecting the growth and development of the fetus. Table 15.2 highlights some of the risks of smoking in pregnancy.

Smoking is the biggest single modifiable risk factor for poor birth outcomes, and a major cause of inequality between the different socio economic groups of mothers and children.

(NHS England, 2019)

Women state that they want to know what the risks are to them and their baby; however, an estimated 25% of women do not disclose that they smoke because they perceive health professionals to be judgemental (RCM, 2019b).

Cigarette packs and television advertisements carry health warnings and photographic evidence relating to the harm that can be inflicted by smoking in pregnancy. Smoking cessation programmes are available in most areas of the United Kingdom and in many other countries around the world. Despite the widespread knowledge and evidence that supports the advice health professionals give to women and families during pregnancy, many women will continue to smoke (Gould et al., 2020; RCM, 2019a, 2019b; NICE, 2010).

The 2018 NHS quarterly statistics indicated that during the second quarter of 2018/19, 10.5% of women were known to be smokers at the time they went into labour. (Gould et al. 2020) While the number of women smoking during pregnancy has declined steadily, the UK Tobacco Control Plan aims to further reduce smoking among pregnant women to 6% by the end of 2022; however, at the current rate of cessation, this figure is unlikely to be achieved. Lange et al. (2018), reporting the findings of a systematic review of 30 years' scientific literature, concluded that there are significant gaps in research, policy and practice on tobacco use and exposure surveillance. It is broadly identified that many of the women who smoke during pregnancy are young and from low socioeconomic backgrounds, and frequently lacking adequate social support (Cook and Cameron, 2015). Notwithstanding, there is a need to counter this trend in younger women; midwives and other health practitioners have an important role to play in this process.

The introduction of e-cigarettes and the practice of 'vaping' has added another layer of complexity to the debate

Continued

CASE SCENARIO 15.5   SMOKING IN PREGNANCY—cont'd

around smoking in pregnancy. There is a perception that vaping is less harmful than smoking and could therefore generate a net public health benefit. E-cigarettes could be viewed as a 'lesser of two evils' compromise for women who wish to continue smoking during pregnancy; however, there is currently no evidence on the safety or otherwise of e-cigarette use during pregnancy in relation to fetal development and pregnancy outcomes (McCubbin et al., 2017; Smoking in Pregnancy Challenge Group, 2017). E-cigarettes still contain nicotine, alongside a range of other toxic substances (Whittington et al., 2018). The idea that e-cigarettes may lead to a reduction in smoking has also been challenged in a meta-analysis in which the authors concluded that the introduction of e-cigarettes is associated with even poorer cessation rates (Kalkhoran and Glantz, 2016), and Whittington et al. (2018) advised that the marketing of e-cigarettes as a safer alternative to tobacco smoking has resulted in increased use in pregnancy.

We need to pay heed to the fact that smoking does not occur in isolation, but is embedded in a larger social context of family and community. The family context of maternal smoking has a huge impact on the woman and her behaviour. Additionally, exposure to second-hand smoke carries a similar risk, albeit a reduced one (Lange et al., 2018). While the evidence suggests that more women give up smoking during pregnancy than at any other time, they are less likely to be successful and more likely to lapse after delivery if someone else in the household smokes. Further education and support is needed, especially among young women, their partners and other family members—and, more importantly, in those who lack social support. Providing advice and support to women to raise their self-esteem, and to reduce the stressors that make giving up smoking a more difficult task, may have greater benefits than more traditional social cessation methods. Several studies and reports (Tong et al., 2016; NICE, 2010; NHS England, 2016) have stressed the increasing importance of preventative work.

In the United Kingdom, the Royal College of Midwives (RCM), in collaboration with the National Centre for Smoking Cessation and Training (NSCST) and Smoking in Pregnancy Challenge Group (2015), ask that midwives should offer routine carbon monoxide screening at every antenatal appointment on an 'opt out' basis, and that all midwives should undertake training in smoking cessation to enable them to provide 'Very Brief Advice' to pregnant women and refer smokers to support services with their consent (RCM, 2019a; 2019b; NICE, 2010). They state that all health professionals caring for women in pregnancy should be aware of, and provide information about, sources of carbon monoxide (smoking, environmental, car fumes, barbeque smoke, second-hand smoke, faulty home appliances [e.g. leaky boilers], lactose intolerance). Particularly when discussing safer sleep, practitioners should highlight the consequences of passive smoking for children in the home, because passive smoking is a major hazard to the health of the millions of children globally who live with smokers (RCP, 2010).

As health professionals, we all have a responsibility to empower women to stop smoking, and to provide information and support to help them achieve a safe and healthy lifestyle for themselves and their baby.

TABLE 15.2	**Increased Risks of Smoking in Pregnancy**		
Mother	**Fetus**	**Newborn Infant**
miscarriage	intrauterine growth	low birth weight
ectopic pregnancy	restriction (IUGR)	sudden infant death syndrome (SIDS)
placenta praevia	fetal hypoxia	asthma and other respiratory conditions
preeclampsia	perinatal mortality	behavioural problems, attention deficit disorders
deep vein thrombosis	birth defects	and hyperactivity
	cognitive and neuro-	stillbirth infections of the ear, nose and throat
	behavioural deficits	learning difficulties
	stillbirth	obesity, diabetes
		childhood cancers
(RCM 2019a; Pineles, 2014)	(Marufu et al., 2015; Mund et al., 2013; RCOG, 2016)	(Lange, 2018; Leigh, 2017; Zacharasiewicz, 2016)

CONCLUSION

Decision-making is complex. A woman's decisions are influenced by her own sociocultural context and emotional, social, environmental, cultural and spiritual perspectives, as well as her attempts to gain some understanding of the brand-new world of her baby. This is not an easy terrain for the midwife or health care professional to navigate as the woman and her partner are making decisions on behalf of their newborn child, which may or may not be time-sensitive and/or have life-altering implications. As midwives and health professionals, we need to draw on appropriate decision-making models and tools that can support our philosophy of partnering with women and families to empower them to feel confident in their decision-making.

KEY POINTS

- Recognize the contested terrain of decision-making.
- Discuss different decision-making theories, models, decision aids and option grids.
- Understand the importance of applying one of these to facilitate shared decision-making.

REFERENCES

Allingham, C., Gillam, L., McCarthy, M., 2018. Fertility preservation in children and adolescents with cancer: pilot of a decision aid for parents of children and adolescents with cancer. JMIR Pediatr. Parent. 1(2) e10463–e10476. doi:10.2196/10463.

Aref-Adib, A., Vlachodimitropoulou, E., Khasriya, E., 2018. UK O&G trainees' attitudes to caesarean delivery for maternal request. J. Obstet. Gynaecol. 38(3), 367–371. doi:10.1080/01443615.2017.1345874

Australian Nursing and Midwifery Accreditation Council (ANMAC), 2014. Midwife: Accreditation Standards. Canberra: Australian Nursing and Midwifery Council.

BabyCentre, 2019. Vitamin K. https://www.babycenter.com.au/a551938/vitamin-k

Benner, P., 1984. From novice to expert: excellence and power in clinical nursing. Addison-Wesley Publishing Company, Menlo Park, CA.

Berry, D., Dienes, Z., 1993. Implicit learning: Theoretical and empirical issues. L. Erlbaum, Hove, UK, p59.

Binns, C., MiKyung, L., Wah , L., 2016. The Long-term public health benefits of breastfeeding. Asia-Pacific Journal of Public Health, 28(1), 7–14

Chodzaza, E., Haycock-Stuart, E., Holloway, A., Rosemary, M., 2018. Cue acquisition: A feature of Malawian midwives decision making process to support normality during the first stage of labour. Midwifery 58, 56–63.

Colman, A., 2006. 'Hypothetico-deductive' In: Colman A (Ed) A Dictionary of Psychology. Oxford Press Online. Oxford University Press, Oxford, UK.

Corben, P., Leask, J., 2018. To close the childhood immunization gap, we need a richer understanding of parents' decisionmaking. Hum. Vaccin. Immunother. 12(12), 3168–3176. doi:10.1080/21645515.2016.1221553.

Declercq, E.R., Sakala, C., Corry, M.P., Applebaum, S., Herrlich, A., 2013. Listening to mothers III: pregnancy and birth. New York: Childbirth Connection.

Douglas, P., Geddes, D. (2018). Practice-based interpretation of ultrasound studies leads the way to more effective clinical support and less pharmaceutical and surgical intervention for breastfeeding infants. Midwifery, 58 p145–155

Downe, S., Finlayson, K., Oladapo, O.T., Bonet, M., Gülmezoglu, A.M., 2018. What matters to women during childbirth: A systematic qualitative review. PLoS ONE. 2018; 13(4), e0194906.

Dreyfus, H.L., Dreyfus, S.E., 1977. Uses and abuses of multi-attribute and multi-aspect model of decision-making. In P. Benner (Ed.), From Novice to Expert. Excellence and Power in Clinical Nursing Practice (Commemorative ed.). Prentice-Hall, New Jersey.

Dreyfus, H.L., Dreyfus, S.E., 1986. Mind over machine – The power of human intuition and expertise in the era of the computer. The Free Press, New York.

Ebert, L., Bellchambers, H., Ferguson, L., Browne, J., 2014. Socially disadvantaged women's views of barriers to feeling safe to engage in decision-making in maternity care. Women Birth 27(2), 132–137. doi: 10.1016/j.wombi.2013.11.003.

Elstein, A., Schwarz, A., 2000. Clinical reasoning in medicine. In: Higgs, J., Jones, M. (Eds.), Clinical reasoning in the health professions. 2nd Edition. Butterworth-Heinemann Ltd, Oxford, UK, pp. 95–106.

Elstein, A., Schwarz, A., 2002. Evidence base of clinical diagnosis: clinical problem sovling and diagnostic secision making: selective seview of the cognitive literature. BMJ 324 (7339), 729–732.

Elstein, A.S., Shulman L.S., Sprafka, S.A., 1978. Medical Problem Solving: An analysis of Clinical Reasoning. Harvard University Press, Cambridge, MA.

Elwyn, G., Durand, M., Song, J.J., 2017. A three-talk model for shared decision making: multistage consultation process. BMJ 359(j4891), 1–7. doi:10.1136/bmj.j4891.

Elwyn, G,, Frosch, D., Thomson, R., Joseph-Williams, N., 2012. Shared decision making: a model for clinical practice. J. Gen. Intern. Med. 27(10), 1361–1367.

Fay, M., Grande, S., Donnelly, K., 2015. Using Option Grids: steps toward shared decision-making for neonatal circumcision. Patient Educ. Couns. 99, 236–242.

Grummer-Strawn, L., Rollins, N., 2015. Summarising the health effects of breastfeeding. Acta Paediatrica supp: https://doi.org/10.1111/apa.13136

Hellerstein, S., Feldman, S., Duan, T., 2015. China's 50% caesarean delivery rate: is it too high? Br. J. Obstet. Gynaecol. 122(2), 160–164. doi:10.1111/1471-0528.12971.

International Confederation of Midwives (ICM), 2005. Partnership Between Women and Midwives. Retrieved from http://www.internationalmidwives.org

International Confederation of Midwives (ICM), 2008. Keeping Birth Normal. http://www.internationalmidwives.org

International Confederation of Midwives (ICM), 2010. Essential Competencies for Basic Midwifery Practice. www.internationalmidwives.org

International Confederation of Midwives (ICM), 2014a. International Code of Ethics for Midwives.

International Confederation of Midwives (ICM), 2014b. Philosophy and Model of Midwifery Care. In. The Netherlands: International Confederation of Midwives.

International Confederation of Midwives (ICM), 2014c. Professional Accountability of the Midwife. In (Vol. Position statement PS20008_014V2014, pp. 2). Geneva: International Confederation of Midwives.

International Confederation of Midwives (ICM), 2017. Definition of the midwife. Retrieved from http://www.internationalmidwives.org

Jefford, E., 2012. Optimal Midwifery Decision-Making during 2nd Stage labour: The intregration of Clinical Reasoning into Practice; (PhD Research), Southern Cross University, New South Wales.

Jefford, E., 2014. The Midwife and Decision-Making Processes: Integration into clinical practice. LAP Lambert, Germany.

Jefford, E., 2020. Midwifery and Decision-Making Theories. In E. Jefford & J. Jomeen (Eds.), *Empowering Decision-Making in Midwifery: A global persepctive*. Routledge, London, pp. 3–14.

Jefford, E., Fahy, K., Sundin, D., 2014. Decision-making theories and their usefulness to the midwifery profession both in terms of midwifery practice and the education of midwives. Int. J. Nurs. Pract. 17, 246–253.

Jefford, E., Fahy, K., 2015. Midwives' clinical reasoning during second stage labour: Report on an interpretive study. Midwifery 31, 519–525. doi:10.1016/j.midw.2015.01.006.

Jefford, E., Fahy, K., Sundin, D., 2014. Decision-making theories and their usefulness to the midwifery profession both in terms of midwifery practice and the education of midwives. Int. J. Nurs. Pract. 17, 246–253.

Jefford, E, Jomeen, J., Martin, C., 2016. Determining the psychometric properties of the Enhancing Decision-making

Assessment in Midwifery (EDAM) measure in a cross cultural context. BMC Pregnancy Childbirth. 19, 95–106. doi:10.1186/s12884-016-0882-3.

Kahneman, D., 2011. Thinking Fast and Slow. Farrar, Straus and Giroux, New York. 2011.

Kapoor V, Douglas P, Hill P et al., 2018. Frenotomy for tongue-tie in Australian children, 2006-2016: an increasing problem. *Med J Austral. 208*(2):88-89. doi: 10.5694/mja17.00438.

Kinniburgh, J.K., Metcalfe, B.A., Razaz, A., Razaz, N., Sabr, Y., Lisonkova, S., 2016. Temporal trends in ankyloglossia and frenotomy in British Columbia, Canada, 2004-2013: a population-based study. *CMAJ Open. 4*(1):E33–E40. doi: 10.9778/cmajo.20150063.

Lawson, A., 2000. The generality of hypothetico-deductive reasoning: making scientific thinking explicit. The American Biology Teacher 62(7), 482–495.

McAndrew, F., Thompson, J., Fellows, L., 2012. The Infant Feeding Survey, 2010. The Health and Social Care Information Centre; UK.

Marinelli, K., Ball, H., Mc Kenna, J., & Blair, P. 2019. An Integrated Analysis of Maternal-Infant Sleep, Breast-feeding, and Sudden Infant Death Syndrome Research Supporting a Balanced Discourse. Journal of Human Lactation 2019, Vol. 35(3) 510–520. HYPERLINK "https://doi.org/10.1177%2F0890334419851797" https://doi.org/10.1177/0890334419851797

Midwifery Council. Te Tatau o te Whare Kahu. 2019. Standards for approval of pre-registration midwifery education programmes and accreditation of tertiary education organisations (3rd Ed). MCNZ, NZ

Miller, S., Bear, R., 2019. Midwifery Partnership. In: Pairman S. Tracy S. Dahlen H & Dixon L (Eds.), Midwifery: Preparation for practice; 4 Edition. Vol. 1. Elsevier, Chatswood, Australia: pp. 299–332.

Mok, H., Stevens, P., 2005. Models of Decision Making. In Raynor, M., Marshall, J., Sullivan, A. (Eds.), Decision Making in Midwifery Practice. Edinburgh: Churchill Livingstone – Elsevier, pp. 53–66.

Mong-Chue, C., 2000. The challenges of midwifery practice for critical thinking. Br. J. Midwifery 8(3), 179–183.

National Childbirth Trust (NCT). 2020 Vitamin K and newborns: what you need to know. https://www.nct.org.uk/labour-birth/after-your-baby-born/vitamin-k-and-newborns-what-you-need-know Reg Charity No (England and Wales): 801395, (Scotland): SC041592. Reg Company No: 2370573.

North Bristol NHS Trust. Vitamin K to Newborn Babies. https://www.nbt.nhs.uk/maternity-services/after-birth/vitamin-k-newborn-babies

Noseworthy, D., Phibbs, S., Benn, C., 2013. Towards a relational model of decision-making in midwifery care. Midwifery 29(7) e42–48.

Nursing and Midwifery Council (NMC), 2009. Standards for pre-registration midwifery education. London: Nursing and Midwifery Council.

Nursing and Midwifery Council (NMC), 2014. Standards for Competence for Registered Midwives. In. London, UK: Nursing and Midwifery Council.

Olza, I., Leahy-Warren, P., Benyamini, Y., Kazmierczak, M., Karlsdottir, S.I., Spyridou, A., et al., 2018. Women's psychological experiences of physiological childbirth: a meta-synthesis. Br. Midwifery J. Open 8(10): e020347.

Office National Statistics (ONS). 2012. Infant Feeding Survey, 2010. https://digital.nhs.uk/data-and information/publications/statistical/infant-feeding-survey/infant-feeding-survey-uk-2010

Sandall, J., Soltani, H., Gates, S., Shennan, A., Devane, D., 2015. Midwife-led continuity models versus other models of care for childbearing women. Cochrane Database Syst. Rev. 4, CD004667. doi: 10.1002/14651858.CD004667.pub5.

Scamell, M., 2016. The fear factor of risk – clinical governance and midwifery talk and practice in the UK. Midwifery 38, 14–20.

Standing, M. (Ed.), 2010. Clinical Judgement and Decision-Making in Nursing and Interprofessional Healthcare.: McGraw-Hill Open University Press, Berkshire, UK.

Thompson, C., Dowding, D., 2009. Theoretical approaches. In: Thompson, C., Dowding, D. (Eds.), Essential Decision Making and Clinical Judgement for Nurses. Churchill Livingstone Elsevier, Edinburgh, pp. 55–77.

Tow, J., 2014. Heal the Mother, Heal the Baby: Epigenetics, Breastfeeding and the Human Microbiome. Breastfeeding Review. Mar; 22(1):7–9.

Vedam, S., Stoll, K., Martin, K., Rubashkin, N., Partridge, S., Thordarson, D., et al., 2017. The Mother's Autonomy in Decision Making (MADM) scale: Patient-led development and psychometric testing of a new instrument to evaluate experience of maternity care. PLoS ONE 12(2), e0171804. doi:10.1371/journal.pone.0171804.

WebMD, 2016. Vitamin K1 ampul – side effects. https://www.webmd.com/drugs/2/drug-93625/vitamin-k-injection/details#side-effects

Wiessinger,D., West, D., & Pitmann, T., 2010. The Womanly Art of Breastfeeding. 8th ed. London:Pinter & Martin.

Wickham, S., 2002. What's Right For Me? Making decisions in pregnancy and birth. AIMS, London.

Vitamin K in the Newborn (Case Study 1)

Ashish, K., Malqvist, M., Rana, N., Ranneberg, L.J., Andersson, O., 2016. Effect of timing of umbilical cord clamping on anaemia at 8 and 12 months and later neurodevelopment in late pre-term and term infants; a facility-based, randomized controlled trial in Nepal. BMC Pediatr. 16(3), 35.

Ashish, K., Rana, N., Malqvist, M., 2017. Effects of delayed umbilical cord clamping vs early clamping on anaemia in infants at 8 and 12 months. a randomized clinical trial. JAMA Pediatr. 17(3), 264–70.

Blackburn, S., 2017. Maternal, Fetal, Neonatal Physiology: A clinical perspective. Fifth ed. Elsevier Saunders, Maryland Heights, MO.

Coffey, P.S., Gerth-Guyette, E., 2018. Current perspectives and practices of newborn vitamin K administration in low- and middle-income countries. Res. Rep. Neonatol. 8, 45–51. https://doi.org/10.2147/RRN.S154652.

Dominguez-Bello, M.G., Costello, E.K., Contreras, M., Magris, M., Hidalgo, G., Fierer, N., et al., 2010. Delivery mode shapes the acquisition and structure of the initial microbiota across multiple body habitats in newborns. Proc. Natl. Acad. Sci. U.S.A. 107(26), 11971–11975. doi: 10.1073/pnas.1002601107.

Enoch, J. (1996). Vitamin K: Is It Necessary? Midwifery Today Childbirth Education. Winter, 40 p28-30

Lippi, G., Franchini, M., 2011. Vitamin K in neonates: facts and myths. Blood Transfus. 9(1), 4–9. doi:10.2450/2010.0034-10.

McDonald, S,J., Middleton, P., Dowswell, T., Morris, P.S., 2013. Effect of timing of umbilical cord clamping of term infants on maternal and neonatal outcomes. Cochrane Database Syst. Rev. 7, CD004074. doi: 10.1002/14651858.CD004074.pub3.

Marcewicz, L.H., Clayton, J., Maenner, M., Odom, E., Okoroh, E., Christensen, D., et al., 2017. Parental refusal of vitamin K and neonatal preventive services: a need for surveillance. Matern. Child Health J. 21(5), 1079–1084. doi:10.1007/s10995-016-2205-8.

Rankin, J., 2017. Physiology in Childbearing. Fourth edn. Elsevier, Edinburgh, UK.

Roman, E., Fear, N.T., Ansell, P., et al., 2002. Vitamin K and childhood cancer: analysis of individual patient data from six case-control studies. Br. J. Cancer. 86(1), 63–69. doi:10.1038/sj.bjc.6600007.

Shearer, M.J., 2009. Vitamin K deficiency bleeding (VKDB) in early infancy. Blood Rev. 23(2), 49–59. doi: 10.1016/j.blre.2008.06.001.

World Health Organization (WHO), 2017. WHO Recommendation of Newborn Health guidelines approved by the WHO Guidelines Review Committee. In: vol. WHO/MCA/17.07. World Health Organization, Geneva, Switzerland, pp.1–26.

Zurynski, Y., Ridley, G., Jalaludin, B., Elliott, E., 2018. 21 Years of surveillance for Vitamin K deficiency bleeding in infants: Policy changes in Australia and international comparisons Arch. Dis. Child. 103(1), A200–A202. doi: org/10.1136/archdischild-2018-rcpch.479.

Wickham, S. (2017). Vitamin K and the Newborn (2nd Ed). Birthmoon Creations, UK. ISBN -13:978-1-9998064-0-8

Tongue-tie (Case Study 2)

Coker-Dekker, O. 'Investigate, measure, think twice before cutting.' New evidence that cutting tongue ties may not help infants to breastfeed. https://www.medela.com/company/news/news/article~medela-com.think-twice-before-tongue-tue~

Douglas, P., Geddes, D. (2018). Practice-based interpretation of ultrasound studies leads the way to more effective clinical support and less pharmaceutical and surgical intervention for breastfeeding infants. Midwifery, 58 p145–155

Ingram, J., Johnson, D., Copeland, M., 2015. The development of a tongue assessment tool to assist with tongue-tie identification. Arch. Dis. Child. Fetal Neonatal Ed. 100(4), F344–F349. doi: 10.1136/archdischild-2014-307503.

Jin, R.R, Sutcliffe, A., Vento, M., 2018. What does the world think of ankyloglossia? Acta Paediatr. 107, 1733–1738. doi:10.1111/apa.14242.

Joseph, K.S., Kinniburgh, B., Metcalfe, A., Razaz, N., Sabr, Y., Lisonkova, S., 2016. Temporal trends in ankyloglossia and frenotomy in British Columbia, Canada, 2004–2013: a population-based study. CMAJ Open 4(1), E33–E40. doi:10.9778/cmajo.20150063.

Kapoor, V., Douglas, P., Hill, P. et al., 2018. Frenotomy for tongue-tie in Australian children, 2006–2016: an increasing problem. Med. J. Aust. 208(2), 88–89. doi: 10.5694/mja17.00438.

Kinniburgh, JK., Metcalfe, B. A. Razaz, A.,Razaz, N., Sabr, Y & Lisonkova, S. (2016). Temporal trends in ankyloglossia and frenotomy in British Columbia, Canada, 2004-2013: a population-based study. CMAJ Open. 4(1):33-E40. doi: 10.9778/cmajo.20150063

Lange, S., Probst, C., Rehm, J., Popova, S. (2018) National, regional, and global prevalence of smoking during pregnancy in the general population: a systematic review and meta-analysis Lancet Global Health, 6 pp. e769–e776

Maldonado, E., López-Gordillo, Y., Partearroyo, T., Varela-Moreiras, G., Martinez-Alvarez, C., Perez-Miguelsanz, J., 2018. Tongue abnormalities are associated to a maternal folic acid deficient diet in mice. Nutrients 10(1), 26. doi: 10.3390/nu10010026.

Messner, A., Lalakea, M., 2000. Ankyloglossia: controversies in management. Int. J. Pediatr. Otorhinolaryngol., 54 (2-3), 123–131. doi: 10.1016/s0165-5876(00)00359-1.

Muldoon, K., Gallagher, L., McGuinness, D., Smith, V., 2017. Effect of frenotomy on breastfeeding variables in infants with ankyloglossia (tongue-tie): a prospective before and after cohort study. BMC Pregnancy Childbirth 17(1), 373. doi:10.1186/s12884-017-1561-8.

National Institute for Clinical Excellence (NICE), 2005a. Division of Ankyloglossia (tongue-tie) for breastfeeding. https://www.nice.org.uk/guidance/ipg149/resources/division-of-ankyloglossia-tongue-tie-for-breastfeeding-pdf-304342237.

National Institute for Clinical Excellence (NICE), 2005b. Overview of Division of ankyloglossia (tongue-tie) for breastfeeding – Guidance. https://www.nice.org.uk/guidance/IPG149.

National Institute for Clinical Excellence (NICE), 2019. Interventional Procedures Overview of Division of Ankyloglossia for Breastfeeding https://www.nice.org.uk/guidance/ipg149/documents/interventional procedures-overview-division-of-ankyloglossia-tonguetie-for-breastfeeding2.

NHS site: https://www.nhs.uk/conditions/tongue-tie/

Walsh, J., Links, A., Boss, E. et al.,2017. Ankyloglossia and lingual frenotomy: national trends in inpatient diagnosis and management in the United States, 1997–2012. Otolaryngol Head Neck Surg. 156(4), 735–740. doi: 10.1177/0194599817690135.

Infant Feeding (Case Study 3)

Edwards, M.E., Jepson, G., McInnes, R.J., 2018. Breastfeeding initiation: An in-depth qualitative analysis of the perspectives of women and midwives using social cognitive theory. Midwifery 57, 8–17. doi:10.1016/j.midw.2017.10.013.

Entwistle, F.M., 2013. The evidence and rationale for the UNICEF UK Baby Friendly Initiative standards. UNICEF UK.

Grummer-Strawn, L., & Rollins, N,. 2015. Summarising the health effects of breastfeeding. Acta Paediatrica supp: https://doi.org/10.1111/apa.13136.

Hoddinott, P., & Pill, R., 2013. A Qualitative Study of Women's Views About How Health Professionals Communicate About Infant Feeding. Health Expert. Dec; 3(4):224-233. doi: 10.1046/j.1369-6513.2000.00108.x

Kramer, M., Chalmers, B., Hodnett, H., Sevkovksaya, Z., Dzikovich, I., Shapiro, S., et al., 2001. Promotion of breastfeeding intervention trial (PROBIT): a randomized trial in the Republic of Belarus. JAMA 285(4), 413–420. doi:10.1001/jama.285.4.413.

McAndrew, F., Thompson, J., Fellows, L., Large, A., Speed, M., Renfrew, M.J., 2012. Infant Feeding Survey 2010, Health and Social Care Information Centre, pp. 111–112.

Office National Statistics. 2012. Infant Feeding Survey, 2010. HYPERLINK "https://digital.nhs.uk/data-and%20information/publications/statistical/infant-feeding-survey/infant-feeding-survey-uk-2010" https://digital.nhs.uk/data-and information/publications/statistical/infant-feeding-survey/infant-feeding-survey-uk-2010

Quigley, M.A., Cumberland, P., Cowden, J.M., Rodrigues, L.C., 2006. How protective is breast feeding against diarrhoeal disease in infants in 1990's England? Arch. Dis. Child. 91(3), 245–250.

Renfrew, M., McFadden, A., Dykes, F., Wallace, L.M., Abbott, S., Burt, S., et al., 2006. Addressing the learning deficit in breastfeeding: strategies for change. Matern. Child Nutr. 2(4), 239–244.

Robinson, B.A., Hartrick Doane, G., 2017. Beyond the latch: A new approach to breastfeeding. Nurse Educ. Pract. 26, 115–117. doi:10.1016/j.nepr.2017.07.011.

Roll, C.L., Cheater, F., 2016. Expectant parents' views of factors influencing infant feeding decisions in the antenatal period: a systematic review. Int. J. Nurs. Stud. 60, 145–155. doi: 10.1016/j.ijnurstu.2016.04.011.

Rollins, N.C., Bhandari, N., Hajeebhoy, N., Horton, S., Lutter, C.K., Martines, J.C., et al., 2016. Why invest, and what it will take to improve breastfeeding practices? Lancet 387(10017), 491–504. doi: 10.1016/S0140-6736(15)01044-2.

Rollnick, S., Miller, W., Butler, C.C., 2008. Motivational interviewing in health care: Helping patients change behaviour, The Guildford Press, New York.

Sheehan, A., Schmied, V., Barclay, L., 2013. Exploring the Process of Women's Infant Feeding Decisions in the Early Postbirth Period. Jul;23(7):989-98.doi: 10.1177/1049732313490075. Epub 2013 May 9

Tricky, H., 2016. Infant Feeding: changing the conversation. NCT Research Perspectives 33.

Sheehan, A,. Schmied, V., & Barclay, L,. 2013. Exploring the Process of Women's Infant Feeding Decisions in the Early Postbirth Period. Jul;23(7):989-98.doi: 10.1177/1049732313490075. Epub 2013 May 9.

Victora, C.G., Aluísio, J.D, Barros, A.J.D, França, G.V.A., Horton, S., Krasevec, J., et al., 2016. Breastfeeding in the 21st century: epidemiology, mechanisms, and lifelong effect. Lancet. 387(10017), 475–90. doi: 10.1016/S0140-6736(15)01024-7.

UNICEF UK, 2018. Having meaningful conversations with mothers: A guide to using the Baby-Friendly signature sheets.

UNICEF UK, 2019. Infant formula and responsive bottle feeding. A guide for parents.

Safe Sleep (Case Study 4)

Ball, H., Howel, D., Bryant, A., Best, E., Russell, C., & Ward-Platt, M,. 2016.Bed-sharing by breastfeeding mothers: who bed-shares and what is the relationship with breastfeeding duration? Acta Paediatrica 105, pp. 628–634

Ball, H.L., Moya, E., Fairley, L., Westman, J., Oddie, S., Wright, J., 2012. Infant care practices related to sudden infant death syndrome in South Asian and White British families in the UK. Paediatr Perinat Epidemiol 26(1), 3–12. doi:10.1111/j.1365-3016.2011.01217.x.

Ball, H., Howel, D., Bryant, A., Best, E., Russell, C., & Ward-Platt, M,. 2016.Bed-sharing by breastfeeding mothers: who bed-shares and what is the relationship with breastfeeding duration? Acta Paediatrica 105, pp. 628–634

Ball, H.L., Ward-Platt, M.P., Heslop, E., Leech, S.J., Brown, K.A., 2006. Randomised trial of infant sleep location on the postnatal ward. Arch. Dis. Child. 91(12), 1005–1010. doi: 10.1136/adc.2006.099416.

Ball, H.L., Volpe, L.E., 2013. Sudden Infant Death Syndrome (SIDS) risk reduction and infant sleep location – Moving the discussion forward. Soc. Sci. Med. 79 (Supp C), 84–91. doi: 10.1016/j.socscimed.2012.03.025.

Bartick, M., Tomori, C., Ball, H.L., 2018. Babies in boxes and the missing links on safe sleep: Human evolution and cultural revolution. Matern. Child Nutr. 14(2), e12544. doi: 10.1111/mcn.12544

Blair, P.S., Sidebotham, P., Berry, P.J., 2006. Major epidemiological changes in sudden infant death syndrome: a 20-year population-based study in the UK. Lancet 367(9507), 314–319. doi: 10.1016/S0140-6736(06)67968-3.

Blair, P., Sidebotham, P., Pease, A., & Flemming, P., 2014. Bed-Sharing in the Absence of Hazardous Circumstances: Is There a Risk of Sudden Infant Death Syndrome? An Analysis from Two Case-Control Studies Conducted in the UK. http://journals.plos.org/plosone/article/asset?id=10.1371%2Fjournal.pone.0107799.PDF PLOS ONE 9(9): e107799.

Blair, P., Sidebotham, P., Pease, A., & Flemming, P., 2014. Bed-Sharing in the Absence of Hazardous Circumstances: Is There a Risk of Sudden Infant Death Syndrome? An Analysis from Two Case-Control Studies Conducted in the UK

Boseley, S., 2009. The truth about sleeping with baby. http://www.theguardian.com/lifeandstyle/2009/oct/16/sudden-infant-death-syndrome-children.

Fetherston, C. M., & Leach, J. S. 2012. Analysis of the ethical issues in the breastfeeding and bedsharing debate. Breastfeeding Review, 20(3), 7–17.

Fetherston, C. M., & Leach, J. S. 2012. Analysis of the ethical issues in the breastfeeding and bedsharing debate. Breastfeeding Review, 20(3), 7–17.

Gettler, L.T., McKenna, J.J., 2011. Evolutionary perspectives on mother-infant sleep proximity and breastfeeding in a laboratory setting. Am. J. Phys. Anthropol. 144(3), 454–62. doi: 10.1002/ajpa.21426.

Hauck, F., Thompson, J., Tanabe, K.O., Moon, R.Y., Vennemann, M.M., 2011. Breastfeeding and reduced risk of sudden infant death syndrome: a meta-analysis. Pediatrics 128(1), 103–110. doi: 10.1542/peds.2010-3000.

Kendall-Tackett, K., Cong, Z., Hale, T.W., 2010. Mother–infant sleep locations and night-time feeding behavior. Clin. Lactation 1(1), 27–30. doi: 10.1891/215805310807011837.

Marinelli, K., Ball, H., Mc Kenna, J., & Blair, P. 2019. An Integrated Analysis of Maternal-Infant Sleep, Breastfeeding, and Sudden Infant Death Syndrome Research Supporting a Balanced Discourse Journal of Human Lactation 2019, Vol. 35(3) 510–520. HYPERLINK "https://doi.rg/10.1177%2F0890334419851797" https://doi.org/10.1177/0890334419851797

McCoy, R., McKenna, J.J., Gartner, L., 2008. ABM clinical protocol #6: guideline on co-sleeping and breastfeeding.

Breastfeeding Medicine: the Official Journal of the Academy of Breastfeeding Medicine 3(1), 38.

Mc Kenna, J., Ball, H., & Gettler, L., 2007. Mother–infant cosleeping, breastfeeding and sudden infant death syndrome: What biological anthropology has discovered about normal infant sleep and pediatric sleep medicine. American Journal of physical Anthropology. https://onlinelibrary.wiley.com/toc/10968644/2007/134/S45 Volume134, IssueS45 p 133–161 https://doi.org/10.1002/ajpa.20736

McKenna, J., 2009. Sleeping With Your Baby: A Parent's Guide To Co-Sleeping. Platypus Media, Washington, D.C.

McKenna, J., McDade, T., 2005. Why babies should never sleep alone: a review of the co-sleeping controversy in relation to SIDS, bedsharing and breast feeding. Pediatr. Respir. Rev. 6(2), 134–152.

Mc Kenna, J., Ball, H., & Gettler, L., 2007. Mother–infant cosleeping, breastfeeding and sudden infant death syndrome: What biological anthropology has discovered about normal infant sleep and pediatric sleep medicine.A merican Journal of physical Anthropology. HYPERLINK "https://onlinelibrary.wiley.com/toc/10968644/2007/134/S45" Volume134, IssueS45 p 133-161 https://doi.org/10.1002/ajpa.20736

McKenna, J.J., Gettler, L.T., 2016. Why it is important to present all the facts about the legitimate functions and affirmed benefits of breast sleeping. Acta Paediatr. 105(6), 715. doi: 10.1111/apa.13372.

Mitchell, E., Thompson, J., Zuccollo, J.,MacFarlane, M.,Taylor, B.,Elder, D.,Stewart, A., Percival,T.,Baker, N., McDonald, G., Lawton, B., Schlaud, M., & Flemming, P. 2017 The combination of bed sharing and maternal smoking leads to a greatly increased risk of sudden unexpected death in infancy: the New Zealand SUDI Nationwide Case Control Study. NZMA 2 June 2017, Vol 130 No 1456 ISSN 1175-8716

Mitchell, E., Thompson, J., Zuccollo, J.,MacFarlane, M.,Taylor, B., Elder, D., Stewart, A., Percival,T., Baker, N., McDonald, G., Lawton, B., Schlaud, M., & Flemming, P. 2017 The combination of bed sharing and maternal smoking leads to a greatly increased risk of sudden unexpected death in infancy: the New Zealand SUDI Nationwide Case Control Study. NZMA 2 June 2017, Vol 130 No 1456 ISSN 1175–8716

Trevathan, W.R., Smith, E.O., McKenna, J.J., 2008. Introduction and overview of evolutionary medicine. Oxford University Press, New York (USA).

HYPERLINK "https://www.goodreads.com/author/show/4713784.Diane_Wiessinger" Wiessinger, D., West, D., & Pitmann, T., 2010. The Womanly Art of Breastfeeding. 8th ed. London:Pinter & Martin.

UNICEF, 2016. Co-sleeping and SIDS: a guide for health professionals. UNICEF.

Smoking in Pregnancy (Case study 5)

Cook, S.M.C., Cameron, S.T., 2015. Social issues of teenage pregnancy. Obstet. Gynaecol. Reprod. Med. 25(9), 243–248.

Gould G.S., Havard A., Ling Li Lim et al. Exposure to Tobacco, Environmental Tobacco Smoke and Nicotine in Pregnancy: A Pragmatic overview of Reviews of Maternal and Child outcomes, Effectiveness of Interventions and Barriers and Facilitators to Quitting. International Journal of Environmental Research. Public Health 2020, 17(6), 2034 https://doi.org/10.3390/ijerph17062034 accessed July 2020

Kalkhoran, S., Glantz, S.A., 2016. E-cigarettes and smoking cessation in real-world and clinical settings: a systematic review and meta-analysis. Lancet Respir. Med. 4(2), 116–128. doi: 10.1016/S2213-2600(15)00521-4.

Lange, S., Probst, C., Rehm, J., Popova, S. (2018) National, regional, and global prevalence of smoking during pregnancy in the general population: a systematic review and meta-analysis Lancet Global Health, 6 pp. e769-e776

Leigh, S., 2017. Parental smoking linked to genetic changes found in childhood cancer. Medical Express https://medicalxpress.com/news/2017-04-parental-linked-genetic-childhood-cancer.html.

Marufu TC, Ahankari A, Coleman T, Lewis S. Maternal smoking and the risk of stillbirth: systematic review and meta-analysis BMC Public Health v15; 2015 https://www.ncbi.nlm.nih.gov/pmc/articles/PMC4372174/ Accessed June 2020

McCubbin, A., Fallin-Bennett, A., Barnett, J., Ashford, K., 2017. Perceptions and use of electronic cigarettes in pregnancy. Health Educ. Res. 32(1), 22–32.

Mund, M., Louwen, F., Klingelhoefer, D., Gerber, A., 2013. Smoking and pregnancy – a review on the first major environmental risk factor of the unborn. Int. J. Environ. Res 10(12), 6485–6499. doi:10.3390/ijerph10126485.

National Centre for Smoking Cessation & Training (NCST). www.ncsct.co.uk

NHS England, 2019. Saving Babies' Lives: A care bundle for reducing perinatal mortality (version 2). https://www.england.nhs.uk/wp-content/uploads/2019/05/saving-babies-lives-care-bundle-version-two.pdf.

National Institute for Clinical Excellence (NICE), 2010. Stopping smoking in pregnancy and after childbirth. https://www.nice.org.uk/guidance/ph26.

NHS England, 2016. Better Births: The National Maternity Review www.england.nhs.uk/ourwork/futurenhs/mat-review.

Pineles, B.L., Park, E., Samet, J.M., 2014. Systematic review and meta-analysis of miscarriage and maternal exposure to tobacco smoke during pregnancy. Am. J. Epidemiol. 179(7), 807–23.

Royal College of Midwives (RCM), 2019a. Position statement: support to quit smoking in pregnancy https://www.rcm.org.uk/media/3394/support-to-quit-smoking-in-pregnancy.pdf

Royal College of Midwives (RCM), 2019b. Very brief advice (VBA) on smoking in pregnancy. RCM i-learn. https://www.ilearn.rcm.org.uk/enrol/index.php?id=259

Royal College of Physicians (RCP), 2010. Passive smoking and children. A report of the Tobacco Advisory Group of the Royal College of Physicians. London: Royal College of Physicians. https://cdn.shopify.com/s/files/1/0924/4392/files/passive-smoking-and-children.pdf?15599436013786148553=

Smoking in Pregnancy Challenge Group, 2015. 'Smoking Cessation in Pregnancy: A Review of the Challenge'. http://ash.org.uk/information-and-resources/reports-submissions/reports/smoking-cessation-in-pregnancy-a-review-of-the-challenge-2/.

Smoking in Pregnancy Challenge Group, 2017. Use of electronic cigarettes in pregnancy: A guide for midwives and other healthcare professionals. http://smokefreeaction.org.uk/wpcontent/uploads/2017/06/eCigSIP.pdf.

Tong, V.T., Farr, S.L., Bombard, J., D ºAngelo, D., Ko, J.Y., England, L.J., 2016. Smoking before and during pregnancy among women reporting depression or anxiety. Obstet. Gynecol. 128(3), 562–70.

Whittington, J.R., Simmons, P.M., Phillips, A.M., Gammill, S.K., Cen, R., Magann, E.F., et al., 2018. The use of electronic cigarettes in pregnancy: a review of the literature. Obstet. Gynecol. Surv. 73(9), 544–549. doi: 10.1097/OGX.0000000000000595.

Zacharasiewicz, A., 2016. Maternal smoking in pregnancy and its influence on childhood asthma. ERJ Open Res. 2(3), 00042-2016. doi:10.1183/23120541.00042-2016.

INDEX

Page numbers followed by *"f"* indicate figures, *"t"* indicate tables, and *"b"* indicate boxes.

step reflex, 30, 31f
stercobilinogen, 210
strabismus, 182
stress, influences on fetal health, 89–90
structural cardiovascular changes following
    birth, 105–106
subaponeurotic (subgaleal) haemorrhage,
    140t
subdural haemorrhage, 140t
sudden infant death syndrome (SIDS), 35,
    36t
    alcohol consumption, 267
    and bedsharing, 267–268
    smoking, 267
    sofa sharing, 268
syndactyly of second and third toes, 31f
syphilis, 73, 199–201t

T

temperature, newborn examination, 9, 11b
teratogens, 64, 67, 87–89, 93–94
terminal apnoea, 124–125, 125f
testes, newborn screening, 251–252
tests for metabolic disorders, 245–247
tetralogy of Fallot, 160, 166–167, 166f
    intracardiac repair, 167
    palliative shunts, 167
thalassaemias
    antenatal screening, 74
    counselling of at-risk couples, 74–75
    diagnostic procedures, 74
theory of newborn jaundice, adaptive
    process, 212
thermoregulation in the newborn, 111–112
three-talk model for shared decision-
    making, 259
    application, 261–263
    vitamin K administration, 261–263
thrifty phenotype, 91
toes, newborn examination, 29–30, 31f
tone of muscles, newborn examination, 11
tongue-tie diagnosis, 263–265, 264f
toxoplasmosis, 199–201t
transient tachypnoea of the newborn, 126
translocation of chromosomes, 42
transposition of the great arteries (TGA)
    (congenital heart condition), 168–169,
    169f
tuberculosis (TB), vaccination, 253
Turner's syndrome, 42, 202–203t
twinning, 52
type two diabetes in children, 91

U

UK immunization programme, 252
ultrasound scans, 78–79
    abnormality detection rates, 78
    dating scans, 72f, 78
    fetal abnormality screening, 78–79
    importance of informed consent, 79
    nuchal translucency (NT) marker, 75
umbilical cord care
    24-hour rooming-in, 236, 237
    embryo development, 60
    evidence-based care, 236
    for the healthy term baby, 236
    'open cord care', 236, 237
    physiology of umbilical cord separation,
        235–236
    proposed guidelines, 236–237
    risk of infection, 235, 236
    for sick/premature baby, 237
    signs of infection (omphalitis), 237
    skin-to-skin contact, 233, 236
umbilical cord clamping at birth
    benefits of delayed cord clamping,
        108–109
    effects of early cord clamping, 102
umbilical cord, newborn examination, 25,
    28f
umbilical hernia, 28f
unconjugated bilirubin, 210
    lipid soluble, 210
unconjugated hyperbilirubinaemia, 223
    breast milk jaundice, 223–224
unconjugated jaundice, 213
    complications, 221–222
undescended testes, 251
United Kingdom National Screening
    Committee (UK NSC), 68
upper extremities, newborn examination,
    21, 21f
urine, newborn examination, 25, 25t, 28
urobilinogen, 210
uterine blood flow, 59
uteroplacental vascular insufficiency, 59b
uterotonics, newborn physiological
    transition, 107
uvea, 177
uveitis, 183

V

vaginal birth, 210–211
varicella zoster virus (chickenpox), infection
    of fetus, 199–201t

ventricular septal defect (VSD), 162–163,
    162f
vernix caseosa, 232
viral infections of fetus, 199–201t
visual acuity, 178–179, 179f
vitamin K
    administration, 261–262b, 261–263
    deficiency bleeding, 261, 262t

W

weight, newborn examination, 35
whole-genome sequencing, diagnostic
    testing, 193–203
workplace, exposure to toxins, 87–89

X

X chromosome, 42–43
    errors in cell division, 42b, 63
    sex-linked inheritance, 46–47, 63

Y

Y chromosome, 42–43
    errors in cell division, 42b, 63
    sex-linked inheritance, 46–47
yolk sac, 57–58

Z

Zika virus, fetus, 199–201t
zygote, definition, 48–49
zygote formation, 48–52
    fertilization, 51–52
    formation of the ovum, 49–52
    gametogenesis, 48–52, 50f
    mitochondrial DNA, 52b
    oocyte penetration by a single
        spermatozoon, 48
    oogenesis, 49–50
    point of conception, 42–43, 48–49, 64
    spermatogenesis, 49
    start of pregnancy, 67
    survival of spermatozoa, 48
    transit of spermatozoa through the
        uterus, 50–51
    twinning, 52